Clinical Cases in General Medicine

3e

T0359469

This book is dedicated to Dilukshi, for your extraordinary patience and support, and to Saesha and Reshmi, for just being your wonderful selves.

NOTICE

Medicine is an ever-changing science. As new research and clinical experience broaden our knowledge, changes in treatment and drug therapy are required. The editors and the publisher of this work have checked with sources believed to be reliable in their efforts to provide information that is complete and generally in accord with the standards accepted at the time of publication. However, in view of the possibility of human error or changes in medical sciences, neither the editors, nor the publisher, nor any other party who has been involved in the preparation or publication of this work warrants that the information contained herein is in every respect accurate or complete. Readers are encouraged to confirm the information contained herein with other sources. For example, and in particular, readers are advised to check the product information sheet included in the package of each drug they plan to administer to be certain that the information contained in this book is accurate and that changes have not been made in the recommended dose or in the contraindications for administration. This recommendation is of particular importance in connection with new or infrequently used drugs.

Clinical Cases in General Medicine

3e

DR SANJAYA SENANAYAKE FRACP,
MAppEpid, MBBS(Hons), BSc(Med)

Specialist in Infectious Diseases
Associate Professor
Australian National University Medical School

Mc
Graw
Hill
Education

Reprinted 2018, 2019, 2024

First published 2005; Second edition 2010; Third edition 2015

Text © 2015 Sanjaya Senanayake

Illustrations and design © 2015 McGraw-Hill Australia Pty Ltd

Additional owners of copyright are acknowledged in on-page credits.

Every effort has been made to trace and acknowledge copyrighted material. The authors and publishers tender their apologies should any infringement have occurred.

Reproduction and communication for educational purposes

The Australian *Copyright Act 1968* (the Act) allows a maximum of one chapter or 10% of the pages of this work, whichever is the greater, to be reproduced and/or communicated by any educational institution for its educational purposes provided that the institution (or the body that administers it) has sent a Statutory Educational notice to Copyright Agency (CA) and been granted a licence. For details of statutory educational and other copyright licences contact: Copyright Agency, 66 Goulburn Street, Sydney NSW 2000. Telephone: (02) 9394 7600. Website: www.copyright.com.au

Reproduction and communication for other purposes

Apart from any fair dealing for the purposes of study, research, criticism or review, as permitted under the Act, no part of this publication may be reproduced, distributed or transmitted in any form or by any means, or stored in a database or retrieval system, without the written permission of McGraw-Hill Australia including, but not limited to, any network or other electronic storage.

Enquiries should be made to the publisher via www.mcgraw-hill.com.au or marked for the attention of the Rights and Permissions Manager at the address below.

National Library of Australia Cataloguing-in-Publication Data

Author: Senanayake, Sanjaya
Title: Clinical cases in general medicine
ISBN: 9781743074503
Notes: Includes index. Includes bibliographical references
Subjects: Medicine—Handbooks, manuals, etc
        Interns (Medicine)—Handbooks, manuals, etc
        Diagnosis—Case studies
Dewey Number: 616

Published in Australia by
McGraw-Hill Education (Australia) Pty Ltd
Level 33, 680 George Street, Sydney NSW 2000
Publisher: Jane Roy
Production Editor: Daisy Patiag
Editor: Rosemary Moore
Proofreader: Pauline O'Carolan
Indexer: Olive Grove Indexing Services
Designer (cover and interior): Miranda Costa
Typeset in 10/12 pt Minion Pro by SR Nova, India
Printed in Australia by Pegasus

Contents

Foreword

Medical students graduate with gaps in their clinical experience—we cannot expect them to have seen and managed all the 'core' clinical problems deemed by specialists. Student-centred, self-directed learning is promoted in both undergraduate and postgraduate medical courses to help students develop learning skills that they can apply when confronted with previously unseen clinical problems during residency.

This textbook provides a means for medical students and junior doctors to broaden their clinical experiences. Dr Senanayake illustrates a range of common clinical problems as the basis for developing clinical reasoning skills and approaches to management. Each case builds on Dr Senanayake's own clinical experiences and is commonly encountered in a teaching hospital. There is a balance between the complexity of a real patient and the opportunities for learning generated by the case.

The cases not only provide a means for dealing with the problem presented, but should also assist medical students and junior doctors in developing generic approaches to clinical problems. The cases also highlight the application of evidence in the management of a clinical problem. Each chapter concludes with a range of learning outcomes to enable readers to assess their progress.

This book will broaden students' virtual clinical experiences and help junior doctors to deal with the clinical problems they missed before graduation.

Philip Jones
Associate Dean (Education)
Faculty of Medicine
University of New South Wales

Preface

The book: What it's all about and how to use it

It is both a humbling and wonderful experience to be writing a preface for the 3rd edition of this book. It would not have been possible without the support of my publisher, McGraw-Hill Australia, and you, the readers. So I thank you both for the opportunity.

This book continues to present clinical problems in the format of problem-based learning scenarios. You, the reader, become the doctor faced with the responsibility of diagnosing and treating the patient described in each scenario. You are presented with 44 common clinical problems that you are likely to face as a doctor on the wards and in the emergency department. These cases cover a variety of medical disciplines, including cardiology, respiratory medicine, gastroenterology, neurology, endocrinology, rheumatology, infectious diseases, nephrology, immunology, vascular surgery, urology, emergency medicine, haematology and oncology. The new chapters cover thyroid disease, acute pyelonephritis, syncope, post-splenectomy sepsis, influenza and skin and soft tissue infections.

As a teacher, I have always found the problem-based approach to learning an effective teaching tool: it engages and challenges both the student and the teacher, and generates debate and discussion. Here, it gives you, the reader, the opportunity to follow each patient from presentation and tackle the diagnostic and management problems that are likely to arise in real life.

This is an Australian book, presenting Australian practices and references where possible. Although doctors here manage many problems in a similar manner to clinicians overseas, sometimes there are differences. The book also aims to provide an insight into the practices and protocols in hospital wards and emergency departments in Australia.

How to best treat patients from non-English-speaking backgrounds and some of the resources available to you in this context are described in Chapter 16. This is an important topic given the diverse ethnic backgrounds of patients and staff in many Australian hospitals.

Each case study begins with a scenario followed by a series of questions that will challenge you to determine the best diagnosis. You are then taken step by step through the treatment options and patient management. Each case study focuses on a specialist area of medicine. There will be times when you want to read more about a topic covered in a chapter (e.g. pulmonary embolism), or learn more about only one aspect of a topic (e.g. the use of V/Q scans in the diagnosis of pulmonary embolism). In either case, the Index will direct you to more information.

At the end of each chapter you will find a list of my references. You may find these useful in your own research. If you are interested in learning more about a particular topic, or are presenting a topic in a tutorial, the extra detail found in these references may be just what you need.

Finally, I hope the touches of humour throughout the book serve as a reminder that you can be a good doctor and still find time to see the lighter side of medicine. Please enjoy!

Sanjaya Senanayake
March 2015

About the author

Sanjaya Senanayake is an Associate Professor of Medicine at the Australian National University (ANU) medical school. He is also a practising infectious diseases physician.

Acknowledgments

When developing the first edition of this book I received valuable feedback from the audience for whom it was written and this formed the basis for subsequent editions including this one. These include Dr Adam Perczuk; Associate Professor James Bell; Associate Professor David Bihari; Dr Peter Boers; Dr Kate Clezy; Associate Professor David Goldstein; Dr Anna Holdgate; Associate Professor Philip Jones; Dr Edward Korbel; Dr Andrew Lennox; Dr Robert Lindeman; Dr Mark Pitney; Associate Professor Stephen Riordan; Dr Paul Roach; Dr Yvonne Shen; and Dr Anna M Story.

Thanks to Dr Eugene BH Loh for providing the electrocardiographs. Thanks also to the Radiology Departments of the Prince of Wales Hospital, Randwick and the Sutherland Hospital, Caringbah for providing radiologic images.

Chapter 1
Mr Nguyen and Mrs Fennech present with chest pain

Scenario

Another long day begins in the Emergency Department. You are asked to see Mr Nguyen, a 47-year-old man with chest pain. You are concerned that he may have an acute coronary syndrome.

Q: What is your approach to a patient with an acute coronary syndrome?

A: As an intern seeing this patient acutely, you must immediately determine whether his acute coronary syndrome is due to an ST-elevation myocardial infarction (STEMI) or a non-ST-segment-elevation acute coronary syndrome (NSTEACS). Both conditions are serious but a STEMI will nearly always require emergency reperfusion.

Q: In a patient with acute chest pain, do you follow the convention of history, examination and investigations?

A: Chest pain is one of the situations where you break with convention.

It is important that a 12-lead electrocardiograph (ECG) is performed within 5 minutes of the patient arriving in the Emergency Department to identify an acute coronary syndrome. Remember that while 'time is money' in the business world, 'time is myocardium' in the world of cardiology.

Scenario

One of the nurses gives you Mr Nguyen's admission ECG, which was performed a few minutes earlier. The ECG demonstrates ST depression in the inferior leads.

Q: Is the 12-lead ECG with ST depression in the inferior leads consistent with a STEMI?

A: No. The ECG criteria for a STEMI are (Acute Coronary Syndrome Guidelines Working Group, 2006):
  - 1 mm ST elevation in 2 contiguous limb leads

- 2 mm ST elevation in 2 contiguous chest leads
- new-onset left bundle branch block (if there are no previous ECGs for comparison, assume that the left bundle branch block is new).

The ST depression in the inferior leads of Mr Nguyen's ECG is not consistent with a STEMI.

Scenario

You take a history from Mr Nguyen. He runs a retail business that keeps him occupied for almost 15 hours a day. He first experienced chest pain about a month ago. He describes it as a dull central ache that occurred while in a meeting. It did not radiate anywhere. That episode was very mild and lasted for about 5 minutes. Between that episode and today's, he has had 2 similar episodes, each occurring at rest and resolving within 5 minutes. Today's episode also occurred during a meeting. It is the same pain but is much more severe, and it goes up into his neck and jaw. He is quite sweaty with it.

His colleagues called an ambulance. It arrived about 10 minutes after the pain began. The paramedics gave him half sublingual glyceryl trinitrate during the trip to the hospital, but this did not alleviate the pain. He was given a further sublingual glyceryl trinitrate on arrival, along with supplemental oxygen, and the pain is now resolving.

Mr Nguyen is a healthy man whose only medical history is an appendicectomy performed 25 years ago. He has never checked his cholesterol and blood sugar levels. He drinks 20 grams of alcohol a day, but does not smoke. His father died of a heart attack at the age of 50.

The physical examination is unremarkable. He is overweight and looks slightly anxious. His heart rate is 85/minute and regular. His blood pressure is 155/85. There is no blood pressure differential between the arms. All peripheral pulses are present. He has no signs of heart failure and no murmurs.

Q: At this stage, is it reasonable to diagnose Mr Nguyen with a NSTEACS?
A: Yes. The recurrent episodes of dull chest ache at rest radiating to his neck and jaw are consistent with pain of cardiac origin. This, in addition to the strong family history of ischaemic heart disease, are consistent with an acute coronary syndrome. The absence of ST elevation or a left bundle branch block on ECG exclude a STEMI; therefore, it is correct to classify his acute coronary syndrome as a NSTEACS.

Q: You order a chest X-ray, which is unremarkable. The nurse is ready to take his blood. What other tests will you order now?

A:
1. troponin (high sensitivity)
2. full blood count
3. electrolytes, urea, creatinine (EUC)
4. coagulation studies.

Q: Mr Nguyen overhears your discussion with the nurse. He anxiously asks, 'I hate blood tests. Do you really need to check my blood sugar if I'm having a heart attack? I'm sure that I'm not diabetic'.

A: Definitely. There are a few reasons to check Mr Nguyen's random blood sugar now and perform a fasting blood sugar test later:

- Up to 14% of people presenting with an acute coronary syndrome will have undiagnosed diabetes mellitus (Conaway *et al.*, 2005).
- The presence of diabetes mellitus in a patient means that his NSTEACS is in the 'high-risk' category (see page 5), thereby affecting management.
- Early identification of diabetes mellitus and its control will be vital to the overall health of the patient in the long term.

Q: Is a single high sensitivity troponin test sufficient to exclude a diagnosis of an acute coronary syndrome (ACS)?

A: As the name suggests, the high sensitivity (hs) troponin test is good at ruling out an ACS if the result is negative. (Remember that sensitive tests exclude a disease if negative whereas specific tests rule in a disease if positive.) Patients have not had a myocardial infarction if (Chew *et al.*, 2011):

1. a single hs troponin more than 6 hours after symptom onset (and in the absence of ongoing pain) is negative OR
2. two hs troponin tests are negative in the patient who presents within 6 hours of the onset of the pain (one test on presentation and the other 3 hours after presentation and at least 6 hours after symptom onset).

Q: Is there any need to check both troponin and CK results? Surely troponin levels alone would be adequate?

A: Serum troponin levels are more sensitive and specific than CK levels. Troponin levels may take up to 8 hours to rise after the onset of symptoms. They may also remain elevated for 5 days (troponin I) or for up to 10 days (troponin T). On the other hand, while it takes a similar period of time to rise, CK will remain elevated for only about 2–4 days. For this reason, it was thought that CK would be more sensitive at detecting reinfarction than troponin; however, there are ever-increasing data supporting the use of troponin for detecting reinfarction (Apple and Murakami, 2005). If this is true, then there would be little, if any, role for CKMB in acute coronary syndromes.

Q: What should you do while waiting for the results of these investigations?

A:

1. **Control the chest pain.** If 2–3 sublingual nitrate tablets have not resolved the pain completely, it would be reasonable to give 2.5 mg aliquots of intravenous (IV) morphine every few minutes until the pain has resolved or until 10 mg in total (4 × 2.5 aliquots) have been given.

2. **Continuous cardiac monitoring or 'serial' 12-lead ECGs every 15 minutes if the pain continues.** (This is vital because a NSTEACS can evolve into a STEMI, thereby necessitating emergency reperfusion. It is important to realise that NSTEACS is the diagnosis that is given to a patient on presentation to hospital. By the time of discharge the NSTEACS would have been further sub-divided into a non-ST-elevation myocardial infarction (NSTEMI) (if elevated cardiac enzymes confirm myocardial necrosis) or unstable angina (if the acute coronary syndrome is not associated with myocardial necrosis). And, as just discussed, during the admission, the NSTEACS can even evolve into a STEMI.

Scenario

After the 2 sublingual nitrates and supplemental oxygen, Mr Nguyen's pain soon settles. The ST depression returns to normal. The duration of the pain was 45 minutes.

Mr Nguyen's chest X-ray is normal. His blood sugar, full blood count, electrolytes, urea and creatinine are likewise all normal. The high sensitivity troponin levels are as follows:

Test	Normal range	Mr Nguyen
Troponin I (hs)	<26 ng/L	10
Troponin I (hs) (6 hours post pain)	<26 ng/L	225*

* Abnormal result.

Q: You inform Mr Nguyen of the troponin result. He asks, 'Are you sure that the troponin result means a heart attack?'

A: Although an elevated hs troponin is highly sensitive (as the name suggests), it isn't very specific. In other words, there are many causes of a raised troponin other than an ACS. Some causes include (White and Chew, 2008):
- cardiac (e.g. blood pressure extremes, arrhythmias, myopericarditis, aortic dissection, hypertrophic cardiomyopathy, aortic valve disease, rheumatoid arthritis, vasculitis, Takotsubo cardiomyopathy)
- infiltrative myocardial diseases (e.g. amyloidosis, sarcoidosis, haemochromatosis)
- traumatic
- miscellaneous (e.g. sepsis, renal failure, pulmonary embolism, severe asthma, critical illness, hypothyroidism).

 But when there's a rise in hs troponin in a patient with Mr Nguyen's clinical and ECG picture, it is reasonable to attribute the rise to an ACS.

Q: Mr Nguyen has had a troponin rise after around 6 hours after the pain resolved. The myocardial necrosis represented by the raised troponin means that even at this stage of the admission, we can further classify the NSTEACS as a NSTEMI.

 Your medical student, Heime, listens on with interest. He then says, 'I'm confused. You've classified NSTEACS into a NSTEMI or unstable angina. But I thought that NSTEACS could be divided into low risk, intermediate risk or high risk. Am I wrong?'

A: No. Heime is right. It is somewhat confusing but NSTEACS can be divided according to either their clinical diagnosis (NSTEMI or unstable angina) or their level of risk. Determining the level of risk of a NSTEACS is useful for determining management early on in the admission. For example (Acute Coronary Syndrome Guidelines Working Group, 2006):
- High risk: aggressive medical management with coronary angiography and devascularisation.
- Intermediate risk: further observation before reclassifying into high risk or low risk.
- Low risk: discharge on upgraded therapy with urgent cardiology follow-up.

Q: Heime digests this piece of information. 'Okay then, so I need to know how to classify a NSTEACS into risk categories to determine management. Is there a short list to remember?'

A: Unfortunately no. There is a comprehensive list of risk factors to be found in our national guidelines (Acute Coronary Syndrome Guidelines Working Group, 2006) but it is extremely long. It is unrealistic to expect you to remember them all; however, the following acronym will cover many of the features of a high-risk NSTEACS. A patient with a NSTEACS and any one of these risk factors will immediately be classified as high risk:

'HEART DOC'

- H – Haemodynamic compromise.
- E – ECG changes (persistent or dynamic ST depression ≥ 0.5 mm, new T-wave depression ≥ 2 mm or transient ST elevation ≥ 0.5 mm in more than 2 contiguous leads).
- A – Arrhythmia (sustained ventricular tachycardia).
- R – Renal (chronic renal failure with GFR <60 mL/min).
- T – Troponin rise (therefore, any patient with a NSTEMI is automatically high risk).
- D – Diabetes mellitus.
- O – Ongoing chest discomfort that is repetitive or prolonged (>10 minutes).
- C – Coronary revascularisation (coronary artery bypass surgery [CABG] at any time or percutaneous revascularisation within 6 months).

Q: Mr Nguyen overhears your conversation with Heime. With some alarm, he says, 'My condition is high risk? What do you mean by that?'

A: The reason for managing low-, intermediate- and high-risk NSTEACS differently is that they have a different prognosis. The 6-month risk of myocardial infarction (MI) or death for NSTEACS is as follows (Acute Coronary Syndrome Guidelines Working Group, 2006):
- low risk: $<2\%$
- intermediate risk: 2–10%
- high risk: $>10\%$

Q: 'That doesn't sound good,' moans Mr Nguyen. 'What can you do?' How will you acutely manage Mr Nguyen's NSTEMI?

A:

1. **Aspirin**. The paramedics have already given aspirin to Mr Nguyen. Aspirin reduces progression to MI and mortality from cardiac disease by about 50%. A long-term daily dose of 75–150 mg would be appropriate.

2. **Clopidogrel**. This is an inhibitor of platelet aggregation. Its mechanism of action is ADP-receptor antagonism. It is a very useful alternative for patients with ischaemic heart disease who cannot tolerate aspirin.

   Clopidogrel use (300 mg loading dose followed by 75 mg daily) in addition to aspirin has been shown to reduce cardiovascular death, MI, stroke and the need for revascularisation. Although these reductions are better than when aspirin is used alone, complications from increased bleeding can occur.

   Therefore, guidelines recommend that clopidogrel should not be used in patients likely to require coronary artery bypass surgery or immediate coronary angiography (Acute Coronary Syndrome Guidelines Working Group, 2006); however, in practical (or 'real-life') terms, it is difficult early in the admission to know whether or not a patient will require immediate angiography or coronary artery bypass surgery. Therefore, you will find that nearly all these patients are given clopidogrel soon after arriving in hospital anyway. The cardiologists will deal with the consequences of this later.

   Clopidogrel is typically prescribed for at least 12 months following an acute coronary syndrome, particularly if coronary artery stenting has been performed.

   Alternatives to clopidogrel with a similar mode of antiplatelet action include prasugrel and ticagrelor (Chew *et al.*, 2011).

3. **IIb/IIIa receptor antagonist**. IIb/IIIa receptors are found on platelets and are central to platelet aggregation in acute coronary syndromes. IIb/IIIa receptor antagonists therefore play a beneficial role in acute coronary syndromes (Bhatt and Topol, 2000).

   Tirofiban, abciximab and eptifibatide are examples of IIb/IIIa receptor antagonists used in Australia. Although very effective, abciximab's expense means that the other two cheaper agents are used more often.

   (There is a recommendation to avoid IIb/IIIa receptor antagonists unless there is recurrent ischaemia despite appropriate medical therapy—see Chew *et al.*, 2011)

4. **Antithrombin therapy for 48–72 hours (IV unfractionated heparin or subcutaneous low molecular weight heparin [LMWH])**.

   The use of antithrombin therapy combined with aspirin reduces the risk of myocardial infarction and death by a relative risk of 44% in patients with unstable angina or NSTEMI (Goodman *et al.*, 2000). In some cases, bivalirudin (a direct thrombin inhibitor) or fondaparinux (an indirect factor Xa inhibitor) can be used instead of heparin (Chew *et al.*, 2011). For details on how to chart antithrombin agents and monitor their effects, read Chapter 32.

5. **Beta-blockers.** These agents result in reduced progression to MI through a reduction in myocardial oxygen requirements from decreased cardiac work.

Q: What do you need to know before commencing Mr Nguyen on a beta-blocker?

A: It is important to know whether he has:
- a history of asthma
- bradycardia or conduction block
- uncontrolled heart failure
- hypotension
- peripheral vascular disease.

Beta-blockers can exacerbate these conditions. You must therefore exercise caution when using them in these situations.

6. **Early invasive therapy.** This includes coronary angiography, percutaneous coronary intervention (PCI) or coronary artery bypass graft surgery.

In high-risk unstable angina patients, early invasive therapy has been shown to have a number of beneficial effects:
a. Reduction in angina symptoms and nitrate requirement.
b. Reduction in subsequent death or MI.
c. Reduction in further hospitalisation.
d. Earlier discharge from hospital.

7. **Test for other cardiac risk factors:**
- fasting blood glucose
- fasting serum lipids (within 24 hours of admission).

Q: Mr Nguyen commences IV heparin/tirofiban therapy. He has no contraindications to beta-blockers, so he starts them also. He continues on aspirin. Heime looks worried. 'Why don't you give him high flow oxygen? I thought everyone with an acute coronary syndrome needs high flow oxygen. And it's so easy to give!'

A: Supplemental oxygen used to be recommended for all patients with suspected ACS; however, it now appears that its benefits are uncertain. In fact, supplemental oxygen may even be harmful! Therefore, only give supplemental oxygen in the setting of ACS to those in shock or with hypoxia (SaO2 < 93%) (Chew *et al.*, 2011).

Q: If Mr Nguyen had further angina despite this therapy, what other IV medication could be used in the short term?

A: IV glyceryl trinitrate could be used as an infusion. However, the infusion dose must be titrated to blood pressure as hypotension can occur.

Q: The cardiologist wants Mr Nguyen to have a coronary angiogram the next day, with a possible angioplasty and stent. How will you gain consent from Mr Nguyen for an angiogram?

A: Any informed consent should involve an explanation of the procedure methods and risks. The incidence of risks provided below and opposite will vary between cardiology units although they shouldn't be too different from each other. You should tell Mr Nguyen the following:

1. A local anaesthetic will be injected into the upper thigh or wrist.
2. An incision will then be made.
3. A catheter will be introduced into the heart through the artery in the groin or wrist.
4. A dye will then be injected through the catheter. This will allow the cardiologist to detect any narrowing in the heart arteries. There will be an odd sensation as the dye is injected, but this is quite normal so there is no need to panic. There is a risk of a severe allergic reaction to the dye. Although this is very uncommon, he must tell you if he has had reactions to contrast dyes in the past.
5. There is a risk of causing a heart attack (1 in 2000), a stroke (1 in 1000) and death (1 in 4000).
6. It is possible to develop bruising and infection at the groin incision. A swelling around the artery (false aneurysm, haematoma or pseudoaneurysm) can also occur.
7. If the cardiologist finds any narrowing of the arteries, they may decide to use a balloon to expand the artery and place a stent to keep it open. As the balloon is opened, there may be some chest pain.
8. The risks of the balloon procedure are a heart attack (1 in 100), stroke and death.
9. He will be awake throughout the procedure.

Q: Mr Nguyen listens to your explanation of the procedure. He is not overly concerned about the risk of MI or stroke. However, he does ask you about the false aneurysm: 'One of my workers had an angiogram. He developed that false aneurysm in the groin. They had to do surgery for that. Will I have to have surgery if I get a false aneurysm?' What do you tell him?

A: Not necessarily. Generally, the steps in managing a pseudoaneurysm include:

- compression
- ultrasound-guided percutaneous thrombin injection (over 90% successful; Krueger *et al.*, 2005)
- surgical repair.

Q: Mr Nguyen is satisfied with your answer and agrees to undergo the coronary angiogram. There is single-vessel disease with 90% narrowing of the right coronary artery. This is amenable to angioplasty and stenting, which the cardiologist performs.

What therapy should be instituted to prevent thrombotic complications of the stent procedure?

A: Mr Nguyen commenced clopidogrel in the Emergency Department. He should continue this for 12 months, in addition to lifelong aspirin.

Scenario

A few days later, you are asked to see another patient with chest pain. Mrs Fennech is a 60-year-old woman who smokes 10 cigarettes a day. She awoke 30 minutes ago feeling sweaty and nauseated, with severe crushing central chest pain. The pain is radiating down her left arm and up to her neck.

A 12-lead ECG was performed within 5 minutes of her arrival at the Emergency Department (see Fig. 1.1).

The ECG demonstrates ≥2 mm of ST elevation in 2 contiguous chest leads (V2-V6) with ST elevation in I and avL. This is consistent with an acute anterolateral myocardial infarction.

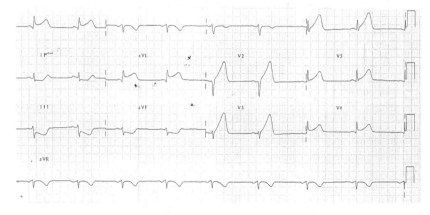

Figure 1.1 Mrs Fennech's 12-lead ECG

The other ECG criteria for MI are:
- 1 mm ST elevation in 2 contiguous limb leads
- new-onset left bundle branch block.

Q: What basic measures should you institute at this stage?

A:

1. **Give supplemental oxygen if hypoxic (oxygen saturation SaO$_2$ < 93%).**
2. **Give 300 mg aspirin (if not already given by the paramedics).** This commonly used medication has a powerful effect against platelets, which are important components of the evolving thrombus in the coronary arteries responsible for the acute STEMI. The early use of aspirin after an acute STEMI reduces the risk of vascular-related death, non-fatal reinfarction and stroke (Anonymous, 1988). In addition, even the 2 forms of revascularisation therapy for acute ST-elevation myocardial infarction (fibrinolysis and percutaneous coronary intervention) result in increased platelet activity which may be detrimental in maintaining patency of the artery (Gawaz *et al.*, 1996; Coller, 1990). Therefore, antiplatelet agents such as aspirin may have an added beneficial effect in the acute treatment of STEMI.
3. **Give clopidogrel (300–600 mg loading dose followed by 75 mg daily).** As with NSTEACS, clopidogrel should be withheld if acute coronary artery bypass surgery is anticipated.
4. **Gain intravenous access and take blood for:**
   a. full blood count
   b. electrolytes, urea, creatinine
   c. coagulation studies
   d. troponin
   e. serum lipids
   f. random blood glucose.

Q: Apart from looking sweaty and unwell, Mrs Fennech's physical examination is unremarkable. In particular, there is no evidence of aortic dissection.

What is your priority now?

A: Remember that 'time is myocardium'. An individual with a STEMI presenting with <12 hours of ischaemic symptoms must be considered for reperfusion therapy. Mrs Fennech would comfortably fit within this window.

In patients with a STEMI, you must quickly decide if they are eligible for reperfusion therapy. There are 2 types of reperfusion therapy: percutaneous coronary intervention (PCI) or fibrinolysis. PCI involves percutaneous transluminal coronary angioplasty (PTCA) with or without stenting.

Q: Is PCI more effective than fibrinolysis for treatment of acute STEMI?

A: Primary angioplasty is associated with fewer deaths, strokes and non-fatal reinfarctions compared to IV thrombolysis (Keeley *et al.*, 2003); however, this is only true if PCI can be provided in a timely fashion. Otherwise fibrinolysis should be used if there are no contraindications. This is discussed further below.

Q: Heime asks, 'How do you know if PCI or fibrinolysis should be given?'

A: A reasonable approach would be (Queensland Health, 2012):

1. If symptom onset <1 hour prior to presentation, consider transfer for immediate PCI within 60 minutes
2. If symptom onset is 1–12 hours prior to presentation, then consider transfer for immediate PCI within 90 minutes
3. If the patient can't be transferred for PCI within the above timeframes, then consider fibrinolysis[1] within 30 minutes

Q: Heime is satisfied with your explanation. 'I have noticed that these guidelines don't mention people presenting more than 12 hours after symptom onset. Is reperfusion a lost cause in these people?'

A: Pretty much. Generally, urgent reperfusion therapy is not recommended in people presenting late unless there is ongoing chest pain.

Q: Unfortunately, you are working in a small peripheral hospital where no angiography facilities are available. You won't be able to transfer Mrs Fennech to a hospital with a dedicated angiography lab for at least 6 hours. She will therefore require thrombolysis. Heime asks, 'So how much better is PCI over fibrinolysis?'

A: Although fibrinolysis is effective, PCI has advantages over it (see table below):

	PCI (%)	Fibrinolysis
Mortality at 4–6 weeks	5	8
Mortality at 6–18 months	5	8
Stroke	<1	2
Reinfarction	3	8
Need for coronary artery bypass surgery	8	13

Source: Adapted from Scottish Intercollegiate Guidelines Network (2013).

---

[1] Some paramedics can even give fibrinolysis in an ambulance.

Q: What do you have to check before Mrs Fennech receives fibrinolysis?
A: You have to ensure that she has no contraindications for fibrinolysis. There are absolute and relative contraindications (Acute Coronary Syndrome Guidelines Working Group, 2006). The absolute contraindications are:
- full-dose GP IIb/IIIa inhibitors with fibrinolytic therapy, especially in the elderly
- active bleeding or bleeding diathesis
- significant closed head or face trauma within the last 3 months
- suspected aortic dissection
- intracerebral haemorrhage anytime previously
- ischaemic stroke within the past 3 months
- known structural cerebrovascular abnormality (e.g. AV malformation)
- known primary or metastatic intracerebral malignancy.

The list of relative contraindications can be found in the National Heart Foundation's 'Guidelines for the management of acute coronary syndromes' (Chew *et al.*, 2011; Acute Coronary Syndrome Guidelines Working Group, 2006). In broad terms, they include people with:
- severe uncontrolled hypertension on presentation or previously
- pregnancy
- concurrent use of anticoagulants
- active peptic ulcer disease
- recent internal bleeding or major surgery
- prolonged or traumatic CPR
- ischaemic stroke more than 3 months earlier
- non-compressible vascular punctures.

It is important to learn this list of contraindications or at least know where to find them at your workplace.

Q: Mrs Fennech has no contraindications for fibrinolysis. What agents are available for use?
A: All fibrinolytic agents work by converting plasminogen to plasmin, which allows fibrinolysis in thrombi. There are 2 broad categories available:
1. streptokinase
2. fibrin-specific fibrinolytics (reteplase, alteplase, tenecteplase).

Q: 'Which group is better?' asks Heime.
A: The table below contrasts the differences between streptokinase and fibrin-specific fibrinolytics (Acute Coronary Syndrome Guidelines

Working Group, 2006). But, in summary, the second-generation fibrin-specific fibrinolytics (reteplase, tenecteplase) are the agents of choice while streptokinase is the least desirable agent to use.

	Streptokinase	Fibrin-specific fibrinolytics
30-day mortality[†]	More	Less (14% difference)
Use in Aboriginal or Torres Strait Islander populations	No	Yes
Can use only once	Yes	No
Lives saved per 1000 patients treated	25	35
Rate-related hypotension	Yes	No
Given as a bolus dose (therefore easier to give)	No	Yes (reteplase, tenecteplase)
Risk of in-hospital stroke[‡]	1–2%	1–2%
Risk of any bleeding events[‡]	around 1%	around 1%

[†]Anonymous (1993).
[‡]Anonymous (1995).
Anonymous (1999).

Q: Heime asks why streptokinase shouldn't be used in Indigenous populations.

A: Indigenous populations, particularly in remote areas of Australia, experience recurrent streptococcal infections. This had led to the generation of relatively high levels of anti-streptokinase antibodies and streptokinase resistance (Urdahl et al., 1996), making streptokinase potentially dangerous and ineffective in these populations. This is also the basis for recommending that streptokinase is never given more than once in any individual.

Q: Your hospital does stock tenecteplase and Mrs Fennech consents to fibrinolysis. Is there any other medication (in addition to the aspirin and clopidogrel) that needs to be given with tenecteplase?

A: Yes. Antithrombin agents (unfractionated IV heparin or subcutaneous LMWH) should be immediately given with the tenecteplase. This recommendation arose because of concerns that reocclusion of the culprit artery can occur after thrombolysis with most of the fibrin-specific fibrinolytics. This is thought to be due to their short half-life and their limited impact on plasma fibrinogen (de Bono *et al.*, 1992).

Q: Heime asks, 'I can prescribe either unfractionated heparin or LMWH. Do you have a preference?'

A: Although there seems to be increased bleeding events with enoxaparin compared to unfractionated heparin, there is an overall clinical benefit if enoxaparin is used for patients with STEMIs (Murphy *et al.*, 2007).

Q: If PCI facilities had been available, should antithrombin agents have also been used?

A: Yes.

Q: At this point, is there anything else that you should arrange?

A: Ideally, Mrs Fennech should be transferred to a hospital with PCI facilities within 90 minutes of completing fibrinolysis (Acute Coronary Syndrome Guidelines Working Group, 2006). This is to ensure that rescue PCI can be performed without delay if necessary. Therefore, it would be worth arranging transport even at this stage.

Q: Soon after the thrombolysis, Mrs Fennech remains asymptomatic and begins to feel better. 'Does this mean the medicine has worked?' asks her anxious husband. How will you decide if reperfusion has successfully occurred?

A: The markers of successful reperfusion include (Acute Coronary Syndrome Guidelines Working Group, 2006):
- symptom relief
- 50% reduction in the ST elevation within 60–90 minutes of fibrinolytic therapy
- resolution of haemodynamic or electrical stability.

Q: What could be done if reperfusion after fibrinolysis is unsuccessful?

A: 'Rescue PCI' can be performed if it is apparent that reperfusion has not been achieved. This is why she needs to be transferred quickly to a hospital with PCI facilities.

Q: Mrs Fennech is transferred to a large teaching hospital with PCI facilities. Two days later, she undergoes a coronary angiogram. It demonstrates diffuse three-vessel disease. Would you recommend coronary artery bypass surgery (CABG)?

A: Indications for CABG in patients with MI are constantly changing as drug therapy and percutaneous intervention improve. Nevertheless, it would currently be reasonable to say that indications for CABG include (Acute Coronary Syndrome Guidelines Working Group, 2006):

- severe three-vessel disease
- left main coronary artery stenosis >50%
- chronic total occlusion not amenable to any other intervention.

Mrs Fennech therefore meets the criteria for CABG and undergoes a triple bypass successfully.

Achievements

You now:

- can classify acute coronary syndromes
- understand the appropriate use of serum cardiac markers
- can competently manage low-risk, intermediate-risk and high-risk NSTEACS
- understand the mechanisms of therapeutic agents in unstable angina
- can gain consent from an individual for coronary angiography and angioplasty
- know the ECG criteria for acute MI
- know the criteria for eligibility for reperfusion therapy
- understand the role of primary and rescue PCI in MI
- know the absolute and relative contraindications for thrombolysis
- know the different types of agents available for thrombolysis
- understand the risks and benefits of thrombolytic agents
- know the role of CABG in MI.

References

Acute Coronary Syndrome Guidelines Working Group (2006), 'Guidelines for the management of acute coronary syndromes', *Medical Journal of Australia*, vol. 184, no. 8 suppl, S1–32.

Anonymous (1999), 'Single-bolus tenecteplase compared with front-loaded alteplase in acute myocardial infarction: The ASSENT-2 double-blind randomised trial. Assessment of the safety and efficacy of a new thrombolytic investigator', *Lancet*, vol. 354, no. 9180, pp. 716–722.

Anonymous (1995), 'Randomised, double-blind comparison of reteplase double-bolus administration with streptokinase in acute myocardial infarction (INJECT): Trial to investigate equivalence. International Joint Efficacy Comparison of Thrombolytics', *Lancet*, vol. 346, no. 8971, pp. 329–336.

Anonymous (1993), 'An international randomized trial comparing four thrombolytic strategies for acute myocardial infarction. The GUSTO investigators', *New England Journal of Medicine*, vol. 329, no. 10, pp. 673–682.

Anonymous (1988), 'Randomised trial of intravenous streptokinase, oral aspirin, both, or neither among 17,187 cases of suspected acute myocardial infarction: ISIS-2. ISIS-2 (Second International Study of Infarct Survival) Collaborative Group', Lancet, vol. 2, no. 8607, pp. 349–360.

Apple, F.S. and Murakami, M.M. (2005), 'Cardiac troponin and creatine kinase MB monitoring during in-hospital myocardial reinfarction', Clinical Chemistry, vol. 51, no. 2, pp. 460–463.

Bhatt, D.L. and Topol, E.J. (2000), 'Current role of platelet glycoprotein IIb/IIIa inhibitors in acute coronary syndromes', Journal of the American Medical Association, vol. 284, no. 12, pp. 1549–1558.

Boersma, E., Maas, A.C., Deckers, J.W. and Simoons, M.L. (1996). 'Early thrombolytic treatment in acute myocardial infarction: Reappraisal of the golden hour', Lancet, vol. 348, no. 9030, pp. 771–775.

Chew, D.P., Aroney, C.N., Aylward, P.E., et al. '2011 addendum to the National Heart Foundation of Australia/Cardiac Society of Australia and New Zealand Guidelines for the management of acute coronary syndromes (ACS) 2006', Heart, Lung & Circulation, vol. 20, no. 8, pp. 487–502.

Coller, B.S. (1990), 'Platelets and thrombolytic therapy', New England Journal of Medicine, vol. 322, no. 1, pp. 33–42.

Conaway, D.G., O'Keefe, J.H., Reid, K.J. and Spertus, J. (2005), 'Frequency of undiagnosed diabetes mellitus in patients with acute coronary syndrome', American Journal of Cardiology, vol. 6, no. 3, pp. 363–365.

de Bono, D.P., Simoons, M.L., Tijssen, J. et al. (1992), 'Effect of early intravenous heparin on coronary patency, infarct size, and bleeding complications after alteplase thrombolysis: Results of a randomised double blind European Cooperative Study Group trial', British Heart Journal, vol. 67, no. 2, pp. 122–128.

Gawaz, M., Neumann, F.J., Ott, I., Schiessler, A. and Schomig, A. (1996), 'Platelet function in acute myocardial infarction treated with direct angioplasty', Circulation, vol. 93, no. 2, pp. 229–237.

Goodman, S.G., Cohen, M., Bigonzi, F. et al. (2000), 'Randomized trial of low molecular weight heparin (enoxaparin) versus unfractionated heparin for unstable coronary artery disease: One-year results of the ESSENCE Study. Efficacy and Safety of Subcutaneous Enoxaparin in Non-Q Wave Coronary Events', Journal of the American College of Cardiology, vol. 36, no. 3, pp. 693–698.

Keeley, E.C., Boura, J.A. and Grines, C.L. (2003), 'Primary angioplasty versus intravenous thrombolytic therapy for acute myocardial infarction: A quantitative review of 23 randomised trials', Lancet, vol. 361, no. 9351, pp. 13–20.

Krueger, K., Zaehringer, M., Strohe, D., Stuetzer, H., Boecker, J. and Lackner, K. (2005), 'Postcatheterization pseudoaneurysm: Results of US-guided percutaneous thrombin injection in 240 patients', Radiology, vol. 236, no. 3, pp. 1104–1110.

Murphy, S.A., Gibson, C.M., Morrow, D.A. et al. (2007), 'Efficacy and safety of the low-molecular weight heparin enoxaparin compared with unfractionated heparin across the acute coronary syndrome spectrum: A meta-analysis', European Heart Journal, vol. 28, no. 17, pp. 2077–2086.

Pfister, M.E. and Andrews, R.T. (2003), 'Bovine thrombin injection for the treatment of iatrogenic arterial pseudoaneurysms: Is it too good to be true?', *Journal of Vascular Surgery*, vol. 37, no. 3, pp. 701–702.

Queensland Government (2012), 'STEMI Management Plan, ST-Elevation Myocardial Infarction for Non-International Cardiac Facilities', available at <http://www.health.qld.gov.au/caru/pathways/docs/pathway_stemi.pdf>.

Schomig, A., Mehilli, J., Antoniucci, D. *et al.* (2005), 'Mechanical reperfusion in patients with acute myocardial infarction presenting more than 12 hours from symptom onset: A randomized controlled trial', *Journal of the American Medical Association*, vol. 293, no. 23, pp. 2865–2872.

Scottish Intercollegiate Guidelines Network (SIGN) (2013), 'Acute coronary syndromes', SIGN publication no. 93, SIGN, Edinburgh, at <www.sign. ac.uk>, accessed 27 October 2014.

Urdahl, K.B., Mathews, J.D. and Currie, B. (1996), 'Anti-streptokinase antibodies and streptokinase resistance in an Aboriginal population in northern Australia', *Australian and New Zealand Journal of Medicine*, vol. 26, no. 1, pp. 49–53.

White, H.D. and Chew, D.P. (2008), 'Acute myocardial infarction', *Lancet*, vol. 372, no. 9638, pp. 570–584.

Chapter 2
Mr Khan presents with chest pain

Scenario

You are in the Emergency Department contemplating what an uneventful shift it has been—nothing but common colds and minor ankle sprains. Then one of the senior nurses rushes towards you, waving a 12-lead ECG: 'We've got a myocardial infarct on an ECG in a man with central chest pain. Can you see him now?' You gratefully agree to see him.

While hurrying towards the man's bed, you examine the ECG (see Fig. 2.1).

Q: The ECG is consistent with an acute inferoposterior MI. Salma, your medical student, tells you that he has no contraindications for thrombolysis. She wants to know if she should get the thrombolytic agent ready. What do you tell her?

A: Although 'time is myocardium', you should not rush into fibrinolysis of the patient until you have taken a good history and examined him properly. You do not want mistakenly to thrombolyse an individual with pericarditis or another condition where this would not be appropriate.

Scenario

Mr Khan is a 52-year-old man who takes a diuretic for a 10-year history of hypertension, but otherwise he has no medical history. He was watching a movie on television when he suddenly developed a sharp, severe pain in his anterior chest. It did not radiate anywhere. He has never had this pain before. The only thing that reduced its severity was half a sublingual glyceryl trinitrate, administered by the paramedics. Even then, however, it did not fully resolve. The pain began 60 minutes ago. You notice that he has a hoarse voice as he talks to you.

You examine him. His heart rate is 95/minute and regular. His blood pressure is 160/95. The jugular venous pressure is not elevated. The apex beat is not displaced and of normal character. Heart sounds are dual, with no murmurs. The respiratory and gastrointestinal examinations are normal.

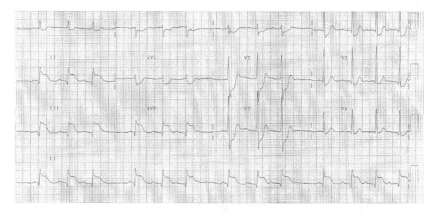

Figure 2.1 12-lead ECG in a man with central chest pain

Q: Is there anything else you need to do as part of the physical examination?

A: Yes, every patient with chest pain must have all peripheral pulses examined and their blood pressure checked in both arms.

Q: You discover that the left radial pulse is slightly weaker than the right. There is also a blood pressure differential between the right arm (160/95) and the left (130/65). Mr Khan's left foot is very cold and the pulses there are much weaker than in the right. A repeat ECG is still consistent with an acute inferior MI.

What is happening?

A: The combination of chest pain, blood pressure differential, an ischaemic foot and ECG changes is consistent with a dissecting aortic aneurysm. Thrombolysis would be potentially fatal in this condition. Once again, you are glad that you routinely check the blood pressure in both arms and examine the peripheral pulses in all patients with chest pain.

Q: Salma tells you that she thought that aortic dissection causes a pain that radiates through to the back. Is this true?

A: It can but not always. Aortic dissection is often a difficult diagnosis to make clinically. Yet it is one that must be made quickly because it has a mortality rate of greater than 25%. One study found that almost 30% of patients were first diagnosed only at postmortem studies (Spittell *et al.*, 1993). The pain can be non-specific but the following are its commonest features (Hagan *et al.*, 2000):

- any pain (96%)
- severe pain or worst ever (91%)
- abrupt onset (85%)

- chest pain (73%)
- ripping pain or tearing pain (51%)
- posterior chest pain or back pain (36% and 53% respectively).

The above list demonstrates that the other classical features of the pain of aortic dissection, namely its ripping character involving the back, are actually not that common at all. Certain individuals, particularly those with Marfan syndrome, can experience painless aortic dissection (Dmowski and Carey, 1999). Therefore, you should not dismiss a diagnosis of aortic dissection in patients who do not report the classical pain.

Q: If this is aortic dissection, should you have heard a murmur?

A: Acute severe aortic regurgitation is one of the most common causes of death in aortic dissection. Aortic regurgitation can occur in up to 50% of cases (Khan and Nair, 2002) although it may only be audible in a smaller proportion: 44% for type A dissections and 12% for type B dissections (Hagan *et al.*, 2000). Type A dissections involve the ascending aorta and type B involves the aorta distal to the left subclavian artery. So, again, do not dismiss the diagnosis because the murmur is not present.

Q: Upon hearing this discussion about her husband, Mrs Khan says, 'But Doctor, you told me that the ECG shows a heart attack. Now you are talking about a dissection or something. And what's wrong with his foot? How can you make sense of all this?'

A: Aortic dissection can lead to a STEMI through a number of mechanisms: compression of a coronary artery by the false lumen of the aneurysm, dissection of a coronary artery or severe hypotension. Even in the absence of a STEMI, about 50% of type A dissections and 20% of type B dissections will be associated with non-specific ST-T wave changes (Dmowski and Carey, 1999).

The differential blood pressure is due to partial compression of 1 or 2 subclavian arteries. The ischaemic foot may be due to femoral artery involvement of the dissection.

Q: Mrs Khan now asks, 'His voice is different too. It is softer and more hoarse. That couldn't be related to this problem, could it?'

A: Actually, it is possible. Extrinsic compression of the recurrent laryngeal nerve by the dissecting aorta can cause vocal cord paralysis by compressing the recurrent laryngeal nerve.

Q: You ask Salma about the best way to diagnose aortic dissection. She replies that a chest X-ray should be performed to look for mediastinal widening. Is she correct?

21

A: The role of a chest X-ray in the diagnosis of aortic dissection is a grey area. Mediastinal widening is the main abnormality but a pleural effusion may be present, indicative of a haemothorax. Salma is right in that anywhere from 60–90% of chest X-rays in acute aortic dissection are abnormal (Erbel *et al.*, 2001); however, this also means that a large proportion may be missed on a chest X-ray. Furthermore, a chest X-ray won't give useful information about other important features of the dissection such as the location of the intimal flap and the extent of the dissection. In other words, even if the chest X-ray is normal, the patient will need another investigation anyway; therefore, in a suspected aortic dissection, it may be worthwhile to skip the chest X-ray and move straight to a more sophisticated test.

Q: Salma then asks, 'Okay, so we won't do the chest X-ray. What do you recommend?'

A: The most useful tests for diagnosing an aortic dissection are shown in the table below.

	Sensitivity (%)	Specificity (%)
Spiral CT	>90[†]	>85[†]
Transoesophageal echocardiogram	99[†]	89[†]
MRI	98[‡]	98[‡]

[†]Erbel *et al.* (2001).
[‡]Nienaber *et al.* (1993).

They all have their advantages and disadvantages and vary in their ability to give ancillary information, such as the location of the intimal flap.

In Australian hospitals, spiral CT with contrast is likely to be the most easily accessible test in a timely fashion in the emergency setting.

Q: A spiral CT demonstrates an extensive aortic dissection (see Fig. 2.2). The intimal flap is in the ascending aorta with the false lumen partially compressing the right coronary artery. The dissection extends down to the left femoral artery. How do you manage the dissection?

A: Call someone! You have done well to make a diagnosis of aortic dissection. Now, however, you should immediately inform the cardiology and cardiothoracic surgery teams, as the mortality from this condition is about 2–4%/hour in the first 12 hours.

The aims of medical treatment are to (Tsai *et al.*, 2005):
- reduce the 'pulsatile load' (dP/dt)

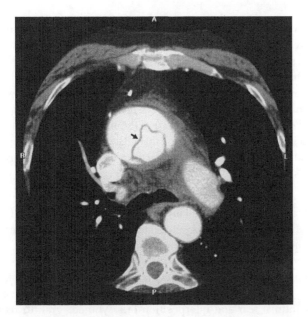

Figure 2.2 CT scan of the chest demonstrating aortic dissection in the ascending aorta (the intimal flap is marked with an arrow)

- reduce systemic hypertension without affecting blood flow to essential organs
- relieve the patient's pain.

Q: The Cardiology Registrar, Bazza, rushes down to see the patient and asks you to commence antihypertensives. Salma asks Bazza which agent should be used and what the target blood pressure is. You welcome her question because you don't know the answer yourself!

A: As discussed above, the blood pressure and heart rate should be lowered to a level that won't compromise perfusion of vital organs. In general, a systolic pressure between 100 mm Hg and 120 mm Hg and a heart rate below 60/minute should be the aim.

Monotherapy with a beta-blocker is appropriate to start with, for example labetalol.

In patients with potential adverse reactions to beta-blockers, a short-acting beta-blocker such as esmolol or calcium antagonists that don't cause reflex tachycardia (verapamil or diltiazem) may be used (Tsai *et al.*, 2005).

If monotherapy isn't successful, vasodilators such as sodium nitroprusside can be added; however, a beta-blocker must be started before the vasodilator, otherwise the reflex release of catecholamines may increase left ventricular ejection force and potentially worsen aortic wall stress (Khan and Nair, 2002).

Of course, in order to achieve and maintain such rigid haemodynamic criteria in such a sick patient, Mr Khan will ideally need monitoring in an Intensive Care Unit (ICU) with an arterial line to provide continuous blood pressure monitoring.

It is also worth remembering that adequate analgesia for this painful condition will also contribute to controlling the heart rate and blood pressure.

Q: You commence a labetalol infusion as the Emergency Department registrar inserts an arterial line and the patient is wheeled to ICU. Mrs Khan wonders whether her husband will need surgery. What do you tell her?

A: In broad terms, patients with type A dissections should undergo surgical repair unless there is a strong contraindication (Khan and Nair, 2002). This generally involves removing entry into the false lumen, excising the intimal tear and interposition of a synthetic graft to repair the aorta. In addition, the aortic valve will need repair or replacement if it is involved in the dissection (Tsai *et al.*, 2005).

Q: The cardiothoracic surgical team review Mr Khan and agree that his type A dissection requires immediate surgery. Mrs Khan is beside herself with anxiety. 'Could my husband die from this?'

A: Absolutely. Acute aortic dissection, even with timely and appropriate treatment, has a high case fatality rate (Tsai *et al.*, 2005).

Type A dissection:

- untreated: 1–2%/hour after symptom onset; 50% at 1 month
- medical treatment only: 50%
- surgical treatment: 15–35%.

Type B dissection:

- if uncomplicated: 10% at 1 month.

Q: 'Is my husband at risk of this terrible thing?'

A: Unfortunately, Mr Khan fits the demographic for the typical patient presenting with a type A aortic dissection, namely a male aged between 50 and 55. Furthermore, he has a chronic history of hypertension, which is found in 62–78% of individuals with dissection.

Other predisposing factors include:
- pregnancy
- cocaine use (due to an acute rise in blood pressure and dP/dt)
- iatrogenic trauma during arterial cannulation
- aortic diseases (Marfan, Turner, Ehlers–Danlos, Loeys–Dietz and Noonan syndromes, to name but a few) (Tsai *et al.*, 2005, Van Laer *et al.*, 2014).

Q: A few days later, you learn that Mr Khan had surgery and is doing well postoperatively. Salma wants to know if he will need ongoing follow-up or should he consider himself cured.

A: Despite this good outcome in the short term, there will always be a risk of recurrence of the aortic dissection and 12–30% of patients will require further surgery in the future; therefore, patients treated for acute aortic dissection will need the following long-term management (Tsai *et al.*, 2005):
- use of a beta-blocker to maintain a healthy blood pressure
- regular clinical and radiological follow-up.

Achievements

You now:
- always examine peripheral pulses and differential blood pressure in patients with chest pain
- know that the absence of classical chest pain to the back or aortic regurgitation does not exclude dissection
- know how to classify aortic dissections as either type A or type B
- know which investigations are useful in diagnosing aortic dissection
- know the role of pharmacotherapy and surgery in treating dissection
- are aware of predisposing factors for aortic dissection.

References

Dmowski, A.T. and Carey, M.J. (1999), 'Aortic dissection', *American Journal of Emergency Medicine*, vol. 17, no. 4, pp. 372–375.

Erbel, R., Alfonso, F., Boileau, C. *et al.* (2001), 'Diagnosis and management of aortic dissection', *European Heart Journal*, vol. 22, no. 18, pp. 1642–1681.

Hagan, P.G., Nienaber, C.A., Isselbacher, E.M. *et al.* (2000), 'The International Registry of Acute Aortic Dissection (IRAD): New insights into an old disease', *Journal of the American Medical Association*, vol. 283, no. 7, pp. 897–903.

Khan, I.A. and Nair, C.K. (2002), 'Clinical, diagnostic and management perspectives of aortic dissection', *Chest*, vol. 122, no. 1, pp. 311–328.

Nienaber, C.A., von Kodolitsch, Y., Siglow, V. *et al.* (1993), 'The diagnosis of thoracic aortic dissection by noninvasive imaging procedures', *New England Journal of Medicine*, vol. 328, no. 1, pp. 1–9.

Spittell, P.C., Spittell, J.A. Jr, Joyce, J.W. *et al.* (1993), 'Clinical features and differential diagnosis of aortic dissection: Experience with 236 cases (1980 through 1990)', *Mayo Clinic Proceedings*, vol. 68, no. 7, pp. 642–651.

Tsai, T.T., Nienaber, C.A. and Eagle, K.A. (2005), 'Acute aortic syndromes', *Circulation*, vol. 112, no. 24, pp. 3802–3813.

Van Laer, L., Dietz, H., Loeys, B. (2014), 'Loeys–Dietz syndrome, 'Advances in experimental medicine and biology', vol. 802, pp. 95–105.

Chapter 3
Mr Winters presents with chest pain

Scenario

It has been a busy day in the Emergency Department. You have seen a woman with pneumonia and 3 elderly people with acute confusion. All have required admission. Just as you are about to take a coffee break, a nurse corners you and says, 'I've got a man with chest pain. He has ECG changes. He may be having an MI. Everyone else is busy. Can you check him out?'

You would rather not miss your well-earned coffee break, but chest pain with ECG changes could be a serious problem. You therefore hurry to see the patient.

Q: Do you tell the nurse to get ready to thrombolyse the patient?

A: Not yet. In Chapter 2 we discussed the importance of balancing the urgency for thrombolysis with a sound clinical assessment. There are conditions presenting with acute chest pain and ECG changes that would not benefit from thrombolysis. In fact, thrombolysis could kill the patient. Such conditions include aortic dissection and acute pericarditis.

You must therefore be efficient but thorough in your clinical assessment of acute chest pain. Your ability to assess this type of pain will naturally improve as you gain experience. In any case, you should always talk to the cardiology department or the medical registrar before thrombolysing a patient.

Q: The patient's name is Mr Winters. He is a 33-year-old courier who is normally healthy. Two years ago he had an arthroscopy after a football injury, but otherwise has been well. He woke up this morning with chest pain.

What do you want to know about the chest pain?

A:
- Where is the pain?
- Does it radiate anywhere?
- What is the character of the pain?

- Does breathing or a change in position exacerbate or relieve the pain?
- What else exacerbates or relieves the pain?
- What were you doing when the pain started?
- Have you ever had this pain before?
- Is the pain constant or intermittent?
- Are any other symptoms associated with the pain?

Scenario

Mr Winters has never had this pain before. He woke up with it this morning (about 6 hours ago). It is central and radiates to his left shoulder. It is definitely worse on inspiration and is sharp in nature. This is the first time he has ever had such pain. He denies other symptoms such as shortness of breath, nausea or sweating. He took a paracetamol tablet with little improvement. He asks you to elevate the head of the bed because lying flat worsens the pain.

Q: Does this seem like chest pain due to an acute coronary syndrome?
A: No. The exacerbation of pain with inspiration and the positional nature of the pain are unusual for an acute coronary syndrome, but would be consistent with acute pericarditis. The site and radiation of the pain are also consistent with acute pericarditis, although these symptoms can also be seen in acute coronary syndromes. (Although it is possible, you would also be less suspicious of an acute coronary syndrome in a 33-year-old man with no known risk factors for ischaemic heart disease.)

Q: What are the most common causes of acute pericarditis?
A: A wide variety of agents can cause acute pericarditis. A mnemonic devised for this is 'Avoid kmart':[1]
- autoimmune disease
- viral (most common)[2]
- other infectious agents (bacteria, fungi)
- idiopathic (probably also viral)
- drugs (hydralazine, phenytoin, isoniazid, rifampicin, penicillin)

---

[1]Please note that this mnemonic is simply the result of the distribution of letters and is not a commentary on the chain of retail stores.
[2]Viral causes include enteroviruses (e.g. coxsackie A or B, echovirus), HIV, influenza, herpes simplex, mumps, chickenpox, Epstein–Barr virus or adenovirus. Patients may recall a recent febrile illness, particularly a respiratory tract illness 10–12 days before the onset of the pain. The absence of such a history does not exclude viral pericarditis, however.

- kidney (renal) failure
- malignancy
- acute MI
- radiotherapy
- trauma (including surgery).

Q: The nurse walks into the room and hands you the 12-lead ECG (see Fig. 3.1).

Lucinda, one of your medical students, is puzzled by the widespread ST elevation. What do you tell her?

	Acute pericarditis	MI	Early repolarisation[*]
ST-segment shape	Concave up	Convex up	Concave up
ST-segment	Many leads	Anatomically distributed leads	Middle/left praecordial leads
ST depression	No	Usually reciprocal ST	No
T-wave inversion[†]	No	At some stage	Maybe
PR segment depression	Yes	No	No
Q waves during evolution	No	Maybe	No
ST/T ratio in lead V6	>0.25	Not applicable	<0.25

[*]Early repolarisation is typically seen in young men. It is a normal variant.
[†]This refers to T-wave inversion in leads with ST-segment elevation.
Source: Adapted from Goyle and Walling (2002) and Marinella (1998).

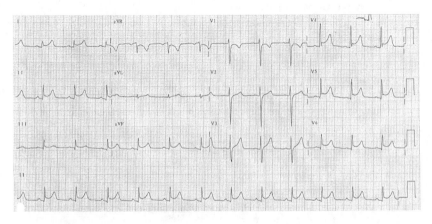

Figure 3.1 Mr Winters's 12-lead ECG

A: The 3 causes of ST elevation that you need to differentiate between are:
1. acute pericarditis
2. MI
3. early repolarisation (refer to the table above).

In most cases, the information gained from the ECG and the clinical picture should be enough to help you differentiate between these conditions.

Scenario

Mr Winters's ECG demonstrates concave up ST-segment elevation in many leads. There is no ST depression. PR-segment depression is present and the ST/T ratio in lead V6 is greater than 0.25. You tell Lucinda that you are satisfied that these ECG findings are consistent with acute pericarditis and are in keeping with the nature of Mr Winters's chest pain.

You now ask your patient about any recent infections. He does recall being unwell 2 weeks ago with a runny nose and sore throat. However, it was a very mild illness that did not bother him and he thought nothing more of it.

Q: You examine Mr Winters. Lucinda wants to know what findings are associated with pericarditis. What do you tell her?

A: The following examination findings may be associated with a diagnosis of pericarditis:
- tachycardia
- hypotension
- pulsus paradoxus (see Chapter 6 for a more detailed explanation of pulsus paradoxus)
- jugular venous pressure abnormalities[3]
- pericardial rub
- Ewart's sign.

Q: What is Ewart's sign?

A: Ewart's sign is a pericardial effusion causing compression of the left lung. It can result in a dull percussion note over the left scapular region.

Q: Lucinda furiously writes down your words of wisdom. She then asks you to explain cardiac tamponade.

---

[3]Tachycardia, hypotension, pulsus paradoxus and jugular venous pressure abnormalities are associated with cardiac tamponade, which is a complication of acute pericarditis.

A: During acute pericarditis, the accumulation of fluid in the pericardial sac can reduce inflow of blood into the ventricles. This can lead to raised intracardiac pressures and reduced cardiac output, which can be fatal.

Q: Lucinda nods and says, 'That's right, I remember now. You get Kussmaul's sign during cardiac tamponade'. Is she right?

A: Yes, but Kussmaul's sign (which is different from Kussmaul's breathing; see Chapter 17) is more commonly found in constrictive pericarditis. This is where a chronic pericarditis results in calcification or thickening of the pericardium. It differs slightly from the acute process of cardiac tamponade.

In normal individuals the jugular venous pulse (JVP) will fall during inspiration. This is easily visible. However, in constrictive pericarditis there is a paradoxical rise in JVP during inspiration. This is Kussmaul's sign and reflects the impaired venous filling.

Q: So what are the JVP abnormalities of acute pericarditis and cardiac tamponade?

A: Uncomplicated acute pericarditis should not be associated with abnormalities of the JVP. But if acute pericarditis is complicated by cardiac tamponade, then the following changes may occur:

- elevated JVP
- prominent x descent.

And note ...

Don't be disheartened if you have never seen an x or y descent in the JVP, prominent or otherwise. Many competent specialists have wondered whether they are myths perpetuated by cardiologists! Cardiologists, however, are adamant that they exist.

Q: On examining Mr Winters, you note that he is tachycardic (110 regular beats/minute) with a blood pressure of 100/60. The JVP is elevated at 6 cm (Lucinda is positive that there is a prominent x descent—you look at her suspiciously). There is no pericardial rub. The examination is otherwise normal. What do you conclude?

A: Mr Winters has a history and ECG consistent with acute pericarditis. The examination findings of hypotension, tachycardia and elevated JVP suggest that the pericarditis has been complicated by cardiac tamponade.

Q: Are you surprised that you could not hear a pericardial rub?
A: Not at all. A pericardial rub is a transient finding that may be present one moment and gone the next. Its presence is useful for diagnosing pericarditis, but its absence should not concern you. Pericardial rubs tend to occur with small pericardial effusions.

A pericardial rub is best heard in the left lower sternal border with the patient sitting forward in full expiration.

Q: You are concerned that Mr Winters has a cardiac tamponade. What should you do?
A: This is potentially a medical emergency. You must now:
- inform the cardiology registrar
- confirm your diagnosis.

Q: How will you confirm the diagnosis of pericardial effusion?
A:

1. **Chest X-ray.** The cardiac shadow will be enlarged if more than 250 mL of fluid has accumulated in the pericardial sac. However, this only confirms the presence of a pericardial effusion. It does not tell you if the effusion is causing cardiac tamponade. Nevertheless, a chest X-ray is a simple investigation that can be performed within minutes in most emergency departments.
2. **Transthoracic (two-dimensional) echocardiogram.** This is a very sensitive, specific and relatively easy way of detecting both pericardial fluid and cardiac tamponade. There are echocardiographic criteria for tamponade, such as right ventricular diastolic collapse and right atrial collapse. It is also possible to estimate the quantity of pericardial fluid on echocardiography.

And note ...

It is also important to note that a transthoracic echo can be helpful in cases where you are not yet sure whether the diagnosis is pericarditis or MI. In MI, you might see localised wall motion abnormalities and no effusion, whereas in pericarditis you might see an effusion without wall motion abnormalities.

3. **CT/MRI.** These imaging modalities may be superior to echocardiography for detecting loculated effusions and pericardial thickening.

Q: You order a mobile chest X-ray. It shows an enlarged cardiac silhouette. While looking at the X-ray, you meet the cardiology registrar, Theo, who has wandered down with the echocardiography machine. Theo performs an echo at the bedside. It demonstrates approximately 600 mL of pericardial fluid with echocardiographic features of tamponade.

Lucinda is surprised by this: 'I thought that you would need much more than 600 mL of fluid in the pericardial space to cause tamponade'. What will the cardiology registrar tell her?

A: The development of tamponade depends on the rate at which fluid accumulates, as well as the quantity. Therefore, according to Braunwald (2002), the rapid accumulation of as little as 200 mL of fluid or the slow accumulation of 2000 mL of fluid can both result in tamponade.

Q: Mr Winters definitely has cardiac tamponade. What must be done now?

A: He requires pericardiocentesis (putting a needle in the pericardial sac to drain the effusion). Even the removal of a small amount of fluid from the pericardial sac can end the tamponade.

It is very unlikely that an intern will be required to perform the pericardiocentesis (at least without supervision). Usually the cardiology registrar or the cardiologist will perform the procedure using local anaesthetic.

Q: Theo explains the situation to Mr Winters, and wants to know if you have taken any blood tests at this stage. You respond in the negative.

Theo replies, 'I am not putting a needle in his pericardial sac without a set of "coags" [coagulation studies] and a platelet count. Please check those as well as other pericarditis bloods'. What blood tests should you order?

A:

1. **Full blood count**. It is important to make sure that the platelet count is not low before any invasive procedure. There may be white cell count abnormalities related to the pericarditis and its cause, but these are likely to be non-specific and unhelpful.
2. **Electrolytes, urea, creatinine and liver function tests**. These tests provide a baseline. In patients where uraemia is a possible cause of pericarditis (which is unlikely in Mr Winters's case), elevated urea and creatinine may be helpful.
3. **Coagulation studies**. The importance of coagulation studies before an invasive procedure was discussed earlier.
4. **Serum troponins**. It is not uncommon for the troponin to be elevated in acute pericarditis due to epicardial involvement. You should not therefore immediately assume that your diagnosis of pericarditis is wrong because the troponin is elevated.

5. **Erythrocyte sedimentation rate (ESR) and C-reactive protein (CRP).** These are non-specific markers of inflammation, but they can be used to monitor treatment.

6. **Antinuclear antibodies.** This is to detect the autoimmune cause of the pericarditis.

7. **Viral serology.** As discussed, viruses are the most common cause of acute pericarditis. But a diagnosis of coxsackie or echovirus pericarditis has no implications for management of the case because it tends to resolve spontaneously. Some specialists therefore might not request serology for these organisms. You should clarify this with the registrar or specialist.

   If you do request serology, make sure you write the name of the organisms on the pathology request form (e.g. 'enteroviral serology'). If you simply write 'viral serology', you will probably receive a call from an angry microbiologist telling you that there are many viruses in the world and they cannot test for them all!

   If the history reveals high-risk sexual behaviour or drug-taking, you should test also for hepatitis B, hepatitis C and HIV. These three viruses definitely can cause a pericardial effusion (Imazio and Adler, 2013) and patients may not recall or may not be forthcoming about a potential exposure. Therefore, it wouldn't be unreasonable to test for these viruses after discussing it with the patient with a pericardial effusion and pericarditis.

8. **Blood cultures if febrile.**

Q: While waiting for the results, Mr Winters complains that he still has the chest pain. 'What can you give me for this pericarditis thing, Doc?'

A: The Therapeutic Guidelines: Cardiovascular (Cardiovascular Expert Group, 2012) suggest a nonsteroidal anti-inflammatory drug (NSAID) e.g. indomethacin 25–50 mg po every 6 hours.

   If the pericarditis doesn't respond, then add colchicine 0.5 mg daily or q12h po for 3 months.

   Another alternative is colchicine. This may be preferable to aspirin or indomethacin in the setting of tamponade.

Q: You commence Mr Winters on 0.5 mg colchicine bd. The results of the blood tests reveal a normal full blood count, coagulation studies, liver function tests with a mildly elevated ESR and CRP. The autoimmune and coxsackie/ echovirus serology will not be available for a few days. The troponin level is normal.

   Theo returns and performs the pericardiocentesis. He drains 550 mL of straw-coloured fluid and leaves a drain in the pericardial sac to prevent the fluid from reaccumulating. He asks you to write the pathology request form for the fluid.

What tests will you order?

A: You should order:

- protein
- Gram stain
- cell count and differential
- cytology (for malignancy)
- culture for coxsackie and echoviruses
- bacterial culture
- tuberculosis polymerase chain reaction and culture (only if at risk for tuberculosis).

Scenario

Theo performs an echo after draining the fluid. You are all pleased (especially Mr Winters) to see that hardly any fluid remains and that the echocardiographic evidence of tamponade has completely resolved. Mr Winters is admitted under the cardiology team.

Q: Not all patients with acute pericarditis will require admission to hospital. What are the indications for admission in cases of acute pericarditis?

A: Goyle and Walling (2002) recommend admission for patients with acute pericarditis in the following circumstances:

- tachycardia
- hypotension
- elevated neck veins
- poor analgesic control
- elevated cardiac enzymes
- pulsus paradoxus[4]
- large pericardial effusion without tamponade (since tamponade can rapidly develop)
- electrical alterans on the ECG.

Scenario

Four days later you go to the cardiology ward to see how Mr Winters is doing. His wife, Sommer, is there and you are pleased to see that they are getting ready to leave the hospital. The pericardial drain was removed

---

[4]Hypotension, elevated neck veins and pulsus paradoxus are features of tamponade.

yesterday and although Mr Winters's pain is still present, the aspirin is keeping it well under control.

Sommer takes out a list of questions and wonders if you can answer them. You tell her that you will try your best.

Q: Can this recur?

A: In the first few months, up to 15% of pericarditis patients will develop a further episode.

Q: What can be done if the fluid and the pericarditis keep recurring?

A: Colchicine can be used for recurrent pericarditis. Corticosteroids have been used, but Fowler and Harbin (1986) note that some patients may become dependent on steroids, which may prolong recovery. Ultimately, if conservative measures fail, the pericardium can be surgically removed.

Q: Even though my husband is feeling a lot better, the nurse said that the ECG this morning was still abnormal. Is that to be expected?

A: Yes. There are classically 4 ECG stages of pericarditis and these can persist for months, even when the illness itself has resolved. As interns seeing patients in the acute setting, you will probably see only those with the ST-elevation stage of the disease (stage 1).

You do not need to learn it, but if you are interested, the following table sets out the 4 stages and their duration.

Stage	ECG appearance	Duration
I	Diffuse ST elevation	Up to 2 weeks
II	ST segments return to baseline; flattening of T-waves	Days to weeks
III	T-wave inversion	Several weeks
IV	Resolution of T-wave inversion	Up to 3 months

Source: Adapted from Marinella (1998).

The Winters are reassured by your answers to their questions. As you watch Mr Winters and his wife Sommer leave the hospital on this warm autumn day with a spring in their step, you reflect on a job well done.

Achievements

You now:
- can recognise the classical pain of acute pericarditis
- know the causes of acute pericarditis

- can use the ECG to differentiate between acute pericarditis, MI and early repolarisation
- know the signs of pericarditis and tamponade
- know which investigations are used to diagnose pericardial tamponade and effusions
- can order appropriate investigations for acute pericarditis
- know the role of pericardiocentesis in tamponade
- know how to treat the pain of acute pericarditis
- can order appropriate tests on pericardial fluid
- know indications for admission for acute pericarditis
- know that there are 4 ECG stages of pericarditis that can last for months.

References

Adler, Y. *et al.* (1998), 'Colchicine treatment for recurrent pericarditis: A decade of experience', *Circulation*, vol. 97, no. 21, pp. 2183–2185.

Braunwald, E. (2002), 'Pericardial disease', in E. Braunwald, A.S. Fauci, D.L. Kasper, S.L. Hauser, D.L. Longo and J.L. Jameson (eds), *Harrison's Principles of Internal Medicine*, McGraw-Hill, New York, pp. 1365–1372.

Cardiovascular Expert Group (2012), *Therapeutic Guidelines: Cardiovascular*, Version 6, Therapeutic Guidelines Ltd, Melbourne.

Fowler, N.O. and Harbin, A.D. 3rd (1986), 'Recurrent acute pericarditis: Follow-up study of 31 patients', *Journal of the American College of Cardiology*, vol. 7, no. 2, pp. 300–305.

Goyle, K.K. and Walling, A.D. (2002), 'Diagnosing pericarditis', *American Family Physician*, vol. 66, no. 9, pp. 1695–1702.

Imazio, M., Adler, Y. (2013), 'Management of pericardial effusion', *European Heart Journal*, vol. 34, no. 16, pp. 1186–1197.

Marinella, M.A. (1998), 'Electrocardiographic manifestations and differential diagnosis of acute pericarditis', *American Family Physician*, vol. 57, no. 4, pp. 699–704.

Chapter 4
Frida presents with palpitations and breathlessness

Scenario

Frida, a 75-year-old woman, presents to hospital with 24 hours of mild shortness of breath. She has noted palpitations on and off for the past 3 days, but has not suffered from chest pain. Her palpable heart rate is 110/minute, her blood pressure is 110/70 and oxygen saturation is at 96% on room air. Her only medical condition is hypertension, for which she has been taking a thiazide diuretic for many months.

The Emergency Department nurse shows you a 12-lead ECG (see Fig. 4.1).

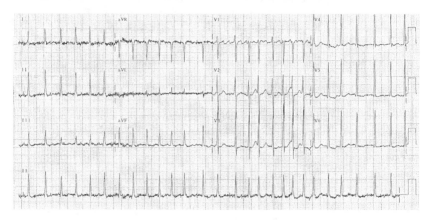

Figure 4.1 Frida's 12-lead ECG

Q: What does the ECG show and what is the most likely diagnosis?

A: The ECG shows atrial fibrillation (AF) with a rapid ventricular response (RVR) of 130. Frida almost certainly has pulmonary oedema due to AF with RVR; however, AF can be precipitated by other conditions that can also cause shortness of breath, for example pulmonary embolism, acute coronary syndrome, pneumonia. You therefore will have to consider causes of AF when treating Frida's condition but this is discussed further below.

Use the 3 Cs to manage patients with AF:
1. cause
2. consequences
3. anticoagulation.

Q: What is the first thing to do for any patient with an arrhythmia?
A: You must decide if Frida requires immediate electrical cardioversion. The criteria include:
- hypotension with signs of hypoperfusion
- severe unresponsive chest pain
- severe heart failure.

You feel that Frida is not sick enough to require immediate electrical cardioversion at this stage.

Q: How will you use the history and examination to evaluate Frida?
A: Try to identify any precipitating factors for the AF. These include (Medi *et al.*, 2007):
- electrolyte abnormalities
- endocrine causes (hyperthyroidism, phaeochromocytoma)
- drugs (alcohol or caffeine)
- PE
- post-surgery
- systemic hypertension
- congestive cardiac failure
- cardiomyopathy
- other causes of atrial dilatation (obesity, obstructive sleep apnoea)
- infiltrative disorders of the atrium (e.g. amyloidosis)
- valvular heart disease (mitral and tricuspid)
- pericarditis or myocarditis
- coronary artery disease
- congenital heart disease (atrial septal defect)
- neurogenic causes (e.g. subarachnoid haemorrhage)
- heightened adrenergic tone (exertion, anxiety).

On examination, look for:
- irregularly irregular pulse and loss of 'a' waves in the jugular venous pressure (consistent with AF)
- valvular heart disease
- cardiomyopathies
- heart failure

- pulmonary hypertension
- features of hyperthyroidism.

Frida's history does not offer further clues as to the cause of the AF, but Frida is certain that she has never experienced palpitations before. Her examination demonstrates an irregularly irregular tachycardia consistent with AF. Her oxygen saturations remain at 96% on room air and her respiratory rate is 20 breaths/minute. The only other abnormality is bibasal coarse inspiratory crackles consistent with pulmonary oedema. Despite this, she looks quite comfortable lying in bed. You conclude that she probably has pulmonary oedema, but is not in severe respiratory distress.

Q: Do you think this is Frida's first episode of AF?

A: It is difficult to be sure. It is certainly her first symptomatic episode of AF. Holter monitor studies have shown that 20% of episodes of paroxysmal AF in the same patient are asymptomatic. It is therefore possible that Frida has had asymptomatic AF previously.

Q: Although you realise that an underlying cause of the AF may not be discovered, what investigations will you order?

A:

1. **Full blood count**. A baseline platelet count is necessary before anticoagulation.
2. **Coagulation studies**. Baseline values will be useful before anticoagulation.
3. **Electrolytes, urea and creatinine (EUC or UEC)**. This might identify electrolyte derangements precipitating AF. It should include calcium, magnesium and phosphate. Because these tests are not part of the routine 'EUC' screen, on the pathology form you must write: EUC Ca^{2+} Mg^{2+} PO_4^{3-}.
4. **Thyroid function tests**. Hyperthyroidism is a cause of AF.
5. **Serial high sensitivity troponins**. AF can occur in the context of coronary artery disease.
6. **Chest X-ray**. This may identify pulmonary oedema, chronic obstructive pulmonary disease, cardiomyopathy, pneumonia or X-ray features of PE (see Chapter 5 for a description of the X-ray features of PE).
7. **12-lead ECG**. You have already seen Frida's ECG. It confirms the diagnosis of AF and allows you to look for any ischaemic changes.
8. **Arterial blood gas**. This allows you to assess how hypoxic Frida is from the pulmonary oedema.

9. **Others.** If there is evidence supporting underlying PE or sepsis, you should further evaluate these diagnoses. For PE this may include investigations such as ventilation-perfusion scans and a helical CT (see Chapter 5). For sepsis, it may include blood cultures and a midstream urine as well as other specimens if clinically appropriate. Note, however, that neither of these investigations should be routinely undertaken in patients with AF.

Q: You organise the appropriate investigations. You feel that Frida is unlikely to be at risk for PE or sepsis, so you don't follow that avenue of investigation.

The chest X-ray is performed quickly. It demonstrates changes consistent with pulmonary oedema. What do you do now?

A: You should treat Frida's pulmonary oedema. This involves treating the pulmonary oedema itself and removing the underlying precipitant (AF with RVR in this case).

Q: How do you treat the pulmonary oedema itself?

A: A well-known mnemonic for the treatment of pulmonary oedema is LMNOP.

L = Lasix (frusemide)
M = Morphine
N = Nitrates
O = Oxygen
P = CPAP (continuous positive airway pressure and position the patient upright).

This does not necessarily reflect the order of the steps you would take, but it is fairly close. For example, the nursing staff would already have initiated oxygen therapy. Remember, however, to be cautious with oxygen therapy in patients with underlying COPD to avoid hypercapnia (see Chapter 7).

1. **Frusemide.** This diuretic exerts its effects in pulmonary oedema through a reduction in preload (through venodilation and diuresis). A reasonable dose would be 20–80 mg intravenously, which can be repeated in 20 minutes if required (Cardiovascular Expert Group, 2012).

   Ask the nursing staff to monitor the urine output to document the degree of diuresis from frusemide. This is very important, but does not necessarily require an indwelling urinary catheter.

   It is worth noting that patients with advanced renal failure will often require much higher doses of frusemide (e.g. 200–250 mg) to achieve a therapeutic response. However, you should consult the medical registrar in such a situation.

2. **Morphine** exerts its effects in pulmonary oedema through a number of mechanisms:

   a. reduction in preload
   b. reduction in afterload and heart rate
   c. reduction in anxiety
   d. reduction in sympathetic nervous system activity.

   The use of morphine to achieve these positive effects must be balanced by its side effects, in particular respiratory depression, hypotension and bradycardia. In fact, Cotter *et al.* (2001) described a study by Sacetti *et al.* (1999) in which it was found that the use of morphine for pulmonary oedema resulted in higher rates of intensive care unit admissions and mechanical ventilation.

   There are no evidence-based guidelines for an optimal dose of morphine in this setting. A reasonable approach would be 1–2 mg IV as a single dose (Cardiovascular Expert Group, 2012).

3. **Nitrates.** Cotter *et al.* (2001) note that nitrates exert their effect in pulmonary oedema through:

   a. reduction in preload
   b. reduction in afterload
   c. possible reduction in myocardial ischaemia.

   In Australia, nitrates for pulmonary oedema will most commonly be administered as a topical patch or an IV infusion.

4. **CPAP** rapidly improves gas exchange and helps avoid intubation in patients with pulmonary oedema (cardiogenic) by reducing airway resistance and decreasing the work of breathing. CPAP can also lower the heart rate.

   The use of 5 cm H_2O CPAP leads to an improvement in both cardiac and stroke volume indices. These indices further improve when the pressure is increased to 10 cm H_2O.

   If CPAP is required in the Emergency Department, it would be reasonable to commence it at 10 cm H_2O (Cardiovascular Expert Group, 2012).

Q: You place Frida on supplemental oxygen. She is given 80 mg IV frusemide. You feel that she is not sick enough to require CPAP at this stage. Very soon, she begins to have a large diuresis and becomes far less breathless. The ECG monitor still shows AF but the ventricular rate has slowed to 95 beats/minute.

Tracy, your medical student, says, 'Now we've got the pulmonary oedema under control, we have to get her out of AF and back into sinus rhythm'. Is Tracy correct?

A: Tracy unwittingly has raised the issue of rate control versus rhythm control in AF. While it might intuitively seem better for a patient to be in sinus rhythm than AF, this is not necessarily the case. In fact, a rhythm control strategy appears to have no survival benefit and may result in more hospitalisations than a rate control approach. The circumstances in which rhythm control may be considered are (January *et al.*, 2014):
- younger patient
- first episode of AF
- difficulty in controlling the rate
- cardiomyopathy due to the tachycardia.

Q: You explain to Tracy that rate control may be enough for Frida. Dr Hart, the on-call cardiologist, reviews Frida and agrees with your assessment. She brings the echocardiography machine with her. Is it worth performing a transthoracic echocardiogram (TTE)?

A: Yes. A TTE will inform you whether Frida has any of the following (January *et al.*, 2014):
- structural heart disease (e.g. mitral valve disease, regional wall hypokinesia suggesting ischaemia)
- heart failure (e.g. reduced left ventricular ejection fraction), which will dictate how cautiously medications like beta-blockers are used
- atrial size.

Q: The TTE is fairly unremarkable. Tracy asks you what drug you want to use to control the rate of Frida's AF. What do you tell her?

A: Beta-blockers are the drug class of choice if there are no contraindications. A nondihyropyridine calcium channel antagonist, such as verapamil or diltiazem, can also be used (Medi *et al.*, 2007). Digoxin and amiodarone are other options, although they are not first-line agents.

Q: What doses of beta-blockers and calcium channel antagonists can be used?

A: IV therapy can be used to rapidly lower the ventricular rate in AF if required (e.g. metoprolol IV 2.5–5 mg bolus over 2 minutes: use up to 3 doses). Then an oral dose is used for maintenance (e.g. metoprolol po 25–100 mg bd, atenolol po 25–100 mg daily, propranolol po 10–40 mg tds or qid, verapamil po 180–480 mg daily, diltiazem po 120–360 mg daily) (January *et al.*, 2014).

Q: The cardiologist agrees that a beta-blocker would be best. Frida is now well enough not to require IV beta-blockers to rapidly lower her heart rate. Dr Hart therefore commences her on metoprolol po 25 mg bd. She then asks you why you didn't choose digoxin as your agent of choice. What do you tell her?

A: Digoxin isn't as effective as beta-blockers in controlling exercise-induced tachycardia (Fuster *et al.*, 2006).

Q: If you had decided to chemically cardiovert Frida, what drugs could you have used?

A: A number of agents can be used, but in Australia you will most commonly encounter amiodarone and sotalol (a beta-blocker).

Q: Is amiodarone relatively free of adverse reactions?

A: Not at all. There are a large number of possible side effects. The most common of these are pulmonary disorders or a variety of thyroid abnormalities.

Pulmonary toxicity (mainly fibrosis and alveolitis) occurs in 1% of patients per year. However, this is generally reversible following the cessation of therapy. Other side effects include bradyarrhythmias, corneal deposits, hepatotoxicity, photosensitivity, neuropathy, nightmares and vivid dreams. Because amiodarone has a long half-life (35–40 days), adverse effects can take a long time to resolve.

In randomised trials, 41% of patients had discontinued amiodarone therapy by 2 years due to adverse reactions; placebo was discontinued in only 27% of patients.

Q: Does Frida need to be anticoagulated?

A: Before answering this question, it is important to understand the relationship between AF and anticoagulation. AF can lead to the formation of left atrial thrombus. Cardioembolism is therefore the major complication of AF. Although left atrial thrombus can embolise anywhere (bowel, legs, etc.), the most feared complication is stroke.

Q: What is the risk of stroke in AF?

A: The risk is 5 times greater than in age-matched controls. The annual risk increases with age: 1.5%/year for ages 50–59 to 23.5%/year for ages 80–89.

Q: What causes of AF are strongly associated with thromboembolism?

A: Patients with AF associated with rheumatic mitral stenosis are 10 times more likely to experience thromboembolism than those with AF of nonvalvular origin.

AF associated with hyperthyroidism is possibly more likely to be associated with thromboembolism than AF in euthyroid states.

Q: Are there independent factors that further increase the risk of stroke in nonvalvular AF?

A: There are a number of risk factors. This has led to the creation of a scoring system called the $CHADS_2$-VAS_c. If a patient has a score ≥ 2, they should receive anticoagulation. This scoring system is fairly easy to remember and makes an easy question for exams! The scoring system is as follows (January *et al.*, 2014):

C: Congestive heart failure – 1 point
H: Hypertension – 1 point
A: Age ≥ 75 – 2 points
D: Diabetes mellitus – 1 point
S: Stroke/TIA/thromboembolic disease – 2 points
V: Vascular disease (prior MI, peripheral arterial disease, aortic plaque) – 1 point
A: Age 65–74 years – 1 point
Sc: Sex category (females only) – 1 point
Frida has a score of 4 (1 point for hypertension, 2 points for her age and 1 point for being female). She therefore should receive oral anticoagulation.

Q: Tracy, the medical student, wants to know what Frida's risk of stroke is. What do you tell her?

A: The annual percentage risk of stroke almost equals the $CHADS_2$-VAS_c score from 0–4, so Frida's score of 4 means that she has a 4% annual risk of stroke (see following table).

$CHADS_2$-VAS_c Score	Approximate annual stroke rate (%)
0	0
1	1
2	2
3	3
4	4
5	7
6	10
7	10
8	7
9	15

Source: Adapted from January *et al.* (2014).

Q: What anticoagulants can she receive (January *et al.*, 2014)?

A: Options for Frida include:
- warfarin at a variable dose (aim for an INR of 2–3)
- dabigatran (direct thrombin inhibitor)*
- rivaroxaban (direct factor Xa inhibitor)*
- apixaban (direct factor Xa inhibitor).*

Q: Frida is commenced on rivaroxaban in addition to the metoprolol. If you had wanted to electrically cardiovert Frida, how would you have done this?

A: The answer to this depends on your method of cardioversion and the duration of the AF (January *et al.*, 2014).

If the AF has been present for < 48 hours, then:
1. cardiovert with or without anticoagulation if the patient has a low thromboembolic risk OR
2. cardiovert with anticoagulation just before or just after the procedure if the patient has a high thromboembolic risk.

If the AF has been present for an unknown duration or ≥ 48 hours, then:
1. anticoagulate for 3 weeks before the cardioversion, and then at least 4 weeks afterwards OR
2. perform a transoesophageal echocardiogram (TOE) with anticoagulation commenced before the TOE (e.g. enoxaparin) and continue anticoagulation for at least 4 weeks post cardioversion.

Q: What should you look for during the TOE if you are planning to electrically cardiovert someone?

A: The presence of any of the following factors during a TOE increases the risk of stroke in AF:
- left atrial appendage thrombus
- spontaneous echo contrast (SEC), a smoke-like haze appearance
- low flow velocities
- complex aortic plaques.

Q: Frida had been relatively healthy till this hospital admission so she is somewhat shell-shocked by recent events. She asks you, 'Doctor, is this "AF" thing common? Because I'd never heard of it till now'.

A: Unfortunately, AF is the most common sustained arrhythmia in the world. One study showed that in people aged ≥ 65 years, the prevalence

---

*These 3 agents, unlike warfarin, don't require therapeutic drug monitoring. But their dose must be adjusted in the presence of renal impairment.

of AF is around 5% (4.6% in women, 6.2% in men) (Medi et al., 2007; Furberg et al., 1994).

Q: Frida has two more questions for you. It appears that Dr Hart stopped her diuretic for hypertension and commenced an ACE inhibitor. 'I thought that my blood pressure was under control so I don't know why she changed it. Do you have any idea?'

A: Although results are conflicting, the use of ACE inhibitors and angiotensin receptor blockers in certain patient groups may reduce the risk of AF (Marott *et al.*, 2014). This could be the basis for Dr Hart's decision.

Q: Frida has a question relates to medications. 'Dr Hart tested my cholesterol and found it to be a bit high. She started me on simvastatin and said it'd also be good for the AF. What did she mean by that? Was she mistaken?'

A: Although the statin class of drugs is used primarily to treat hypercholesterolaemia, it also appears to reduce the risk of recurrence of AF in lone fibrillators who have been successfully cardioverted (Siu et al., 2003).

Q: Your medical student listens with interest before asking, 'Is the risk of stroke from paroxysmal AF the same as for chronic AF?'

A: Yes. Paroxysmal AF is as dangerous as chronic AF in terms of risk for strokes.

Q: If the risk of the stroke is the same, why do we bother classifying AF into subgroups?

A: AF can be classified in the following ways:
- paroxysmal: AF that lasts for < 7 days (due to intervention or spontaneous reversion)
- persistent: AF that lasts for > 7 days
- longstanding persistent: AF that lasts for > 12 months
- permanent
- nonvalvular: AF in the absence of a prosthetic heart valve, rheumatic mitral stenosis or a mitral valve repair.

  The type of AF can predict responses to therapy. For example, there are better outcomes with catheter ablation in paroxysmal AF compared to persistent AF (January et al., 2014).

Q: Apart from pharmacological and electrical cardioversion, are there any other methods for treating AF?

A: Catheter ablation techniques can be used to achieve rhythm control. Although there are a number of techniques (e.g. AV node ablation, pacemaker insertion), the major technique is pulmonary vein isolation (Shukla and Curtis, 2014).

Achievements

You now:
- know the 3 Cs of managing AF
- realise that some patients with AF may need immediate electrical cardioversion
- are familiar with the $CHAD_2$-VAS_c score
- appreciate that many episodes of AF are asymptomatic
- can order correct investigations for a patient with AF
- know the 'LMNOP' of managing pulmonary oedema
- know the common side effects of amiodarone
- understand the role of anticoagulation in preventing thromboembolism in AF
- know the TOE features that increase risk of stroke in AF
- know the role of catheter ablation techniques in the treatment of AF.

References

Anonymous (1997), 'Effect of prophylactic amiodarone on mortality after acute myocardial infarction and in congestive heart failure: Meta-analysis of individual data from 6500 patients in randomised trials', Amiodarone Trials Meta-Analysis Investigators, *Lancet*, vol. 350, no. 9089, pp. 1417–1424.

Cardiovascular Expert Group (2012), *Therapeutic Guidelines: Cardiovascular*, Version 6, Therapeutic Guidelines Ltd, Melbourne.

Cooper, J.M., Katcher, M.S. and Orlov, M.V. (2002), 'Implantable devices for the treatment of atrial fibrillation', *New England Journal of Medicine*, vol. 346, no. 26, pp. 2062–2068.

Cotter, G. et al. (2001), 'Pulmonary edema: New insight on pathogenesis and treatment', *Current Opinion in Cardiology*, vol. 16, no. 3, pp. 159–163.

Esberger, D., Jones, S. and Morris, F. (2002), 'ABC of clinical electrocardiography: Junctional tachycardias', *British Medical Journal*, vol. 324, no. 7338, pp. 662–665.

Ezekowitz, M.D. and Netrebko, P.I. (2003), 'Anticoagulation in management of atrial fibrillation', *Current Opinion in Cardiology*, vol. 18, no. 1, pp. 26–31.

Furberg, C.D., Psaty, B.M., Manolio, T.A., Gardin, J.M., Smith, V.E. and Rautaharju, P.M. (1994), 'Prevalence of atrial fibrillation in elderly subjects (the Cardiovascular Health Study)', *American Journal of Cardiology*, vol. 74, no. 3, pp. 236–241.

Fuster, V., Ryden, L.E., Cannom, D.S. et al. (2006), 'ACC/AHA/ESC 2006 guidelines for the management of patients with atrial fibrillation: A report of the American College of Cardiology/American Heart Association Task Force on Practice Guidelines and the European Society of Cardiology Committee for Practice Guidelines (Writing Committee to Revise the 2001 guidelines for the management of patients with atrial fibrillation), developed in collaboration with the European Heart Rhythm Association and the Heart Rhythm Society', *Circulation*, vol. 114, no. 7, e257–354.

January, C.T., Wann, L.S., Alpert, J.S., *et al.* (2014), '2014 AHA/ACC/HRS guideline for the management of patients with atrial fibrillation', *Journal of the American College of Cardiology*, doi: 10.1016/j.jacc.2014.03.022.

Khairy, P. and Nattel, S. (2002), 'New insights into the mechanisms and management of atrial fibrillation', *Canadian Medical Association Journal*, vol. 167, no. 9, pp. 1012–1020.

L'Her, E. (2003), 'Noninvasive mechanical ventilation in acute cardiogenic pulmonary edema', *Current Opinion in Critical Care*, vol. 9, no. 1, pp. 67–71.

Madrid, A.H., Peng, J., Zamora, J. *et al.* (2004), 'The role of angiotensin receptor blockers and/or angiotensin converting enzyme inhibitors in the prevention of atrial fibrillation in patients with cardiovascular diseases: Meta-analysis of randomized controlled clinical trials', *Pacing and Clinical Electrophysiology*, vol. 27, no. 10. pp. 1405–1410.

Marott, S.C., Nielsen, S.F., Benn, M., Nordestgaard, B.G (2014), 'Antihypertensive treatment and risk of atrial fibrillation: a nationwide study', *European Heart Journal*, vol. 35, no. 18, pp. 1205–1214.

Medi, C., Hankey, G.J. and Freedman, S.B. (2007), 'Atrial fibrillation', *Medical Journal of Australia*, vol. 186, no. 4, pp. 197–202.

Sacetti, A., Ramoska, E., Moakes, M.E., McDermott, P. and Moyer, V. (1999), 'Effect of ED management on ICU use in acute pulmonary edema', *American Journal of Emergency Medicine*, vol. 17, no. 6, pp. 517–574.

Shukla, A. and Curtis, A.B. (2014), 'Avoiding permanent atrial fibrillation: treatment approaches to prevent disease progression', *Vascular Health and Risk Management*, vol. 10, pp. 1–12.

Siu, C.W., Lau, C.P. and Tse, H.F. (2003), 'Prevention of atrial fibrillation recurrence by statin therapy in patients with lone atrial fibrillation after successful cardioversion', *American Journal of Cardiology*, vol. 92, no. 11, pp. 1343–1345.

Wyse, D.G. (2003), 'Rhythm versus rate control in atrial fibrillation', *Journal of Cardiovascular Electrophysiology*, vol. 14, no. 9 (suppl.), S35–39.

Wyse, D.G., Waldo, A.L., DiMarco, J.P. *et al.* (2002), 'A comparison of rate control and rhythm control in patients with atrial fibrillation', *New England Journal of Medicine*, vol. 347, no. 23, pp. 1825–1833.

Chapter 5
Annika presents with breathlessness and haemoptysis

Scenario

Annika, a 45-year-old woman, presents to the Emergency Department with a 24-hour history of shortness of breath and coughing up small amounts of blood. Two weeks ago she was discharged from hospital with a home rehabilitation plan after having hip surgery 3 weeks ago.

Q: What is your major concern?

A: Although there are a number of causes of shortness of breath to exclude, the most likely cause of dyspnoea and haemoptysis in the postoperative setting is pulmonary embolism (PE).

Scenario

You take a more extensive history. This reveals that Annika has a past history of hypertension, for which she takes a thiazide diuretic. She has no other risk factors for ischaemic heart disease and had never been to hospital prior to her hip surgery. The surgery was for a fracture that occurred during a motorcycle accident. She suffered no other serious injuries. She drinks 10 grams of alcohol a day.

Annika had been completely well up until 24 hours ago, when she noticed that she was short of breath walking around the house. The shortness of breath has remained the same, but today she started coughing up small amounts of bright red blood. Naturally, she was worried and came to hospital for assessment.

Q: What other features of the history would support a diagnosis of PE?

A: These features would include:
- presence of a sharp chest pain that is worse on inspiration
- history of not receiving deep venous thrombosis (DVT) prophylaxis (although receiving DVT prophylaxis is not 100% efficacious in preventing thromboembolism)

- DVT during her admission for hip surgery
- previous history or family history of thromboembolism
- history of smoking
- history of hypertension (which this patient has)
- use of oral contraceptive pill
- history of immobility.[1]

Q: What features on physical examination would support a diagnosis of PE?

A: The diagnosis would be supported by the presence of:
- tachycardia (non-specific)
- hypoxia on oxygen pulse oximetry
- fever (non-specific)
- signs of right ventricular dysfunction such as bulging neck veins with prominent 'v' waves, parasternal heave, a palpable and loud pulmonary component of the second heart sound and a systolic murmur at the left lower sternal edge louder on inspiration
- swollen tender calf consistent with DVT.

Q: This patient is tachycardic with an oxygen saturation on room air of 93%, but otherwise has no other positive findings. You are still convinced that PE is the most likely diagnosis. What criteria can you use to guide you?

A: The '2-level Wells score' is a useful diagnostic tool to diagnose PE. The criteria are as follows (National Institute for Health and Clinical Excellence, 2014):
- Clinical signs and symptoms of DVT – 3 points
- An alternative diagnosis is less likely than PE – 3 points
- Heart rate >100 beats per minute – 1.5 points
- Immobilisation for >3 days or surgery in the previous 4 weeks – 1.5 points
- Previous DVT/PE – 1.5 points
- Haemoptysis – 1 point
- Malignancy (on treatment, treated in the last 6 months, or palliative) – 1 point

(PE likely if > 4 points, PE unlikely if 4 points or less.)

---

[1] Smoking, hypertension and use of an oral contraceptive pill are risk factors for PE.

Q: Annika has a 2-level Wells score of 7 (an alternative diagnosis is less likely than PE, tachycardia, surgery in the previous 4 weeks, haemoptysis) which makes PE likely. What should you do from here?

A: Annika should undergo a CT pulmonary angiogram (CTPA) immediately or be anticoagulated if a delay in the CTPA is anticipated (National Institute for Health and Clinical Excellence, 2014).

A multirow-detector CTPA has a sensitivity of >95% in detecting lobar, segmental and centrally located PE. The sensitivity falls for small, distal, subsegmental PE (Huisman and Klok, 2013).

Q: What if Annika's 2-level Wells score was 4 or less, making PE unlikely?

A: In that case, a D-dimer should be performed. If the D-dimer is elevated, then a CTPA should be performed. If the D-dimer is not elevated, no further testing for PE is required (National Institute for Health and Clinical Excellence, 2014).

The rationale for this is that the D-dimer is a fibrin breakdown product that is elevated in DVT disease, PE and a number of inflammatory disorders. A D-dimer therefore has a poor positive predictive value, but a strong negative predictive value in the diagnosis of PE. In simple terms, this means that a negative D-dimer suggests that PE is unlikely.

Q: Although CTPA testing is usually available, the machine has broken down and is being serviced. What would be the next best imaging test that Annika should undergo?

A: **V/Q radionuclide scan.** Although CTPA is the preferred diagnostic test for PE, the V/Q scan can be useful, especially in those patients where CTPA may be risky or contraindicated (e.g. renal failure, allergy to contrast). There are 4 possible results:

1. normal scan
2. low probability scan
3. intermediate probability scan
4. high probability scan.

And note ...

Junior doctors often assume that a normal scan and a low probability scan are the same thing. They are not. The PIOPED study (Anonymous, 1990) demonstrated that a normal scan means that PE is very unlikely, but 6% of 'low probability' patients had a PE. A high probability scan result also has a very good positive predictive value (i.e. there is a high likelihood that the patient has a PE). However, only 41% of patients with PE in a large study had a high probability scan. In other words, it is not a very sensitive test, but it is very specific. Most lung scans are reported as intermediate or low probability. A study of a subset of the PIOPED study (1990) demonstrated that 22% of patients with an intermediate probability scan had pulmonary emboli.

High probability or normal scan results are therefore helpful in diagnosing PE. However, do not let a low or intermediate probability scan dismiss a diagnosis of PE if your instincts tell you otherwise.

Q: What other tests might be useful in the meantime?

A: While the following tests won't diagnose PE, they can contribute to Annika's care in a number of ways:

1. **Full blood count**. This will demonstrate if anaemia is causing or contributing to the dyspnoea. An elevated white cell count might point to an infective or inflammatory cause of the dyspnoea such as pneumonia, but this is non-specific. It is also important to know the baseline platelet value if you are going to anticoagulate Annika with heparin. Heparin can lead to 'heparin-induced thrombocytopaenia'.

2. **Arterial blood gas**. The Prospective Investigation of Pulmonary Embolism Diagnosis (PIOPED) study (Anonymous, 1990) demonstrated that arterial oxygen levels and the alveolararterial gradient are poor diagnostic tools in PE (see Chapter 25). Furthermore, a normal arterial blood gas does not rule out a diagnosis of PE. Therefore, apart from demonstrating that the patient is hypoxaemic and providing a baseline value, an arterial blood gas is not useful in differentiating PE from other causes of dyspnoea. Similarly, Stein *et al.* (1991) found that 26% of patients with PE had a partial pressure of arterial oxygen ≥80 mm Hg while 14% had an alveolar–arterial gradient ≥20 mm Hg.

3. **Serial high sensitivity troponin levels**. Elevated serum troponin levels can occur in acute PE and may be a marker of adverse outcomes; therefore, an initially elevated troponin level does not necessarily indicate an acute coronary syndrome. But the duration of troponin elevation in PE tends to be far less than in an acute coronary syndrome, that is, 40 hours versus 10–14 days (Horlander and Leeper, 2003).

4. **ECG**. The ECG is not a sensitive or specific test for diagnosing acute PE. Ullman *et al.* (2001) found that 15–27% of ECGs in

people with PE are normal. The ECG tends to be abnormal in those people with submassive or massive PE. Twenty-one ECG changes have been associated with PE, including some of the following:

a. sinus tachycardia with non-specific ST and T-wave changes (the most common finding)

b. T-wave inversion V1-4 (possibly secondary to right coronary artery compression from right ventricular overload)

c. partial right bundle or right bundle branch block

d. S1Q3T3 (S-wave in lead I, Q-wave and T-wave inversion in lead V3; this is a classical ECG picture for PE, but is very rare. It represents acute cor pulmonale)

e. new-onset AF or flutter (which can be a consequence of PE further adding to the dyspnoea caused by the PE itself).

5. **Chest radiograph.** A normal CXR in a dypsnoeic patient supports a diagnosis of PE. Nevertheless, there are some X-ray changes particular to PE:

a. Westermark's sign—focal oligaemia (i.e. reduced vascular markings)

b. Hampton's hump—a peripheral wedge-shaped density above the diaphragm

c. Palla's sign—an enlarged descending right pulmonary artery.

Very importantly, nuclear medicine physicians will often approve a lung scan (V/Q scan) only if a chest X-ray has been performed within the past 24 hours.

Other non-diagnostic but useful blood tests include:

6. **Coagulation studies.** Baseline values will be useful before anticoagulating this patient.

7. **Electrolytes, urea and creatinine.** The dose of low molecular weight heparins will need to be reduced in the presence of significant renal failure.

Echocardiography. The role of echocardiography in acute PE is still not completely clear. It has a poor sensitivity of only around 40% (Goldhaber, 1998) but might guide therapeutic decisions such as the need for thrombolysis (Hamilton-Craig et al., 2008). The echocardiographic changes seen in acute PE tend to reflect right ventricular pressure overload. A specific appearance is known as McConnell's sign in which motion of the right ventricular apical wall remains normal despite hypokinesis of the free wall (Goldhaber, 1998).

Q: Annika has a normal full blood count and troponin level. Her arterial blood gas demonstrates hypoxaemia with an arterial oxygen of 70 mm Hg. The A–a gradient is elevated, at 30 mm Hg. The D-dimer is also elevated. Her ECG demonstrates sinus tachycardia but no ischaemic changes. The CXR is unremarkable. These findings support your diagnosis of PE.

She is taken to her V/Q scan. One of the nurses asks, 'If she couldn't have the V/Q scan or the CTPA for some reason, are there any other ways to see a PE?'

A:
1. **MRI angiography.** Although few centres in Australia provide this service, it appears promising, with sensitivities of 90–100% and specificities of 60–73% in different studies.
2. **Pulmonary angiography (the 'gold standard').** Although pulmonary angiography has an excellent sensitivity and specificity of more than 95%, it is rarely used in Australia nowadays as a diagnostic tool for PE as the procedure itself has a mortality rate of 0.5% and a complication rate of 2–6%. It has been superseded by the less invasive CTPA.
3. **Venous ultrasonography.** Given that a pulmonary embolus arises from DVT, it is worth evaluating a patient for it. Again, however, this test is useful only if it is positive in demonstrating DVT. A negative result should not dissuade you from a diagnosis of pulmonary embolus. Even bilateral venography in patients with angiographically proven PE can produce a negative result.

Q: Annika's V/Q scan comes back as high probability for PE with multiple V/Q mismatches, confirming your clinical diagnosis.

What are V/Q mismatches?

A: This is not as complicated as it sounds! McCabe *et al.* (1991) described the 2 parts to a lung scan:
1. ventilation (V) scan
2. perfusion (Q) scan.

The perfusion scan is obtained through the injection of radionuclide-labelled albumin. The ventilation scan is obtained through the inhalation of various radio-labelled gases. In PE, the embolus to the artery affects perfusion. However, the ventilation should not be affected. As a result, there is normal V but abnormal Q, hence a 'V/Q mismatch'.

Sometimes the report will mention 'matched V/Q defects'. There are a number of causes here, but pneumonia and atelectasis are the most common. In the case of pneumonia, ventilation is affected because of consolidation of lung tissue. In response to the hypoxia from the pneumonia, local vasoconstriction occurs. Perfusion is therefore reduced. As a result, both V and Q are reduced, hence a 'matched V/Q defect'.

Q: So a single V/Q mismatch equals a high probability lung scan?

A: It is not as simple as that. There are a number of criteria for a high probability lung scan. In broad terms, they are based on:

- number of V/Q mismatches
- size of the V/Q mismatches
- whether or not the chest X-ray is normal.

Q: One of the medical students in the Emergency Department has been looking on with interest. She asks, 'Should you do a thrombophilia screen before you anticoagulate the patient'.
What is a thrombophilia screen?

A: In fact, there is technically no such thing as a 'thrombophilia screen' and haematologists may take exception to use of the term! What the medical student is referring to are certain defects in the coagulation pathway that predispose to thromboembolism. The presence of such defects might influence the duration of the patient's therapy (e.g. rather than the conventional 6 months, lifelong therapy may be required). Furthermore, the presence of such defects may prompt future avoidance of certain medications (e.g. oral contraceptives, which can be procoagulant).

If looking for coagulation disorders, it would be reasonable to ask for the following tests:

- factor V Leiden (most common defect)
- homocysteine (high levels)
- prothrombin G20210A
- antithrombin III, proteins C and S (deficiency)
- antiphospholipid antibodies, lupus anticoagulant.

However, the thrombophilia screen is not a routine test in PE. Anyway, this may not be the best time to test Annika for these disorders since false positive results may occur in the acute phase of PE and while subsequently being anticoagulated. Also, in cases where there is an obvious cause for the PE (a so-called 'provoked' PE), the screen is unnecessary (National Institute for Health and Clinical Excellence, 2014). Given that Annika's PE most likely resulted from her orthopaedic surgery, it would therefore be reasonable to skip the screen. Nevertheless, screening for these coagulation disorders should be performed on patients presenting with recurrent thromboembolic events or where thromboembolic events occur with no clear precipitants.

Q: The medical registrar is called to the wards for a cardiac arrest. She leaves you with an instruction to anticoagulate the patient. Should you use IV unfractionated heparin or subcutaneous low molecular weight heparin (LMWH), for example enoxaparin?

A: LMWH is probably better than IV unfractionated heparin in haemodynamically stable patients with acute PE, assuming that there are none of the usual contraindications to LMWH. (National Institute for Health and Clinical Excellence, 2014; Quinlan *et al.*, 2004; van Dongen *et al.*, 2004). (For detailed information on anticoagulating patients, see Chapter 32.) Fondaparinux is another parenteral alternative to LMWH but is not as widely used in Australian hospitals (National Institute for Health and Clinical Excellence, 2014).

Q: Annika asks you how long she will need oral anticoagulant therapy. What do you tell her?

A: In a patient like Annika with her first episode of provoked PE, at least 3 months of therapy would be reasonable. In those with an unprovoked PE, a duration over 3 months should be considered, depending on their risk of bleeding (National Institute for Health and Clinical Excellence, 2014).

Nazario *et al.* (2002) refer to guidelines quoted by Hyers *et al.* (2001) on this issue:

- Most patients: continue treatment for more than 3 months (usually 6 months).
- First event with a reversible or time-limited risk factor:[2]continue treatment for more than 3 months.
- First episode of idiopathic venous thromboembolism: continue treatment for more than 6 months.
- Recurrent idiopathic venous thromboembolism or a continuing risk factor: continue treatment for more than 12 months (usually lifelong).[3]
- Symptomatic isolated calf thrombosis: continue treatment for 6–12 weeks (although opinions differ on this).

If anticoagulation is not possible, perform serial imaging over the next 10–14 days to monitor for proximal extension.

---

[2]These factors include surgery (as with Annika), immobilisation, trauma and the use of oestrogen.

[3]Continuing risk factors include cancer, antithrombin deficiency and anticardiolipin antibody syndrome.

Q: 'I hate needles and blood tests', says Annika. 'Is there an alternative to the injections and warfarin?'

A: Rivaroxaban is an oral anti-Xa inhibitor that can be commenced without using heparin. In Australia, it has been approved for treating PE (Department of Health, 2013).

Scenario

Despite the guidelines, duration of therapy will often vary between institutions and physicians. You therefore tell Annika that she will require at least 3 months of warfarin therapy.

While you are writing up the enoxaparin, the nurse looking after this patient calls you urgently. The patient has acutely deteriorated after complaining of sudden severe inspiratory chest pain. She suddenly became tachypnoeic, her oxygen saturation dropped to 81% on room air and her blood pressure dropped to 75/40 with a simultaneous rise in heart rate to 120/minute. She is peripherally shut down but is alert. You give her a bolus dose of IV fluid and order an urgent 12-lead ECG and mobile CXR.

The mobile CXR does not demonstrate a pneumothorax and is unremarkable. The 12-lead ECG simply shows sinus tachycardia.

Q: What is the likely explanation of Annika's deterioration and what can you do?

A: She has most likely suffered from a second but much larger pulmonary embolism leading to haemodynamic instability. She could die.

The first thing to do is call a cardiac arrest ('code blue' in some centres). As an intern, you are not expected to deal with this situation alone. In fact, even a senior doctor would call a cardiac arrest under these circumstances.

If Annika has no contraindications, thrombolysis with a tissue plasminogen activator can be used for the patient with PE and haemodynamic instability (National Institute for Health and Clinical Excellence, 2014). The main risk is major haemorrhage, in particular intracerebral haemorrhage. Alternatively, Annika could undergo an embolectomy, either with an open surgical procedure or using a transvenous catheter.

Q: Annika receives thrombolysis without complications and improves. She subsequently is anticoagulated with rivaroxaban, but still gets recurrent PE. Annika has been looking up the Internet and wonders about a caval filter (also discussed in Chapter 32). Is this a reasonable option?

A: Yes, it is. A caval filter (or 'inferior vena caval filter' or 'IVC filter') is a gadget placed percutaneously into the IVC to prevent propagation of thrombus from distal sites to the lungs. It does not have to be permanently placed there and can be removed at a future date. The indications for a caval filter include people with PE who have contraindications to anticoagulation or those who continue to suffer embolic events despite good anticoagulation—Annika would fall into the latter category.

Q: Annika wonders how safe caval filters are and whether they are likely to fail.

A: They are relatively effective—recurrent emboli only occur in 2–5% of people with filters. Complications are usually associated with long-term use and include IVC perforation, migration of the filter and circulatory problems due to IVC thrombosis (Hamilton-Craig *et al.*, 2008).

Q: What is the potential long-term complication of recurrent PE?

A: Pulmonary hypertension (PH) that can lead to severe dyspnoea.

Q: Although there are a number of treatments for PH of any cause, is there any specific treatment for PH caused by recurrent PE?

A: Pulmonary thromboendarterectomy, but it has a mortality rate of up to 10%.

Achievements

You now:
- know the best tests to diagnose PE and their limitations
- know how to use the 2-level Wells score to guide you to or away from a diagnosis of PE
- know how long to anticoagulate patients with PE in different settings
- know how to order a basic thrombophilic screen
- know the role of thrombolysis in treating PE.

References

Anonymous (1990), 'Value of the ventilation/perfusion scan in acute pulmonary embolism: Results of the prospective investigation of pulmonary embolism diagnosis (PIOPED). The PIOPED Investigators', JAMA, vol. 263, no. 20, pp. 2753–2759.

Department of Health (2013), 'Rivaroxaban (PE), tablets, 15mg and 20mg, Xarelto - March 2013', Pharmaceuticals Benefits Scheme, at <www.pbs.gov.au/info/industry/listing/elements/pbac-meetings/psd/2013-03/rivaroxaban-pe>, accessed 5 November 2014.

Diffin, D.C. *et al.* (1998), 'Effect of anatomic distribution of pulmonary emboli on interobserver agreement in the interpretation of pulmonary angiography', *American Journal of Roentgenology*, vol. 171, no. 4, pp. 1085–1089.

Erdman, W.A. *et al.* (1994), 'Pulmonary embolism: Comparison of MR images with radionuclide and angiographic studies', *Radiology*, vol. 190, no. 2, pp. 499–508.

Gefter, W.B. *et al.* (1995), 'Pulmonary thromboembolism: Recent developments in diagnosis with CT and MR imaging', *Radiology*, vol. 197, no. 3, pp. 561–574.

Goldhaber, S.Z. (1998), 'Pulmonary embolism', *New England Journal of Medicine*, vol. 339, no. 2, pp. 93–104.

Goldhaber, S.Z. *et al.* (1997), 'A prospective study of risk factors for pulmonary embolism in women', *JAMA*, vol. 277, no. 8, pp. 642–645.

Goldhaber, S.Z., Visani, L. and De Rosa, M. (1999), 'Acute pulmonary embolism: Clinical outcomes in the International Cooperative Pulmonary Embolism Registry (ICOPER)', *Lancet*, vol. 353, no. 9162, pp. 1386–1389.

Goodman, L.R. and Lipchik, R.J. (1996), 'Diagnosis of acute pulmonary embolism: Time for a new approach', *Radiology*, vol. 199, no. 1, pp. 25–27.

Hamilton-Craig, C.R., McNeill, K., Dunning, J., Walters, D.L., Slaughter, R. and Kermeen, F. (2008), 'Treatment options and strategies for acute severe pulmonary embolism', *Internal Medicine Journal*, vol. 38, no. 8, pp. 657–667.

Horlander, K.T. and Leeper, K.V. (2003), 'Troponin levels as a guide to treatment of pulmonary embolism', *Current Opinion in Pulmonary Medicine*, vol. 9, no. 5, pp. 374–377.

Huisman, M.V., Klok, F.A. (2013), 'How I diagnose acute pulmonary embolism', *Blood*, vol. 121, no. 22, pp. 4443–4448.

Hull, R.D. *et al.* (1983), 'Pulmonary angiography, ventilation lung scanning, and venography for clinically suspected pulmonary embolism with abnormal perfusion lung scan', *Annals of Internal Medicine*, vol. 98, no. 6, pp. 891–899.

Hyers, T.M. *et al.* (2001), 'Antithrombotic therapy for venous thromboembolic disease', *Chest*, vol. 119, no. 1 (suppl.), pp. 176S–193S.

Johnson, M.S. (2002), 'Current strategies for the diagnosis of pulmonary embolus', *Journal of Vascular & Interventional Radiology*, vol. 13, no. 1, pp. 13–23.

Lesser, B.A. *et al.* (1992), 'The diagnosis of acute pulmonary embolus in patients with chronic obstructive pulmonary disease', *Chest*, vol. 102, no. 1, pp. 17–22.

McCabe, J.L., Grossman, S.J. and Joyce, J.M. (1991), 'Ventilation-perfusion scintigraphy', *Emergency Medicine Clinics of North America*, vol. 9, no. 4, pp. 805–825.

National Institute for Health and Clinical Excellence (2014), 'Venous thromboembolic diseases: the management of venous thromboembolic diseases and the role of thrombophilia testing', NICE clinical guideline 144 (published 2012, reviewed 2014), at <guidance.nice.org.uk/cg144>, accessed 31 October 2014.

Nazario, R., Delorenzo, L.J. and Maguire, A.G. (2002), 'Treatment of venous thromboembolism', *Cardiology in Review*, vol. 10, no. 4, pp. 249–259.

Quinlan, D.J., MacQuillan, A., Eikelboom, J.W. *et al.* (2004), 'Low-molecular-weight heparin compared with intravenous unfractionated heparin for treatment of pulmonary embolism: A meta-analysis of randomized, controlled trials', *Annals of Internal Medicine*, vol. 140, no. 3, pp. 175–183.

Stein, P.D., Fowler, S.E., Goodman, L.R. *et al.* (2006), 'Multidetector computed tomography for acute pulmonary embolism', *New England Journal of Medicine*, vol. 354, no. 22, pp. 2317–2327.

Stein, P.D., Terrin, M.L., Hales, C.A. *et al.* (1991), 'Clinical, laboratory, roentgenographic, and electrocardiographic findings in patients with acute pulmonary embolism and no pre-existing cardiac or pulmonary disease', *Chest*, vol. 100, no. 3, pp. 598–603.

The Prince of Wales Hospital Haematology Unit (2002), Section 13: Thrombotic Disorders and their Therapy, at <www.sesinfo/powh/Documents/Haematology/pdf/13Thrombosis.pdf>.

Ullman, E., Brady, W.J., Perron, A.D., Chan, T. and Mattu, A. (2001), 'Electrocardiographic manifestations of pulmonary embolism', *American Journal of Emergency Medicine*, vol. 19, no. 6, pp. 514–519.

van Dongen, C.J., van den Belt, A.G., Prins, M.H. and Lensing, A.W. (2004), 'Fixed dose subcutaneous low molecular weight heparins versus adjusted dose unfractionated heparin for venous thromboembolism', *Cochrane Database of Systematic Reviews*, 4: CD 001100.

Chapter 6
An asthmatic woman presents with shortness of breath

Scenario

It has been an unusually easy day in the Emergency Department, with few patients to be seen. You remark to everyone, 'It has been really quiet today'. Your comment leads to groans and the shaking of heads in disappointment.

Q: What have you done wrong?

A: You have said the 'Q' word. Emergency staff are highly superstitious when it comes to the word 'quiet'. They believe that uttering it will lead to a large influx of patients—and most doctors who have worked in Emergency Departments would agree!

Scenario

Sure enough, a nurse comes over to tell you that a young woman has shortness of breath and needs to be seen right away. While walking to the patient's bed, he tells you that the patient is 22 years old and has a known history of asthma. She looks quite unwell.

Q: What is going to be the most likely cause of shortness of breath in this patient?

A: Common things happen commonly. Therefore, in a young woman with shortness of breath and a history of asthma, the most likely cause of her breathing difficulty will be asthma! Nevertheless, you need to keep an open mind when you talk to, examine and investigate her to rule out other causes of dyspnoea. Occasionally, a less likely diagnosis will appear.

Q: What is the first step?

A: Before undertaking a full history and physical examination in an asthmatic, it is important to make an initial clinical assessment to assess severity, in order to determine whether invasive or non-invasive

ventilatory assistance is required. Important clues suggesting the need for ventilatory assistance include:
- inability to talk due to breathlessness
- agitation or reduced level of consciousness
- central cyanosis
- rapid, shallow breathing
- silent chest
- hypotension
- bradycardia.

Q: Kylie is able to talk in phrases and is not cyanosed. She tells you that she has had asthma for 10 years and this feels like a typical attack. Her oxygen saturation on room air is 92% and her respiratory rate is 24/minute. She has widespread wheeze in her chest.
　Would you do anything else before taking a detailed history and examining her fully?

A: Kylie is hypoxic on room air and is tachypnoeic with widespread wheeze. Acute asthma is very likely here. It would therefore be reasonable to give her salbutamol and supplemental oxygen while you take a history and examine her.

Q: Although you take a detailed medical history exploring all aspects of her illness, what do you want to know specifically about Kylie's asthma?

A: You want to know:
- the year in which her asthma was diagnosed
- what treatment she currently takes for asthma and if she is compliant with that treatment
- whether she has an 'asthma plan'
- whether or not she measures her peak expiratory flow (PEF) normally and during this illness
- what treatment she has used during this illness
- if her exercise tolerance has deteriorated during this illness
- if there was an infective precipitant to this episode
- whether there is a past history of severe and sudden exacerbations*
- if there has been prior intubation for asthma (prior admission to an intensive care unit)*
- if there have been 2 or more admissions to hospital for acute asthma in the past year*
- if there have been repeated visits to the Emergency Department for acute asthma within a year*

- if there has been hospitalisation or Emergency Department visit for asthma in the past month
- current or recent use of systemic corticosteroids*
- if she uses more than 2 canisters per month of inhaled short-acting beta-2-agonists*
- requires ≥3 classes of asthma medications
- her underlying psychiatric or psychosocial illness*
- if she is of low socioeconomic status*
- if she is a rural dweller*
- if she uses illicit drugs*
- if there are other comorbidities, such as pulmonary or heart disease*
- if there is difficulty perceiving airway obstruction or its severity.*

Q: Although you will perform a complete physical examination, what signs in particular will concern you with regard to Kylie's asthma?

A:

	Mild	Moderate	Severe	Impending respiratory arrest
Talks in	Sentences	Phrases	Words	
Respiration rate	Increased	Increased	>30	
AMU/SSR[†]	Often not used	Commonly used	Usually used	Paradoxical chest/ abdominal movement
Heart rate	<100	100–120	>120	Bradycardia
Pulsus paradoxus	Absent, <10 mm Hg	If present, 10–25 mm Hg	Often present, >25 mm Hg	Absence suggests fatigue
Wheeze	End expiratory	Loud throughout expiratory	Loud in inhalation and expiratory	Absent

[†]AMU/SSR—accessory muscle use/suprasternal retraction.
Source: Siwik *et al.* (2002).

---

*These points are recognised as risk factors for death from asthma (Respiratory Expert Group, 2015; Siwik *et al.*, 2002).

Q: What is the pulsus paradoxus?

A: Normally there is a systolic reduction in blood pressure during inspiration that is <10 mm Hg. Pulsus paradoxus refers to a reduction in blood pressure during inspiration >10 mm Hg.

There are a number of conditions associated with pulsus paradoxus, the 2 most important being acute asthma (moderate–severe) and cardiac tamponade.

Q: You want to find out if your patient has pulsus paradoxus. What do you do?

A: Apply a sphygmomanometer cuff to the patient's arm. Inflate the cuff above the systolic pressure and slowly deflate until the peak systolic pressure of expiration is heard. Continue to deflate the cuff slowly until you note the first systolic pressure occurring throughout both inspiration and expiration. The difference between these 2 values should be <10 mm Hg.

Scenario

The patient tells you that she normally only uses a salbutamol puffer once or twice a day. She has been hospitalised twice in the past year for asthma, but has never required intubation or admission to intensive care. She was last hospitalised 6 months ago. She has not been on prednisone recently. Her GP recommended a steroid puffer, but she doesn't think she needs it. This episode started 3 days ago with a runny nose. Two days ago she became short of breath. This gradually worsened despite using her puffer up to 6 times a day.

On examination, Kylie is speaking in phrases. Her respiratory rate is 24/minute with accessory muscle use and her heart rate is 110/minute. Her blood pressure is 110/60 with a pulsus paradoxus of 12 mm Hg. She has widespread wheeze throughout expiration. The remainder of the examination is normal.

Q: What is your diagnosis?

A: Kylie has a history and examination consistent with moderately severe asthma. The precipitant is probably a viral upper respiratory tract infection reflected by her runny nose.

Q: Are there any basic tests you can quickly undertake to assess further the severity of Kylie's asthma attack?

A: The following table shows the use of pulse oximetry, arterial blood gases, forced expiratory volume in 1 second (FEV1) and PEF to indicate the severity of an acute asthma attack. (The FEV1 is better than the PEF unless Kylie has a record of her PEFs.)

	Mild	Moderate	Severe
Best or predicted PEF or FEV1	>80%	50–80%	<50%
SaO_2 room air	>95%	91–95%	<91%
PaO_2 room air	Normal	>60 mm Hg	<60 mm Hg
$PaCO_2$ room air	<42 mm Hg	<42 mm Hg	=42 mm Hg

Source: Siwik et al. (2002).

Q: What other tests would you order and why?

A:

1. **Full blood count.** A rise in neutrophils could support a precipitating respiratory tract infection.
2. **Electrolytes.** Beta-2-agonists can lead to low potassium, magnesium or phosphate levels.
3. **Theophylline level.** This test is required if the patient is taking theophylline.
4. **Chest X-ray.** This is a simple test that can exclude the presence of pneumonia, pneumothorax, atelectasis or pneumomediastinum, all of which can be associated with asthma.

    Some centres will tell you that a chest X-ray only needs to be performed if the patient does not respond to initial therapy for asthma in the Emergency Department.

Q: Kylie's PEF is 55% predicted and her SaO_2 on room air is 95%. Her arterial blood gas reveals a PaO_2 of 75 mm Hg and $PaCO_2$ of 38 mm Hg. Her FBC, electrolytes and chest X-ray are all normal. The investigations support your clinical assessment of moderately severe asthma. How do you manage Kylie's asthma?

A:

1. **Supplemental oxygen by nasal prongs or mask to maintain SaO_2 >94%.**
2. **Inhaled short-acting beta-2-agonists (such as salbutamol, albuterol).**
3. **Systemic corticosteroids.** Corticosteroids play a beneficial role in acute asthma because they reduce length of hospital admission, short-term risk of relapse and mortality.

4. **Anticholinergics.** The use of anticholinergics (commonly ipratropium) in conjunction with short-acting beta-2-agonists is beneficial in severe episodes of acute asthma. Given that our patient has only moderately severe disease, there is no need to use ipratropium at this stage.

5. **Other measures for severe asthma.** Although these do not apply in this case, other measures include:
   a. IV beta-agonist therapy such as IV salbutamol
   b. IV aminophylline
   c. IV magnesium sulfate
   d. non-invasive positive pressure ventilation
   e. mechanical ventilation.

Q: The nurse asks you whether she should give salbutamol through a nebuliser or a spacer. What do you tell her?

A: Use a metered dose inhaler (MDI) plus spacer instead of a nebuliser in the setting of an acute asthma attack; however, a nebuliser may have to be used if the patient can't tolerate the MDI plus spacer (Newman *et al.*, 2002; Idris *et al.*, 1993; Respiratory Expert Group, 2015).

Details on dosing can also be found in the Therapeutic Guidelines: Respiratory (2015) which should be available on your hospital's intranet or as a hard copy in the Emergency Department. Another useful guide online is the Australian Asthma Handbook (National Asthma Council Australia, 2014) (www.asthmahandbook.org.au). With regards to Kylie's moderately severe asthma, the recommendation is for 4–10 inhalations of 0.1 mg salbutamol via an MDI plus spacer every 1–4 hours or a 5 mg salbutamol nebuliser every 1–4 hours (patients with severe asthma will require continuous nebules or more frequent dosing (3 treatments every 20 minutes in the hour). Because beta-2-agonists commonly cause a tachycardia, you should monitor the patient's heart rate during continuous therapy.

Q: The nurse says, 'I guess you'll want an IV steroid rather than oral therapy since it will work more effectively'. What is your response?

A: Oral therapy is in fact as good as IV steroid therapy unless there are concerns about aspiration or reduced gastrointestinal absorption.

Q: What dose of corticosteroid would you give?

A: If you decide to administer IV hydrocortisone, give 100 mg every 6 hours. For oral therapy, the Therapeutic Guidelines: Respiratory (2015) recommend 37.5–50 mg/day prednisolone.

Q: Kylie receives continuous salbutamol nebules over an hour and a single dose of 50 mg prednisolone. You do not think that her runny nose and absence of fever warrant the use of antibiotics. The nursing staff want to know if Kylie can go home so they can use the bed for another patient. How do you decide?

A: Easy! You need to assess whether Kylie has had a good, partial or poor response to your therapy. A good response would be indicated by:
- PEF or FEV1 $\geq$ 70% predicted or best
- no distress and normal respiratory examination
- the response is sustained for an hour.

A partial response would be indicated by:
- PEF or FEV1 $\geq$ 50% but <70%
- mild to moderate symptoms.

A poor response would be indicated by:
- PEF or FEV1 <50%
- $PCO^2 \geq$ 42 mm Hg
- severe symptoms and signs.

If Kylie has had a good response, she can be discharged on a combination of short-acting beta-2-agonists and a course of prednisone. If she has only a partial or poor response, she will probably need to be hospitalised. It would be reasonable at this stage to add ipratropium nebules to the beta-2-agonist nebules.

Scenario

Kylie does feel somewhat better after this treatment. Nevertheless, her PEF is 60% and she is still breathless, with scattered expiratory wheeze. You therefore decide that she has had only a partial response to therapy and requires hospitalisation.

She is admitted under a respiratory physician and is transferred to the respiratory ward. You like to follow up on patients that you have treated in the Emergency Department, so you wander up to the respiratory ward 2 days later to see how Kylie is faring. She recognises you immediately and says she is much better, and is soon to be discharged. She thanks you for your help.

Q: Kylie also says that this asthma attack really scared her, and she wants to know what she can do to stop this from happening again. What do you tell her?

A: She is asking you about secondary prevention of further attacks of acute asthma. Conservative measures include stopping smoking, reducing weight if overweight, having an annual influenza vaccination and avoiding allergens (e.g. certain foods and animals). Treating other underlying conditions that may precipitate asthma is also important. These could include gastro-oesophageal reflux and postnasal drip.

Most teaching hospitals in Australia have an asthma educator. The role of this health professional is to see all asthma patients during or after discharge and educate them about their illness.

The asthma educator, often in conjunction with the treating team, will also help the patient to create an 'asthma action plan'. The aim of such a plan is to teach patients to know when their asthma is worsening, and what to do when this happens (e.g. increase puffer dose, see their GP, go to hospital). Each asthma plan is individualised. For example, some patients with troublesome asthma will be told to check their peak flow measurement at home every day. Others, with milder asthma, will be told to check it whenever they develop an upper respiratory tract infection.

Medications for asthma should be used in the following order (National Asthma Council Australia, 2014):

1. **Short-acting beta-agonists** (e.g. inhaled salbutamol or terbutaline) are good for acute mild attacks at home or to prevent exercise-induced asthma. They should be taken only when required and do not have to be taken regularly.

2. **Inhaled corticosteroids** should be added at a low dose when:
   - a person with newly diagnosed asthma has mild symptoms that occur ≥ twice a month OR
   - the person has been awoken by asthma at night at least once in the previous month OR
   - the person has symptoms < twice per month but required oral corticosteroids in the past 2 years for an acute flare-up of asthma OR
   - the person has ever required artificial ventilation or intensive care admission for asthma.

   Low doses of inhaled corticosteroids can provide significant benefits with only small risks of long-term side effects.

3. **Combination inhaled corticosteroids/long-acting beta-agonists** (e.g. fluticasone/salmeterol or fluticasone/eformoterol) can be used if the patient also has frequent daytime symptoms. An alternative to this is medium-high dose inhaled corticosteroids plus a short-acting beta-agonist. The long-acting beta-agonists reduce exacerbations of asthma and improve asthma control better than short-acting beta-agonists.

4. **Theophylline (a methylxanthine that inhibits phosphodiesterase)** is not as effective as long-acting beta-agonists. Toxicity and interactions with numerous medications limit its use.

5. **Prednisolone and steroid-sparing agents** cause numerous side effects that must be weighed against the benefits.

Q: Kylie asks you what you know about leukotriene antagonists (e.g. montelukast and zafirlukast)?

A: In adults, they can be used as an alternative to the combination of regular low-dose inhaled corticosteroids and prn short-acting beta-agonists (National Asthma Council Australia, 2014).

There is an association between leukotriene antagonists and Churg–Strauss syndrome (a vasculitis associated with asthma). However, it is unclear whether these medications unmask the disease or actually precipitate it.

Q: Kylie says that the respiratory physician outlined a similar management plan. When she discovered that Kylie had been using her salbutamol puffer at least once a day for the past 6 months, she decided to add a low-dose inhaled corticosteroid. She will review Kylie as an outpatient towards the end of the prednisone course.

Your patient has had prednisone before. She does not enjoy taking tablets and wonders if she can stop them suddenly, without weaning the dose over weeks.

A: The use of prednisone can suppress the body's intrinsic production of glucocorticoids. Therefore, if prednisone is suddenly ceased before the body has time to recommence producing adequate amounts of glucocorticoids, a potentially life-threatening 'Addisonian crisis' can occur. The gradual reduction in the dose gives the body time to slowly increase its own glucocorticoid production to adequate levels by the time the taking of prednisone is ceased.

Nevertheless, the Therapeutic Guidelines: Respiratory (2015) state that prednisone can be ceased after the treatment course of 5–10 days.

References

Idris, A.H., McDermott, M.F., Raucci, J.C., Morrabel, A., McGorray, S. and Hendeles, L. (1993), 'Emergency department treatment of severe asthma: Metered-dose inhaler plus holding chamber is equivalent in effectiveness to nebulizer', *Chest*, vol. 103, no. 3, pp. 665–672.

National Asthma Council Australia (2014), 'Australian asthma handbook—quick reference guide', Version 1.0, National Asthma Council Australia, Melbourne, at <www.asthmahandbook.org.au>, accessed 4 November 2014.

Newman, K.B., Milne, S., Hamilton, C. and Hall, K. (2002), 'A comparison of albuterol administered by metered-dose inhaler and spacer with albuterol by nebulizer in adults presenting to an urban emergency department with acute asthma', *Chest*, vol. 121, no. 4, pp. 1036–1041.

Respiratory Expert Group (2015), *Therapeutic Guidelines: Respiratory*, Version 5, Therapeutic Guidelines Ltd, Melbourne.

Siwik, J.P., Nowak, R.M. and Zoratti, E.M. (2002), 'The evaluation and management of acute, severe asthma', *Medical Clinics of North America*, vol. 86, no. 5, pp. 1049–1071.

Tattersfield, A.E. *et al.* (2002), 'Asthma', *Lancet*, vol. 360, no. 9342, pp. 1313–1322.

Chapter 7
A man with chronic obstructive pulmonary disease presents with breathlessness and an abdominal mass

Scenario

It is winter and very cold. The chill seems to pervade even the heated Emergency Department. You have seen so many patients with pneumonia in the past week that you have lost count of them. Welcome to winter! You pick up the next patient card: it is a 65-year-old man with chronic obstructive pulmonary disease (COPD) who presents with shortness of breath.

Q: What do you do?
A: You must first make a brief clinical assessment to see if he requires urgent non-invasive or invasive ventilatory assistance.

Scenario

Mr van Stein is a thin man. He talks in phrases and tells you that he has emphysema. His oxygen saturation on room air is 92% and his respiratory rate is 22 breaths/minute. His heart rate is 100/minute and blood pressure is 140/70. His temperature is 37.8 °C.

You do have sufficient time to take a full history and examination, so you take a history regarding his presentation. He tells you that in the past 4 days he has experienced increasing shortness of breath and is now breathless at rest. This has been associated with a worsening of his usual chronic cough, which is productive with more sputum than usual that is a deep yellow colour. He has felt hot and shivery with this illness.

Q: What questions do you ask Mr van Stein about his COPD?
A: You need to know:
- when his COPD was first diagnosed
- the name of the doctor (if he has one) who manages his COPD
- his normal exercise tolerance
- whether he uses puffers or nebulisers
- whether he is dependent on corticosteroids

- his use of domiciliary oxygen
- his history of smoking or ongoing smoking.

Scenario

Mr van Stein tells you that he has smoked a packet of cigarettes a day for 40 years. He still smokes, but has cut down to half a packet a day. He was first diagnosed with COPD 4 years ago, after being investigated for shortness of breath on mild exertion. Although his GP referred him to a respiratory physician, he did not attend because he was afraid he would be told to stop smoking!

Mr van Stein does not take any medication for his condition. Normally, he can walk 100 metres on a flat surface before becoming breathless. This has deteriorated in the past 6 months. He usually has a cough productive of grey sputum in the morning.

His examination findings reveal hyperexpanded lungs that are tympanitic to percussion. Auscultatory findings reveal diffusely reduced vesicular breath sounds with wheeze and prolonged expiration. You incidentally note that he has an abdominal aortic aneurysm (AAA) of approximately 4.0 cm.

Q: What is your diagnosis?

A: Mr van Stein meets the case definition for an acute exacerbation of COPD, namely a 'change in the patient's baseline dyspnoea, cough and/or sputum that is beyond normal day-to-day variations, is acute in onset and may warrant a change in regular medication in a person with underlying COPD' (Global Initiative, 2006). The examination findings are also typical for COPD. You suspect that infection is the likely precipitant.

Q: Is infection a common cause of acute exacerbations of COPD?

A: Yes. Infections, left ventricular failure, pulmonary embolism and air pollution are all recognised precipitants of an exacerbation of COPD (Abramson *et al.*, 2014).

Q: What investigations will you order?

A:
1. Arterial blood gas on room air
2. full blood count
3. electrolytes, urea, creatinine
4. blood cultures
5. sputum cultures
6. bedside spirometry

7. chest X-ray to identify various causes of his deterioration (e.g. pulmonary oedema, pneumothorax, pneumonia)
8. 12-lead ECG.

Q: After you have taken blood and ordered the other investigations, Mr van Stein looks longingly at the oxygen mask and says, 'I would love some oxygen to help my breathing'. His oxygen saturation is 92% on room air. Is there any information you would like to know before giving him supplemental oxygen?

A: Yes, some patients with COPD need a degree of hypoxia to stimulate their respiratory drive. Their arterial blood gas often demonstrates CO_2 retention (high $PaCO_2$). If these individuals are given high-flow oxygen, their oxygen level rises. They then lose their hypoxic drive and die.

You must therefore check the $PaCO_2$ in the blood gas before administering oxygen therapy and 1–2 hours after commencing oxygen therapy. Table 9.13 in the Therapeutic Guidelines: Respiratory (Respiratory Expert Group, 2015) provides a guide of how to use supplemental oxygen in the setting of CO_2 retention. These guidelines will probably be available online on your hospital's intranet or be available in the Emergency Department as a hard copy.

And note ...

It is not uncommon to see 'CO_2 retainers' with COPD receive high-flow oxygen with disastrous and unnecessary consequences. Please avoid this by checking the $PaCO_2$ on an arterial blood gas before and after commencing oxygen therapy. At the same time, if a patient is profoundly hypoxic and extremely unwell, supplemental oxygen should be given urgently. The arterial blood gas can be taken afterwards.

Q: Your patient's results are as follows:

Test	Result	Test	Result
pH	7.36	EUC	Normal
pO_2	65	Liver function	Normal
pCO_2	39	ECG	Normal
Haemoglobin (130–180 g/L)	160	Chest X-ray	Hyperinflation
White cell count (3.5–11 × 10⁹/L)	14 (80% neutrophils)	FBC	Neutrophilia
Platelets (150–450 × 10⁹/L)	180	FBC	Normal

Q: How do you interpret them?

A: Mr van Stein is hypoxic but does not retain CO_2. His white cell count is elevated with a neutrophilia. This is consistent with a bacterial infection being responsible for the exacerbation of his COPD. Hyperinflated lung fields with flattened diaphragms are typical of COPD.

Q: What is your management strategy for the acute exacerbation of COPD?

A:

1. **Supplemental oxygen.** Keep Mr van Stein's oxygen saturation around 95%. Repeat an arterial blood gas while on supplemental oxygen to see if he is retaining CO_2.
2. **Inhaled bronchodilators.** A combination of a short-acting beta-agonist (e.g. salbutamol) and an anticholinergic such as ipratropium is appropriate. Delivery of bronchodilators via a metered dose inhaler (MDI) with spacer is as effective as a hand-held nebuliser (Global Initiative, 2006).
3. **Systemic corticosteroids.** The use of corticosteroids in patients hospitalised with an exacerbation of COPD can reduce the length of hospital admission, improve the FEV1 and reduce the chance of relapse. Use oral corticosteroids (prednisolone 40–50 mg/day) for up to 2 weeks (Abramson *et al.* 2014); however, if there are problems with absorption or concerns about aspiration, use IV hydrocortisone 100 mg every 6 hours until prednisolone can be safely used orally.
4. **Antibiotics.** Antibiotic therapy is not recommended for all patients with an acute exacerbation of COPD. The groups likely to benefit from antibiotic therapy are those with (Global Initiative, 2006):
   - increased sputum purulence, increased sputum production and increased dyspnoea (best evidence) OR
   - increased sputum purulence AND EITHER increased sputum production or increased dyspnoea OR
   - an exacerbation so severe it requires assisted non-invasive or invasive ventilation.

   If Mr van Stein continues to deteriorate despite these measures, non-invasive ventilatory assistance using positive pressure 'BIPAP' and finally intubation can be used.

Q: Mr van Stein improves over the next 3 days in hospital. His sputum identifies a heavy growth of Moraxella catarrhalis.

   Is this surprising?

A: No. In people with COPD, *M. catarrhalis*, Streptococcus pneumoniae and Haemophilus influenzae are the most commonly isolated organisms from the lower airways (Global Initiative, 2006). In fact, one can't even be sure if the isolation of *M. catarrhalis* from sputum is due to infection or colonisation.

Q: It is apparent from the history you took from Mr van Stein in the Emergency Department that he has no long-term management plan for his COPD.
What do you do?

A: The first thing to do when Mr van Stein is feeling almost back to normal is to undertake baseline lung function tests.

Q: What would you expect his lung function tests to demonstrate?

A: In COPD, the lung function tests should demonstrate an obstructive picture (low forced expiratory volume in 1 second/forced vital capacity, or FEV1/FVC ratio).

Q: What other conditions give rise to obstructive lung function tests?

A: Asthma and bronchiectasis.

Q: What conditions commonly give rise to restrictive lung function tests (high FEV1/FVC ratio)?

A: You should consider the following:
- interstitial lung disease
- obesity
- chest wall deformities
- pneumothorax and pleural effusions.

Q: Mr van Stein has an FEV1/FVC ratio of 65%, which is consistent with COPD. The FEV1 is apparently 60% of predicted. What regular treatment would you recommend?

A: The following table provides a guideline to treating people with differing severities of COPD. The individual modalities are discussed in more detail on the following pages.

STAGE (all stages will have FEV1/FVC <0.7)	I: Mild	II: Moderate	III: Severe	IV: Very severe
FEV1 (% of predicted)	>80%	50–79%	30–49%	<30%
Smoking and other risk factor reduction	Yes	Yes	Yes	Yes
Influenza and 23-valent pneumococcal vaccines	Yes	Yes	Yes	Yes

STAGE (all stages will have FEV1/FVC <0.7)	I: Mild	II: Moderate	III: Severe	IV: Very severe
Short-acting beta-agonists as needed	Yes	Yes	Yes	Yes
Long-acting beta-agonists	No	Yes	Yes	Yes
Pulmonary rehabilitation	No	Yes	Yes	Yes
Inhaled corticosteroid	No	No	Yes*	Yes*
Supplemental oxygen	No	No	No	Yes[†]
Surgical options	No	No	No	Consider

* Add inhaled corticosteroids if there are repeated exacerbations.
† Supplemental oxygen is usually only provided if strict criteria are met (see overleaf).
Source: Adapted from the Global Initiative (2006).

1. **Smoking cessation**. This is an important, cost-effective measure that can:
   1. reduce the decline in FEV1 over time (Anthonisen *et al.*, 2002; Anthonisen *et al.*, 1994)
   2. reduce the mortality from various causes in those with airway obstruction (Anthonisen *et al.*, 2005).
   Cessation can be assisted through counselling, nicotine replacement and medications.
2. **Bronchodilators**. These include:
   - short-acting inhaled beta-agonists (e.g. salbutamol)
   - long-acting inhaled beta-agonists (e.g. salmeterol, eformoterol)
   - inhaled anticholinergics (e.g. ipratropium)
   - oral phosphodiesterase inhibitors (e.g. theophylline)
   - newer drugs such as phosphodiesterase 4 inhibitors and a long-acting anticholinergic (tiotropium).[1]
   Overall, these medications improve symptoms and may improve exercise performance and lung function; however, they do not reduce mortality or affect the course of disease.
3. **Home oxygen**. The Thoracic Society of Australia and New Zealand (McDonald *et al.*, 2014) recognises the benefits of long-term continuous oxygen therapy (>18 hours/day) by means of oxygen concentrators and cylinders. The society recommends that such oxygen therapy should be provided to those with:
   - PaO_2 of 55 mm Hg or less OR

---

[1]Tiotropium improves FEV1.

- PaO_2 of 56–59 mm Hg in the presence of hypoxic organ damage (e.g. polycythaemia, pulmonary hypertension or right heart failure).

    There are also criteria for nocturnal oxygen therapy and intermittent oxygen (see the online resource).

    Mr van Stein, however, would have to stop smoking before accessing domiciliary oxygen. Otherwise the combination of fire and oxygen could be disastrous!

4. **Inhaled corticosteroids.** Inhaled corticosteroids have a limited role in the long-term management of COPD. They have not been shown to influence the natural history of the disease. In patients with moderate to severe COPD, they may reduce the number of acute exacerbations. They can lead to a small improvement in FEV1.

5. **Pulmonary rehabilitation.** This is an exercise and education program directed at individuals with various forms of chronic respiratory disease, including COPD. An important aspect of this program is that it addresses extrapulmonary issues such as depression, social isolation and muscle wasting which can contribute to the severity of their COPD in a number of ways.

    Some of the benefits of pulmonary rehabilitation in COPD include (Global Initiative, 2006):
    - reduced sensation of breathlessness
    - improved exercise capacity
    - reduced number of hospital admissions
    - reduced length of stay in hospital
    - improved health status.

6. **Influenza and pneumococcal vaccine.** Annual influenza vaccination administration reduces hospitalisation rates in individuals with chronic respiratory disease. In certain groups (all COPD patients $\geq$ 65 years or those less than 65 years with an FEV1 <40% predicted) the 23-valent pneumococcal vaccine is also recommended (Global Initiative, 2006).

7. **Exercise training, education and self-management, psychosocial support and breathing exercises** (in selected COPD patients) are other non-operative modalities that can be used (Abramson *et al.*, 2014).

8. **Lung–volume reduction surgery (LVRS).** LVRS involves removal of part of the lungs in order to reduce hyperinflation, thereby increasing efficiency of respiratory muscles and elastic recoil pressure of the lungs (Global Initiative, 2006). This can

lead to improved survival, increased work capacity and better health-related quality of life although it mainly seems to benefit individuals with upper-lobe disease and a low baseline exercise capacity (Naunheim *et al.*, 2006).

9. **Lung transplantation.** Other surgical measures such as bullectomy can improve symptoms.

Q: The respiratory physician commences Mr van Stein on inhaled short-acting and long-acting beta-agonists in addition to arranging immunisation against influenza and pneumococcus.

You had not forgotten that you found an AAA when you first examined Mr van Stein in the Emergency Department. However, you wanted to make sure his exacerbation of COPD was under control before you investigated the AAA further. Now that he is much better, you order an abdominal ultrasound, which reveals a 4.2 cm infrarenal AAA. Mr van Stein is slightly alarmed by the finding: 'My brother had one of those tummy aneurysms. Does it run in families?' What is your response?

A: Up to 20% of first degree relatives of people with AAAs will develop an AAA so there is an increased risk in families; however, there are other risk factors for a AAA. Mr van Stein has been smoking a pack of cigarettes a day for 40 years. The strongest independent risk factor for the presence of AAAs is smoking. Some 90% of individuals with AAAs have a history of smoking. In addition, former smokers have a lower risk of aneurysm rupture or death from an aneurysm rupture than current smokers (Powell and Greenhalgh, 2003). This is another reason why Mr van Stein should give up smoking. Being male and having cardiovascular comorbidities such as hypertension, hypercholesterolaemia, other aneurysms and atherosclerosis would also increase his risk of developing an AAA (Robinson *et al.*, 2013).

Q: Mr van Stein asks, 'Does it matter if I've got a swollen aorta in my tummy?'

A: You explain that if it ruptures, it will rapidly kill up to 90% of people. Emergency surgery in that setting still results in up to 40% mortality (Robinson *et al.*, 2013).

Q: Mr van Stein is startled by these figures. 'Well, let's operate and fix it now!'

A: No. Elective repair of aneurysms is only beneficial for large AAAs, defined as >5.5 cm for males and >5 cm for females. The 12-month risk of rupture of Mr van Stein's 4.2 cm AAA is only about 1% (Robinson *et al.*, 2013; Hirsch *et al.*, 2006).

Q: Will Mr van Stein need screening?

A: Yes. Even though Australia doesn't have formal screening guidelines, unlike some other countries, Mr van Stein would benefit from regular screening ultrasounds. The intervals between screening vary according to the size of the AAA: from every 3 months to every 2 years. For Mr van Stein's 4.2 cm AAA, screening every 12 months would be appropriate (Robinson *et al.*, 2013; Hirsch *et al.*, 2006).

Q: If the AAA required repair, how could it be performed?

A: Broadly, there are two options: an open repair or an endovascular aneurysm repair (EVAR). The open repair has a mortality around 1–8%. On the other hand, the EVAR has a lower morbidity and mortality than an open repair, although not all AAAs are suitable for an EVAR (Robinson *et al.*, 2013).

Q: One year later, you find yourself in the lift with the respiratory physician who looked after Mr van Stein. After an awkward silence, you inquire about your former patient's progress. The respiratory physician says that Mr van Stein is still smoking 2–3 cigarettes a day, and that his breathlessness is worsening despite compliance with pharmacotherapy.

What are the likely causes of deteriorating breathlessness in a patient with COPD?

A: Although any cause of dyspnoea may be responsible, the most likely causes are:

- worsening COPD itself
- pulmonary hypertension (PH)
- age-related loss of lung function.

Q: What role does PH play in COPD?

A: PH is a complication of COPD that can result in cor pulmonale (hypertrophy of the right ventricle followed by dilatation and ultimately failure). Hypoxic vasoconstriction of the pulmonary vasculature is the best-known cause of PH in COPD, although, in reality, it is a multifactorial process. PH is a sign of severity in COPD and is associated with a more adverse outcome than those without it. PH in COPD is defined by a mean pulmonary artery pressure at rest >25 mm Hg on right heart catheterisation (Abramson *et al.*, 2014); however, early on, the raised pulmonary artery pressures can occur only with exertion and not at rest. Therefore, some COPD patients will suffer symptoms from PH that won't be detected on a cardiac catheterisation (which is naturally performed at rest) (Hida *et al.*, 2002).

Q: What are the symptoms and signs of PH?

A: Symptoms include breathlessness, peripheral oedema, syncope and chest pain. Signs include a raised jugular venous pressure with prominent 'a' waves, parasternal heave, palpable and loud pulmonary component of the second heart sound and pulmonary regurgitation.

Unfortunately, the symptoms are inconsistent and the signs can be masked by the hyperinflated lungs of COPD patients. In other words, it can be a very difficult diagnosis to make clinically. Nevertheless, always be suspicious of PH in patients with COPD whose breathing deteriorates. Even a diagnosis of PH in COPD through investigations can be difficult.

Q: Are any investigations helpful in diagnosing PH?

A: Yes. The following investigations would be helpful in this diagnosis:

1. **Arterial blood gas**. Hypoxia (PaO_2 <60 mm Hg) and/or CO_2 retention ($PaCO_2$ >40 mm Hg) are predictive of PH in COPD.
2. **Full blood count**. Chronic hypoxaemia can lead to polycythaemia, represented by an elevated haematocrit. Polycythaemia can increase pulmonary artery pressures.
3. **Electrocardiography**. Non-specific changes can occur and include:
   a. right axis deviation
   b. right bundle branch block
   c. tall R in V1
   d. deep S in V6
   e. P pulmonale (tall P wave).
4. **Radiology**. A pulmonary artery/aorta ratio >1 on CT chest is suggestive of possible PH (Abramson *et al.*, 2014). Also, a diameter wider than 16 mm of the right descending pulmonary artery on a plain chest X-ray in COPD patients is more than 90% accurate in predicting PH.
5. **Echocardiography**. Pulsed Doppler echocardiography is useful.
6. **Radionuclide angiography and thallium myocardial scintigraphy**.
7. **Magnetic resonance imaging**.
8. **Right-sided cardiac catheterisation**. This is the gold standard for diagnosis. Nevertheless, it is an invasive investigation and is therefore less likely to be used.

Q: How do you treat the PH in COPD patients?

A: This is a difficult area and it is important to realise that therapeutic modalities used for other forms of PH are not necessarily going to work for PH due to COPD. The mainstays of treating PH due to COPD are (Abramson *et al.*, 2014; Hida *et al.*, 2002):

1. **optimising treatment of the COPD itself**
2. **long-term continuous oxygen therapy (>15 hours/day)**
3. **diuretic therapy for right heart failure** (to reduce peripheral oedema and hepatic congestion); however, excessive diuretics can cause metabolic alkalosis, which in turn can reduce respiratory drive
4. **non-invasive ventilation or vasodilators** (e.g. non-dihydropyridine calcium antagonists, ACE inhibitors) may have a role in certain situations.

References

Abramson, M., Crockett, A.J., Dabscheck, E., *et al.* (2014), 'The COPDX Plan: Australian and New Zealand guidelines for the management of chronic obstructive pulmonary disease', Version 2.38, at <www.copdx.org.au/images/stories/pdf/The_COPD-X_Plan_Version_2.38_June_2014.pdf>, accessed 21 November 2014.

Anthonisen, N.R., Connett, J.E., Kiley, J.P. *et al.* (1994), 'Effects of smoking intervention and the use of an inhaled anticholinergic bronchodilator on the rate of decline of FEV1: The Lung Health Study', *Journal of the American Medical Association*, vol. 272, no. 19, pp. 1497–1505.

Anthonisen, N.R., Connett, J.E. and Murray, R.P. (2002), 'Smoking and lung function of Lung Health Study participants after 11 years', *American Journal of Respiratory and Critical Care Medicine*, vol. 166, no. 5, pp. 675–679.

Anthonisen, N.R., Skeans, M.A., Wise, R.A. *et al.* (2005), 'The effects of a smoking cessation intervention on 14.5-year mortality: A randomized clinical trial', *Annals of Internal Medicine*, vol. 142, no. 4, pp. 233–239.

Frith, P., Mckenzie, D. and Pierce, R. (2001), 'Management of chronic obstructive pulmonary disease in the twenty-first century', *Internal Medicine Journal*, vol. 31, no. 9, pp. 508–511.

Global Initiative for Chronic Obstructive Lung Disease (2006), 'Global strategy for the diagnosis, management and prevention of chronic obstructive pulmonary disease', at <www.who.int/respiratory/copd/GOLD_WR_06.pdf>, accessed 14 May 2009.

Hida, W. *et al.* (2002), 'Pulmonary hypertension in patients with chronic obstructive pulmonary disease: Recent advances in pathophysiology and management', *Respirology*, vol. 7, no. 1, pp. 3–13.

Hirsch, A.T., Haskal, Z.J., Hertzer, N.R. *et al.* (2006), 'ACC/AHA 2005 Practice guidelines for the management of patients with peripheral arterial disease (lower extremity, renal, mesenteric, and abdominal aortic): A collaborative report from the American Association for Vascular Surgery/Society for

Vascular Surgery, Society for Cardiovascular Angiography and Interventions, Society for Vascular Medicine and Biology, Society of Interventional Radiology, and the ACC/AHA Task Force on Practice Guidelines (Writing Committee to Develop Guidelines for the Management of Patients with Peripheral Arterial Disease): Endorsed by the American Association of Cardiovascular and Pulmonary Rehabilitation; National Heart, Lung, and Blood Institute; Society for Vascular Nursing; TransAtlantic Inter-Society Consensus; and Vascular Disease Foundation', *Circulation*, vol. 113, no. 11, e463–654.

MacNee, W. and Calverley, P.M. (2003), 'Chronic obstructive pulmonary disease 7: Management of COPD', *Thorax*, vol. 58, no. 3, pp. 261–265.

Maloney, J.P. (2003), 'Advances in the treatment of secondary pulmonary hypertension', *Current Opinion in Pulmonary Medicine*, vol. 9, no. 2, pp. 139–143.

McDonald, C.F., Whyte, K., Jenkins, S., *et al.* (2014), 'Adult domiciliary oxygen therapy: clinical practice guideline', The Thoracic Society of Australia and New Zealand, at <www.thoracic.org.au/imagesDB/wysiwyg/OxygenGuidelines_March2014_FINAL.pdf>, accessed 6 November 2014.

Naunheim, K.S., Wood, D.E., Mohsenifar, Z. *et al.* (2006), 'Long-term follow-up of patients receiving lung-volume-reduction surgery versus medical therapy for severe emphysema by the National Emphysema Treatment Trial Research Group', *Annals of Thoracic Surgery*, vol. 82, no. 2, pp. 431–443.

Nichol, K.L. *et al.* (1994), 'The efficacy and cost effectiveness of vaccination against influenza among elderly persons living in the community', *New England Journal of Medicine*, vol. 331, no. 12, pp. 778–784.

Powell, J.T. and Greenhalgh, R.M. (2003), 'Clinical practice: Small abdominal aortic aneurysms', *New England Journal of Medicine*, vol. 348, no. 19, pp. 1895–1901.

Respiratory Expert Group (2015), *Therapeutic Guidelines: Respiratory*, Version 3, Therapeutic Guidelines Ltd, Melbourne.

Robinson, D., Mees, B., Verhagen, H. and Chuen, J. (2013), 'Aortic aneurysms: screening, surveillance and referral', *Australian Family Physician*, vol. 42, no. 6, pp. 364–369.

Chapter 8
Mrs Mason presents with haematemesis

Scenario

You are sitting in the Emergency Department's tearoom watching the final episode of *The Voice*. The senior nurse walks in and interrupts your viewing: 'A 44-year-old woman has been vomiting blood. She looks pretty pale. All the other doctors are busy. We need your help'.

Q: Do you tell the nurse to give you a few minutes, as the show is almost over?

A: Haematemesis is a life-threatening medical emergency with a mortality of about 10% (Hegade *et al.*, 2013). You must go immediately. You will have to catch up with *The Voice* later.

Q: You greet the patient, Mrs Mason. The senior nurse is right—she is very pale. There is a bowl next to her that probably contains 200 mL of blood with a coffee ground appearance. The nurse says that she vomited about 5 minutes ago.
What is your next step?

A: Mrs Mason could suffer a massive haematemesis at any moment and die in front of you. Before progressing further, you must do the following:

1. **Check her baseline blood pressure and heart rate to assess her haemodynamic status**. The nursing staff would almost certainly have done this the moment Mrs Mason arrived in the Emergency Department, but you should make sure it has been done. Also check the oxygen saturation. If Mrs Mason is suffering from massive haematemesis, her airway may become compromised and need protection.

2. **Obtain IV access as soon as possible, using 2 large-bore cannulae.**

3. **Commence IV fluids.**

4. **Take blood.**

5. **Insert a urinary catheter to monitor urine output.**

Q: What blood tests will you order and why?
A:
  1. **Full blood count.** You need to assess her degree of anaemia.
     Look for underlying thrombocytopaenia as a possible cause.
  2. **Group and hold.** The patient will almost certainly need a transfusion.

And note ...

A 'group and hold' is quicker than ordering a 'cross-match'.
  3. **Coagulation studies.** This will test her INR and APTT. Any
     abnormalities in coagulation could have contributed to the
     bleeding and may be amenable to correction.
  4. **Electrolytes, urea, creatinine and liver function.** You will
     often see an elevated urea in upper gastrointestinal bleeding.
     Nevertheless, this is a non-specific finding that does not point
     you towards an underlying diagnosis. But abnormal liver function
     tests may raise the possibility of underlying chronic liver disease,
     making the possibility of oesophageal varices more likely.

     Mark the blood form 'URGENT—GIT bleed' (or something
     similar) to get the tests done quickly. It is also worth calling the
     laboratory to inform them of the urgency of these test results.

Q: The nurse questions you about the IV fluids you asked for: 'Do you
want crystalloid or colloid? At what rate should the fluid be given?'
What do you tell her?
A: Crystalloids include fluids such as dextrose and normal saline. Colloids
are a more expensive alternative and include albumin, dextran, gelatins
and starches. There has been controversy for many years about which
group is superior in critically ill patients. But a meta-analysis (Perel
and Roberts, 2007) concluded that there was no survival benefit from
using colloids over the less expensive crystalloids; therefore, you can
feel justified in using crystalloids to resuscitate Mrs Mason. However,
since it is still a controversial issue, don't be surprised if more senior
doctors still use colloids in this setting.

Q: You order 1 litre of normal saline and ask for it to be given at the
maximum rate (known as 'Stat!' in modern American medical dramas).
Mrs Mason's blood pressure is 100/60. She is tachycardic (110/minute)
and saturating at 98% on room air. You have inserted 2 large-bore IV
cannulae and sent off the appropriate blood tests. Now you can take a
history and examine her in more depth.
What are the likely causes of haematemesis?

A: The causes of haematemesis include (Hegade *et al.*, 2013):
- peptic ulcer disease (the most common cause) – 36% of cases
- Mallory–Weiss tear – 2%
- oesophageal/gastric varices – 11% (see Chapter 11 for more information on the management of variceal bleeding)
- oesophagitis – 9%
- gastric erosions
- cancer – 4%.

Q: What are the relevant factors in Mrs Mason's history?
A: In this case, the relevant factors would be:
- number of episodes and quantity of haematemesis
- presence of melaena (black tarry stool due to the presence of altered blood)
- any abdominal pain
- symptoms of anaemia
- previous history of peptic ulcer disease or chronic liver disease
- use of any ulcerogenic medications
- alcohol history.

Q: What is a Mallory–Weiss tear? What history will make you suspicious of this diagnosis?
A: This is a tear, usually around the gastro-oesophageal junction, resulting from the stress induced by coughing or vomiting. The clue to the diagnosis is that the haematemesis was preceded by retching, coughing or blood-free vomiting. The majority of Mallory–Weiss tears will resolve spontaneously.

Q: What common medications can cause peptic ulcer disease?
A: Aspirin can be a cause. Likewise, non-steroidal anti-inflammatory drugs (NSAIDs) are associated with a two- to three-fold increase in the risk of significant gastrointestinal bleeding.

Scenario

Mrs Mason tells you that she has felt weak for the past 3 days. Her bowel motions have been black for the past 2 days. The haematemesis occurred only today and was not preceded by non-bloody vomiting. She has had 3 bloody vomits in the past 4 hours and feels very unwell.

She denies using aspirin or NSAIDs. She has no known history of peptic ulcer disease and is otherwise healthy. She drinks 10 grams of alcohol a day and does not binge drink. Her blood pressure has risen to 110/70 with the IV fluids, but she remains tachycardic and very pale. The remainder of the physical examination is unremarkable.

Q: The phone rings. It is the laboratory. They inform you of the following blood results:

Test	Measure	Test	Measure
Haemoglobin	67 g/L	Urea	12 mM
Mean cell volume	85 fL	Electrolytes and creatinine	Normal
White cell count	8×10^9/L	Coagulation studies	Normal
Platelets	190×10^9/L	Liver function tests	Normal

How do you interpret these results?

A: Mrs Mason has an alarmingly low haemoglobin (normal Hb 115–165 g/L), which is normochromic and normocytic consistent with an acute gastrointestinal bleed. Her normal platelet count and normal coagulation studies make a bleeding disorder much less likely. As mentioned earlier, elevated urea in the context of an acute gastrointestinal bleed is not surprising.

Q: At this stage, how would you manage Mrs Mason?
A:

1. She should be nil by mouth.
2. She needs a blood transfusion.
3. She should be in the resuscitation room and have continuous heart rate and blood pressure monitoring.
4. She needs a stool chart.
5. Inform a more senior Emergency Department doctor of this patient as well as the gastroenterology registrar.

Q: What about an endoscopy?

The Blatchford score is a useful tool to determine this. A score of > 0 is almost 100% sensitive in identifying severe bleeding. Conversely, those with a score of 0 can be discharged without an endoscopy. The table below demonstrates the Blatchford score variables, the presence of any of which would give a score of > 0 and therefore require the patient to have an endoscopy. Mrs Mason certainly has a score > 0 (it is 12) and therefore she should undergo an urgent endoscopy. In this setting, an endoscopy within 24 hours of presentation is ideal (Hegade *et al.*, 2013).

Blatchford score variable	Level for score > 0
Systolic BP	≥ 100 mm Hg
Blood urea	≥ 6.5 mmol/L
Haemoglobin (males)	≥ 12 g/dL
Haemoglobin (females)	≥ 10 g/dL
Heart rate	≥ 100 beats/minute
Melaena	Present
Syncope	Present
Hepatic disease	Present
Cardiac failure	Present

Source: Adapted from Hegade *et al.*, (2013)

Would you start an anti-ulcer medication now?

A: Although proton-pump inhibitors (PPIs) are very useful after endo-scopic management of the acute upper GI bleed, the role of PPIs before an endoscopy is controversial (Hegade *et al.*, 2013).

Q: Over the phone, the gastroenterology registrar tells you not to start PPIs before the endoscopy. You chart 3 units of packed red cells (packed cells) for a blood transfusion. The nurse asks you, 'Don't you need to give platelets with the blood transfusion?' What is your response?

A: The nurse is concerned about a dilutional coagulopathy. This can occur during a massive and rapid transfusion since packed cells contain no platelets or clotting factors. When patients are about to receive a mas-sive transfusion, this will lead to a hospital activating their 'massive transfusion protocol'. This may vary from one institution to another. One approach would be (National Blood Authority, 2012):

- Every 30–60 minutes, check the full blood count, coagulation screen, ionised calcium and arterial blood gases.
- Aim for temperature > 35 degrees Celsius; pH > 7.2; base excess < −6; lactate < 4 mM, ionised calcium > 1.1 mM; platelets > 50×10^9/L; PT/APTT < 1.5 normal, INR ≤ 1.5; fibrinogen > 1g/L.
- Transfuse platelets if the platelet count is less than 50×10^9/L (<100×10^9/L for intracerebral bleeding).
- Transfuse fresh frozen plasma (FFP) 15 mL/kg if INR > 1.5.
- Transfuse 3–4 g cryoprecipitate if serum fibrinogen is < 1 g/L.

- Consider recombinant factor VIIa as a final measure, that is, surgical and other interventional avenues have been exhausted and the bleeding continues in the presence of a coagulopathy.
- Consider the use of tranexamic acid in the presence of trauma.

Q: In patients with heart failure, what precautions might you take during a blood transfusion?

A: In such patients, the concern is that the packed cell transfusion will result in fluid overload and pulmonary oedema. Two ways to limit these complications are:

1. transfusing at a slow rate (1 unit of packed cells over 4 hours instead of 1 hour). Obviously, this will have to be titrated to the urgency of the patient's requirement for the packed cells
2. administering frusemide between units of packed cells (e.g. 20–40 mg IV between units).

However, your patient is 44 years old and has no history of heart failure. Therefore, you can transfuse the packed cells as fast as necessary and not worry about giving frusemide.

Q: The gastroenterology registrar arrives and your patient is soon taken to the endoscopy theatre. What is the role of endoscopy in this setting?

A: Haemostasis can be achieved and mortality reduced. Patients at high risk of recurrent bleeding can be identified and monitored carefully after endoscopy.

Q: What about using endoscopy as an opportunity to biopsy the ulcer in this situation?

A: Although endoscopy is commonly used to biopsy ulcers in elective situations, a biopsy probably would not be performed in the setting of an acute upper gastrointestinal bleed. The immediate priorities are to stop the bleeding and assess the risk of rebleeding.

Patients will often return long after (e.g. 6–8 weeks) they have recovered from the bleed for a repeat endoscopy. A biopsy can be performed at that time.

Q: How can active bleeding be controlled?

A: There are a number of techniques available, although the 3 common ones are injection (often with epinephrine), thermocoagulation and mechanical therapy (e.g. using endoscopic clips). They are often used in combination (e.g. with injection being followed by thermocoagulation) (Hegade *et al.*, 2013).

Q: What are the endoscopic signs that there is high risk of rebleeding and why is this important?

A: The signs include (Hwang *et al.*, 2012):

- actively bleeding ulcer (approaches 100% rate of rebleeding)
- non-bleeding visible vessel (up to 50% rate of rebleeding)
- non-bleeding adherent clot (8–35% rate of rebleeding)
- ulcer oozing (10–27% rate of rebleeding if no other stigmata)
- flat spots (8% rate of rebleeding)
- clean-based ulcers (<3% rate of rebleeding).

Some 15% of cases suffer from recurrent bleeding after endoscopy. The mortality rate in these cases is high. It is therefore worth closely monitoring high-risk patients in a high-dependency or an intensive care unit.

Q: A duodenal ulcer with an adherent clot at its base is seen. There is no active bleeding. Mrs Mason is sent to the high-dependency unit post endoscopy. Should she receive PPIs at this point?

A: Yes, definitely. Once endoscopic haemostasis has been achieved, the use of an IV PPI for 72 hours reduces rebleeding and mortality (Hegade *et al.*, 2013). The Therapeutic Guidelines: Gastrointestinal (Gastrointestinal Writing Group, 2011) recommends an IV PPI (esomeprazole, omeprazole or pantoprazole), all of which can be given as a bolus dose of 80 mg followed by an infusion of 8 mg/hour.

Q: Mrs Mason responds well to therapy and is discharged after 5 days. She returns for a follow-up gastroscopy in 6 weeks. The duodenal ulceration is reduced, but still present. The registrar takes biopsies. What is he looking for?

A: He is testing for Helicobacter pylori and malignancy.

Q: What is the role of *H. pylori* in peptic ulcer disease?

A: The majority of gastric (70–80%) and duodenal ulcers (>95%) are caused by this bacterium (Hegade *et al.*, 2013).

Q: Is *H. pylori* associated with any other diseases?

A: Yes. They include the following:

- gastritis
- mucosal-associated lymphoid tissue (MALT) lymphoma[1]
- gastric cancer.

---

[1]It is interesting to note that simply eradicating *H. pylori* will lead to resolution of gastric MALT lymphoma in 70–80% of cases!

Q: Two Australians, Barry Marshall and Robin Warren, played a pivotal role in the discovery of the association between *H. pylori* and peptic ulcer disease (Marshall and Warren, 1984). For their achievements, they were awarded the Nobel Prize in Physiology or Medicine in 2005 (Aussie Aussie Aussie – Oi Oi Oi!).
What does Barry Marshall have in common with two famous figures from medical history, John Hunter and Daniel Carrion?

A: In order to prove the association between *H. pylori* and gastritis, Barry Marshall ingested *H. pylori* to induce disease. John Hunter infected himself with syphilis and gonorrhoea for scientific purposes. Daniel Carrion, a medical student, infected himself with Bartonella bacilliformis and demonstrated that 2 separate clinical diseases (verruga peruana and Oroya fever) had the same cause. Unfortunately, Daniel Carrion died from his experiment, but the disease was named after him (Carrion's disease).

Q: How is *H. pylori* diagnosed?

A: *H. pylori* is diagnosed by non-invasive methods including:
1. **Urea breath test**. This test utilises the urease activity of *H. pylori*. Its sensitivity and specificity is more than 90% and it is good for diagnosis and follow-up after treatment. But you do need to wait more than 4 weeks after therapy before retesting to avoid false negative results.
2. **Stool antigen**. This test has a sensitivity of 89–98% and specificity of more than 90%. It is good for diagnosis and follow-up after treatment. In this case you need to wait more than 8 weeks after therapy before retesting to avoid false negative results.
3. **Serology** has a sensitivity and specificity similar to the urea breath test. It has only limited use in following the success of therapy.
   Invasive methods of diagnosis (which apply to our patient) include:
   a. **Urease test on biopsy specimen**. This test is both rapid and cheap. Its sensitivity is 79–100% and specificity is 92–100%. False negatives can occur with active or recent bleeding or in the presence of antibiotic or antisecretory treatment.
   b. **Histologic examination of biopsy specimens**.

Q: The biopsy urease test is positive, confirming the presence of *H. pylori*. What benefits are there in treating Mrs Mason and what regimen would you prescribe?

A: You know that eradication of *H. pylori* dramatically reduces the rate of recurrence of peptic ulcer disease.

There are various combinations you could prescribe for Mrs Mason. These usually involve 2 or 3 drugs, generally a PPI with 2 antibiotics.

In Australia, 7-day combination treatment packs, containing clarithromycin, omeprazole and amoxycillin, are available from pharmacies (gastroenterologists refer to them as 'triple therapy').

The Therapeutic Guidelines: Gastrointestinal (2011) recommend the following 7-day regimen as the first line of therapy:

- clarithromycin 500 mg bd AND
- omeprazole or esomeprazole 20 mg bd AND
- amoxycillin 1 g bd.

In patients that are hypersensitive to penicillin, metronidazole 400 mg bd can be substituted for amoxycillin.

Mrs Mason improves in hospital and is discharged on a 7-day course of omeprazole, clarithromycin and amoxycillin. A urea breath test 6 weeks later confirms eradication of *H. pylori*.

Achievements

You now:

- can perform an initial assessment and resuscitation of patients with acute GIT haemorrhage
- order appropriate investigations in acute GIT haemorrhage
- distinguish between crystalloid and colloid fluids and their role in acute GIT haemorrhage
- can chart packed cells for a blood transfusion
- understand the causes of haematemesis
- can take a focused history of the patient with an acute upper GIT haemorrhage
- know the typical presentation of patients with Mallory–Weiss tears
- can direct appropriate ongoing monitoring and treatment of such a patient
- appreciate the role of pharmacotherapy in acute GIT haemorrhage
- appreciate the role of endoscopy as a therapeutic, prognostic and diagnostic tool
- know the disease processes attributed to *H. pylori*
- know how to diagnose *H. pylori* and treat it with 'triple therapy'.

References

Choi, P.T. *et al.* (1999), 'Crystalloids vs. colloids in fluid resuscitation: A systematic review', *Critical Care Medicine*, vol. 27, no. 1, pp. 200–210.

Conlong, P. (1998), 'Practical advice on treating haematemesis', *Hospital Medicine*, vol. 59, no. 11, pp. 851–855.

Conrad, S.A. (2002), 'Acute upper gastrointestinal bleeding in critically ill patients: Causes and treatment modalities', *Critical Care Medicine*, vol. 30, no. 6, S365–368.

Gastrointestinal Writing Group (2011), *Therapeutic Guidelines: Gastrointestinal*, Version 5, Therapeutic Guidelines Ltd, Melbourne.

Hegade, V.S., Sood, R., Mohammed, N. and Moreea, S. (2013), 'Modern management of acute non-variceal upper gastrointestinal bleeding', *Postgraduate Medical Journal*, vol. 89, no. 1056, pp. 591–598.

Hwang J.H., Fisher, D. A., Ben-Menachem, T., *et al.*, (2012), 'The role of endoscopy in the management of acute non-variceal upper GI bleeding', *Gastrointestinal Endoscopy*, vol. 75, no. 6, pp. 1132–1138.

Lau, J.Y. and Chung, S. (2000), 'Management of upper gastrointestinal haemorrhage', *Journal of Gastroenterology and Hepatology*, vol. 15 (suppl.), pp. G8–12.

Leontiadis, G.I., Sharma, V.K. and Howden, C.W. (2006), 'Proton pump inhibitor treatment for acute peptic ulcer bleeding', *Cochrane Database of Systematic Reviews*, 1: CD002094.

Marshall, B.J. and Warren, J.R. (1984), 'Unidentified curved bacilli in the stomach of patients with gastritis and peptic ulceration', *Lancet*, vol. 1, no. 8390, pp. 1311–1315.

National Blood Authority (2012), 'Patient blood management guidelines: Module 1. Critical bleeding massive transfusion: Quick reference guide', at <www.blood.gov.au/system/files/documents/pbm-module-1-qrg.pd>, accessed 7 November 2014.

Office of the Chief Health Officer (2008), 'Massive transfusion guideline', ACT Health, CED08–072.

Perel, P. and Roberts, I. (2007), 'Colloids versus crystalloids for fluid resuscitation in critically ill patients', *Cochrane Database of Systematic Reviews*, 4: CD 000567.

Schierhout, G. and Roberts, I. (1998), 'Fluid resuscitation with colloid or crystalloid solutions in critically ill patients: A systematic view of randomised trials', *British Medical Journal*, vol. 316, no. 7136, pp. 961–964.

Suerbaum, S. and Michetti, P. (2002), 'Helicobacter pylori infection', *New England Journal of Medicine*, vol. 347, no. 15, pp. 1175–1186.

Walt, R.P. *et al.* (1992), 'Continuous intravenous famotidine for haemorrhage from peptic ulcer', *Lancet*, vol. 340, no. 8827, pp. 1058–1062.

Chapter 9
Timothy presents with acute abdominal pain

Scenario

It has been a very busy shift in the Emergency Department. Each patient has been complicated. You pick up the next patient's card with a certain amount of dread. You see that Timothy is a 50-year-old man with 6 hours of abdominal pain.

Q: What is your approach?
A: First check the patient's blood pressure, heart rate, oxygen saturation and temperature to ensure that he is stable. Then take a history and examine him.

Scenario

Timothy is in obvious discomfort, but has normal observations apart from a heart rate of 105 regular beats a minute. He tells you that although he is usually healthy, he awoke this morning with upper abdominal pain that has gradually worsened. It is constant and severe and does not radiate. He is nauseated and has vomited once. There was no blood in the vomit. His most recent bowel motion was last night and it was normal. He has passed flatus today. He has not experienced any difficulty in the passage of urine. He has never had this pain before and never wants to experience it again!

An examination reveals a tachycardia and tender epigastrium without guarding. There are no masses and bowel sounds are present. The remainder of the physical examination is normal.

Q: What investigations do you perform and why?
A:
1. **Erect chest X-ray**. This is to check for subdiaphragmatic air (indicating a perforated viscus) or lower lobe pneumonia.

2. **12-lead ECG and high sensitivity troponins.**[1] These are to check for acute MI.
3. **Erect and supine abdominal X-rays.** These are taken to check for:
   a. acute bowel obstruction—more than 2–3 air-fluid levels, localised dilatation of bowel
   b. ileus—more than 2–3 air-fluid levels, widespread dilatation of bowel
   c. gastroenteritis—more than 2–3 air-fluid levels, no dilatation of bowel
   d. pancreatitis—'sentinel loop' of dilated bowel adjacent to the pancreas; a non-specific finding.
4. **Liver function tests to look for:**
   a. acute hepatitis
   b. acute cholangitis.

These may assist with aetiology or in ascertaining the severity of certain conditions (discussed later in this chapter).

And note ...

Students often expect only the transaminases (AST, ALT) to be elevated in acute hepatitis, and the gamma glutamyl transferase (GGT) and alkaline phosphatase (ALP) to remain normal. They expect the opposite to be true in acute cholangitis. However, often all of the liver enzymes are elevated in both conditions. But even then, GGT and ALP are often more elevated than the transaminases in acute cholangitis, while the converse is true in acute hepatitis. You would also expect bilirubin to be elevated in both conditions.

Specialists love to show liver function tests to medical students and interns and ask for their interpretation. If a pattern is present, you can sound polished by saying, 'All the liver enzymes are elevated, but hepatocellular injury predominates, suggesting acute hepatitis' or 'All the liver enzymes are elevated, but an obstructive pattern predominates, suggesting acute cholangitis'.

5. **Amylase and lipase.** These tests are done to check for acute pancreatitis.

---

[1]Medical students often forget that lower lobe pneumonia and acute coronary syndromes are uncommon but extremely important causes of acute abdominal pain and tenderness. Overlooking STEMI or NSTEMI in this situation by forgetting such a simple test as an ECG can be disastrous.

6. **Full blood count, urea, creatinine, electrolytes, troponin, calcium and blood sugar.**[2] Although these tests are rarely diagnostic, they do provide a baseline and can be indices of severity for certain conditions (discussed later in the chapter). However, the presence of a metabolic acidosis (reduced serum bicarbonate) would support ischaemic bowel or diabetic ketoacidosis (acidosis associated with hyperglycaemia) as possible causes of the abdominal pain.

7. **Dipstick urinalysis.** This tests for acute pyelonephritis (white cells and nitrites present) and renal colic (microscopic haematuria). It is a simple bedside test that is worth doing even though your patient's epigastric pain is unlikely to represent either of these conditions. If the urinalysis is abnormal, the specimen should be sent for formal microscopy and culture.

Q: The ECG, chest X-ray and abdominal X-rays are all unremarkable. Cardiac enzymes, urea, creatinine, urinalysis and electrolytes likewise are all normal. The white cell count is mildly elevated, at 14×10^9/L with a neutrophilia. The liver function tests are normal apart from an aspartate aminotransferase (AST) of 70 U/L (<40 normally). The serum amylase is 900 IU/L (normal <130) and serum lipase is 300 (normal <50).

What is your diagnosis?

A: The markedly elevated amylase and lipase in the setting of acute upper abdominal pain suggest a diagnosis of acute pancreatitis. Although classical acute pancreatitis pain radiates through to the back, this does not always occur in clinical practice.

Q: Your medical student, Allie, asks, 'Don't we need a CT scan to confirm a diagnosis of acute pancreatitis?'

A: In order to make a diagnosis of acute pancreatitis, 2 of the following 3 criteria must be met (Banks et al., 2012):

1. **abdominal pain consistent with acute pancreatitis** (acute severe persistent epigastric pain that often radiates to the back)
2. **serum lipase or amylase at least 3 times the upper limit of normal**
3. **characteristic radiologic evidence of acute pancreatitis** (typically on a contrast-enhanced CT but also potentially on MRI or transabdominal ultrasonography).

---

[2]In women of childbearing age with acute abdominal pain, do not forget to ascertain a menstrual history and take blood for a qualitative beta-HCG to exclude an ectopic pregnancy.

To answer Allie's question, we don't need a CT scan because the patient's pain in combination with the markedly elevated lipase and amylase are sufficient to make a diagnosis of acute pancreatitis.

Q: Allie has heard that peptic ulcer disease can elevate serum amylase. She wonders how reliable the test is. What do you tell her?

A: She has raised the issue of the specificity of serum amylase in diagnosing acute pancreatitis. Serum amylase is not 100% specific for acute pancreatitis and can be elevated in other conditions.

Q: 'So the serum lipase is the better test?' she asks you.

A: Overall yes, but this needs to be explored further. The newer serum lipase assays are now regarded as the primary diagnostic marker of acute pancreatitis since it is greater than 90% sensitive in detecting this condition.

However, when it comes to specificity, both serum lipase and amylase can be elevated due to other conditions (see the table below) although the degree of elevation in these other conditions is quite low. In other words, if either test is elevated more than three-fold the upper limit of normal, then acute pancreatitis is the likely cause (Cappell, 2008).

	Serum amylase	Serum lipase
False positives*	Renal failure	Renal failure
	Variety of intra-abdominal conditions	Intestinal perforation/inflammation
	Salivary gland inflammation	
	Macroamylasaemia	
False negatives	Acute pancreatitis from hypertriglyceridaemia	
	Delayed presentation[†]	
	Acute-on-chronic alcoholic pancreatitis	

*The false positive elevations are usually only mild; therefore, levels greater than 3 times the upper limit of normal are probably due to acute pancreatitis.
[†]In acute pancreatitis, serum amylase returns to normal within 2–3 days whereas serum lipase can remain elevated for 1–2 weeks.
Source: Adapted from Cappell (2008), Table of false positive and false negative results with serum lipase and amylase in acute pancreatitis.

Q: What do you do now?

A: Given that a diagnosis of acute pancreatitis is likely, it is important to:

- assess the severity of the condition
- initiate treatment
- find an underlying cause.

Q: You ask your medical student to assess the severity of your patient's pancreatitis. 'Looks pretty severe to me' is the inspired reply.
Can you think of a more objective way to assess the severity of this condition?

A: In broad terms, acute pancreatitis can be divided into 3 categories: mild, moderately severe and severe, based on the presence of organ failure and local/systemic complications (see table below). Examples of local complications include peripancreatic collections causing fever, neutrophilia and abdominal pain. An example of a systemic complication is acute pancreatitis exacerbating a pre-existing comorbidity (e.g. ischaemic heart disease or chronic lung disease). Regarding organ failure, scoring systems have been developed to identify its presence e.g. the Modified Marshal Scoring System for Organ Dysfunction (Banks *et al.*, 2012).

As you can see from the variables in the table below, assessing the severity of the acute pancreatitis is not a single evaluation limited to admission, but an ongoing assessment by the treating team. It is important to identify sick patients because people with severe disease from early in their admission have mortality rates up to 50% (Banks *et al.*, 2012). People with mild disease have mortality rates of <5%.

	Local or systemic complications	Organ failure that resolves within 48 hours	Organ failure persisting for more than 48 hours
Mild	No	No	No
Moderately severe	Yes*	Yes*	No
Severe		No	Yes

Source: Adapted from Banks *et al.* (2012).
* For moderately severe disease, the presence of either organ failure OR local/systemic complications is sufficient.

Similarly, Ranson's criteria involves a score based on indices at admission and during the first 48 hours. It is another index of severity in acute pancreatitis.

On admission	During the initial 48 hours
Age > 55	Absolute decrease in haematocrit >10%
White cell count > 16 000/mm3	Increase in blood urea nitrogen > 5 mg/dL (1.8 mmol/L)
Blood glucose > 11.1 mmol/L (200 mg/dL)	Serum calcium < 2 mmol/L (8 mg/dL)
Serum LDH > 350 IU/L	Arterial PO2 < 60 mm Hg
Serum AST > 250 IU/L	Base deficit > 4 mmol/L Fluid sequestration > 6 litres

Source: Adapted from Baron and Morgan (1999).

Q: Allie determines that Timothy most likely has mild acute pancreatitis. She recommends an initial management plan for him of remaining nil by mouth, having analgesia and IV fluids. Does this sound reasonable?

A: Yes.

1. **Analgesia.** The Therapeutic Guidelines: Gastrointestinal (Gastrointestinal Writing Group, 2011) recommend morphine (2.5–5 mg IV) or fentanyl (50–100 micrograms) as initial doses with further doses titrated to effect.
2. **Nil by mouth/IV fluids.**
3. **Nasogastric tube (optional in mild disease).**

Most patients with mild disease will recover within 2–3 days.

Q: Timothy improves with the analgesia and IV fluids. He and his wife are concerned about why this has happened to him. 'I heard Oprah interviewing an alcoholic who had pancreatitis. I'm most certainly not an alcoholic!'

A: You explain to the patient and his wife that:

- 80% of cases of acute pancreatitis are due to gallstones or excessive alcohol use
- 10% occur due to a number of uncommon or rare causes[3]
- 10% are idiopathic (of unknown cause).

As Timothy gives a history of drinking only 10 grams of alcohol a day with no binge drinking, the most likely cause is gallstones.

---

[3]These uncommon causes include medications, trauma, operations or procedures, hypertriglyceridaemia, hypercalcaemia, autoimmune disease, infections, scorpion bites and Crohn disease.

Q: Are there any test results that would support your diagnosis that Timothy is not a heavy drinker of alcohol?

A: Often the mean cell volume and GGT are elevated in people who drink heavily. These tests are normal in your patient, suggesting that he is not a heavy drinker.

Q: Your medical student correctly states that the sensitivity and specificity of MCV and liver function tests to identify chronic heavy users of alcohol are not great. She recalls a more recent blood test that is a good marker of chronic alcoholism, but she can't remember its name. Can you assist her?

A: She is probably referring to carbohydrate-deficient transferrin (CDT). It is available in some Australian hospitals. But while CDT has a very good specificity of about 90%, it has a poor sensitivity; therefore, other tests, such as ethyl glucuronide in hair with a better sensitivity than and similar specificity to CDT, may be more reliable markers (Morini *et al.*, 2009).

Q: 'How about a CT abdomen?' asks your medical student.

A: If the purpose of further imaging is to identify gallstones as the cause of Tim's pancreatitis, then an ultrasound would be the easier and more sensitive test. The role of CT abdomen in acute pancreatitis is to determine the severity of pancreatitis and extent of necrosis. It is usually reserved for those patients who present with severe disease or don't improve after a few days of treatment. In fact, the CT appearance has led to the development of a severity index which has prognostic implications in acute pancreatitis (Cappell, 2008). The other role of CT abdomen early in the presentation is to look for other causes of an acute abdomen if the diagnosis of acute pancreatitis is not certain.

Q: You send Timothy for an abdominal ultrasound. He returns with a normal study. Was your diagnosis of gallstone pancreatitis wrong?

A: You are probably still correct. Unfortunately, ultrasound has a sensitivity of only 70% in gallstone pancreatitis. It would therefore be worth repeating the test in a few weeks.

Q: Your patient wants to know if he needs any invasive investigations right now. What do you tell him?

A: He has mild acute pancreatitis and will recover in the next 2–3 days. Therefore, unless he develops cholangitis from choledocholithiasis, he is unlikely to require any invasive investigations immediately. Nevertheless, he may need a cholecystectomy in the near future.

Immediate or early invasive intervention has been of benefit in acute pancreatitis where:

- patients with severe acute pancreatitis are undergoing endoscopic retrograde cholangiopancreatography (ERCP) and sphincterotomy within 72 hours of admission
- patients with infected (not sterile) pancreatic necrosis are undergoing necrosectomy (removal of necrotic pancreatic tissue).

Q: What is the tragic irony of an ERCP?

A: Although an ERCP can be used in the treatment of acute pancreatitis, the procedure itself can precipitate the condition. Think of the 'Rule of Fives': acute pancreatitis complicates about 5% of ERCPs and 5% of these cases are severe (Cappell, 2008).

Q: What is a pseudocyst?

A: A pancreatic pseudocyst is a collection of fluid not lined by true epithelium that develops around the pancreas in the first month after an episode of acute pancreatitis. The most common presentation is upper abdominal pain with a palpable mass in the upper abdomen. The serum amylase is often elevated. Although the pseudocysts will spontaneously resolve in up to 40% of cases, they should be followed by ultrasound or CT scanning to monitor progress.

To avoid complications, it is suggested that pseudocysts be drained when they are 5–6 cm in diameter, or when they fail to resolve within a certain period of time. Complications include infection, rupture and haemorrhage, which can be life threatening.

Achievements

You now:

- can order appropriate investigations for an acute abdomen
- can remember that lower lobe pneumonia and acute MI can cause an acute abdomen
- can remember to order beta-HCG in women of child-bearing age with an acute abdominal pain
- know the limitations of plasma amylase and lipase in acute pancreatitis
- can classify the severity of acute pancreatitis
- can manage acute pancreatitis
- know the causes of acute pancreatitis
- know markers of chronic alcohol abuse
- understand the limitations of ultrasound in diagnosing choledocholithiasis (duct stones)

- know the indications for invasive therapy in acute pancreatitis
- know what a pseudocyst is and how to manage it.

References

Banks, P.A., Bollen, T.L., Dervenis, C., *et al.* (2012), 'Classification of acute pancreatitis 2012: Revision of the Atlanta classification and definitions by international consensus', *Gut*, vol. 62, no. 1, pp. 102–111.

Baron, T.H. and Morgan, D.E. (1997), 'The diagnosis and management of fluid collections associated with pancreatitis', *American Journal of Medicine*, vol. 102, no. 6, pp. 555–563.

Baron, T.H. and Morgan, D.E. (1999), 'Acute necrotizing pancreatitis', *New England Journal of Medicine*, vol. 340, no. 18, pp. 1412–1417.

Beckingham, I.J. and Bornman, P.C. (2001), 'Acute pancreatitis', *British Medical Journal*, vol. 322, no. 7286, pp. 595–598.

Cappell, M.S. (2008), 'Acute pancreatitis: Etiology, clinical presentation, diagnosis and therapy', *Medical Clinics of North America*, vol. 92, no. 4, pp. 889–923.

Gastrointestinal Writing Group (2011), *Therapeutic Guidelines: Gastrointestinal*, Version 5, Therapeutic Guidelines Ltd, Melbourne.

Morini, L., Politi, L., Acito, S., Groppi, A. and Polettini, A. (2009), 'Comparison of ethyl glucuronide in hair with carbohydrate-deficient transferrin in serum as markers of chronic high levels of alcohol consumption', *Forensic Science International*, Epub ahead of print 1 May 2009, oi:10.1016/j. forsciint.2009.04.003.

Sakorafas, G.H. and Tsiotou, A.G. (2000), 'Etiology and pathogenesis of acute pancreatitis: Current Concepts', *Journal of Clinical Gastroenterology*, vol. 30, no. 4, pp. 343–356.

Smotkin, J. and Tenner, S. (2002), 'Laboratory diagnostic tests in acute pancreatitis', *Journal of Clinical Gastroenterology*, vol. 34, no. 4, pp. 459–462.

Villatoro, E., Bassi, C. and Larvin, M. (2006), 'Antibiotic therapy for prophylaxis against infection of pancreatic necrosis in acute pancreatitis', *Cochrane Database of Systematic Reviews*, 4: CD002941.

Chapter 10
Anoushka presents with bloody diarrhoea

Scenario

You are the gastroenterology intern. You have been sent down to the Emergency Department to clerk a new admission. The young woman has been referred by her GP, who writes:

> Thank you for seeing Anoushka P., a 22-year-old university student with diarrhoea that is occasionally bloody. She previously has been well. The results of a stool specimen showed the following:
>
> white cells: numerous
> red cells: numerous
> culture: no growth.
>
> She has been unable to attend university this week and does not look well. Could you please investigate this further?
>
> Thank you and regards,
>
> Dr Edna Zhivago

Q: What disease process does the presence of numerous white cells in the stool specimen suggest?

A: Colitis, for which there are a number of causes, including:
- inflammatory bowel disease (IBD; Crohn disease and ulcerative colitis)
- infective colitis
- pseudomembranous colitis
- ischaemic colitis
- microscopic colitis.

Q: From the few details in the GP's letter, which causes of colitis in the preceding list are unlikely in Anoushka?

A: Microscopic colitis typically causes watery diarrhoea without blood. Anoushka is having bloody diarrhoea, so microscopic colitis is unlikely.
  Ischaemic colitis tends to affect older individuals with predisposing factors such as atherosclerosis, congestive heart failure, shock or aortoiliac

surgery. At 22, Anoushka is therefore also unlikely to be suffering from this condition. Nevertheless, it is worth remembering that ischaemic colitis can affect young people with vasculitis or hypercoagulable states, as well as young women taking the oral contraceptive pill.

Scenario

You take a history. Anoushka developed diarrhoea about a week ago. She has about 7 bowel motions a day. Half the motions are associated with bright red blood in the toilet bowl. There has been no mucus in the stools. She has no abdominal pain or vomiting. She has noticed chills and sweats in the past week, and had a fever of 38 °C when she checked it yesterday. Her appetite is also less than usual. She has been extremely healthy till now. She does not smoke and drinks 10 grams of alcohol a week.

Regarding causes of her diarrhoea, she denies any travel outside her home city for the past 5 years. She does not take the oral contraceptive pill and has not had any antibiotics recently. She has not eaten any unusual foods and no one in her household has a diarrhoeal illness. There is no family history of IBD.

On examination, Anoushka looks unwell. Her heart rate is 105/minute and regular. Her blood pressure is 100/60 and she has a fever of 38.2 °C. She has very mild epigastric and left-sided abdominal tenderness. There are no signs of peritonism and no masses. The rectal examination reveals dark red blood. The remainder of the examination is normal.

The physical examination has not provided you with any extra information about the cause of Anoushka's colitis. However, it has confirmed that she is unwell.

Q: What investigation will Anoushka ultimately require?
A: The most useful investigation will be a colonoscopy, or at least a flexible sigmoidoscopy. However, at this stage, it would be worth ordering some preliminary investigations.

Q: What preliminary investigations should you order?
A:
1. Full blood count
2. electrolytes, urea and creatinine
3. liver function tests
4. ESR, cRP[1]

---

[1] The full blood count, electrolytes, urea and creatinine, liver function tests, ESR and cRP will not assist in diagnosis, but will provide baseline values that can be followed throughout Anoushka's illness.

5. examination of 3 stool specimens (not just 1) for microscopy/ culture/sensitivity/ova/cysts/parasites (write 'M/C/S OCP' on the pathology request form)
6. iron studies, B12 and folate (she may be nutritionally deficient due to malabsorption, bloody diarrhoea, IBD, etc.)
7. plain abdominal X-rays.

Q: What is the significance of pANCA and ASCA?

A: pANCA refers to perinuclear-staining antineutrophil cytoplasmic antibodies, which are more common in IBD than in the general population. Nevertheless, there are a number of pANCA-positive conditions directed against different antigens. ASCA is also more common in IBD.

The following table (from Friedman and Blumberg, 2002) shows the prevalence of pANCA and ASCA in ulcerative colitis, Crohn disease and ulcerative colitis with sclerosing cholangitis.

	Crohn disease	Ulcerative colitis	Ulcerative colitis with PSC*	General population
pANCA	10%	70%	82%	3%
ASCA	70%	15%		5%

* PSC—primary sclerosing cholangitis.
Source: Friedman and Blumberg (2002).

However, pANCA and ASCA aren't part of the routine diagnostic work-up for IBD (Mowat *et al.*, 2011).

Q: How might the plain X-rays assist you?

A: In early IBD, a plain radiograph might be completely normal. Nevertheless, it may be possible to see:
- thickened bowel wall
- dilated bowel (e.g. in toxic megacolon or proximal to a stricture)
- narrowed segments of bowel (strictures).

In ischaemic colitis, though unlikely in this patient, you might see:
- mild diffuse bowel dilatation
- gasless abdomen
- 'thumbprinting' due to bowel wall thickening
- 'sawtoothing' due to multiple ulcerations of the colonic wall
- tubular narrowing
- free air within the abdominal cavity or air within the bowel wall or in the portal venous system (signs of severe ischaemic disease).

CT scanning of the abdomen can be helpful in differentiating ulcerative colitis, Crohn disease and ischaemic colitis. However, you may be reluctant to give oral contrast to such a sick patient.

Q: Anoushka's initial results are as follows:

Measure	Normal range	Result
Haemoglobin	130–180 g/L	110*
Mean cell volume	80–100 fL	82
White cell count	3.5–11 × 10^9/L	14*
Platelet count	150–450 × 10^9/L	182
Sodium	135–145 mmol/L	137
Potassium	3.6–5.1 mmol/L	4.1
Chloride	95–107 mmol/L	98
Bicarbonate	22–32 mmol/L	25
Urea	2.9–7.1 mmol/L	4
Creatinine	60–110 μmol/L	90
Calcium	2.25–2.58 mmol/L	2.25
ESR	mm/hour	78*
Albumin	33–48 g/L	30*
cRP	<5 mg/L	180*

* Abnormal results.

The plain abdominal radiograph is normal.
How do you interpret these results?

A: Anoushka has a normochromic normocytic anaemia, a neutrophilia, a raised ESR and cRP and hypoalbuminaemia. Given her age and history, she most likely has acute infective colitis or IBD.

Her preliminary blood results are consistent with both these diagnoses, but are not helpful in differentiating between the two. The normal X-ray does not exclude either diagnosis.

Q: What organisms can cause an acute infective colitis?
A: Some causes are:
- *Shigella*
- *Salmonella*
- *Campylobacter*
- enteropathogenic *Escherichia coli*

- *Yersinia*
- *Neisseria gonorrhoea* (usually causes a proctitis without diarrhoea)
- amoebic colitis
- tuberculosis.

Q: How will you differentiate between these 2 diagnoses and why is it important to do so?

A: Examination of the stool samples should exclude common infective causes. If no pathogens have been isolated from 3 stool specimens over 3 separate days, it would be reasonable to make a provisional diagnosis of IBD.

A severe episode of IBD requires IV corticosteroid therapy. IV corticosteroid is an agent you would be very reluctant to give if you still suspected an acute infection! It is therefore important to exclude infective colitis as a diagnosis before commencing this therapy.

Until then, you should do the following:

1. Keep Anoushka nil by mouth.
2. Institute IV fluids.
3. Closely monitor the urine output. This may require inserting a urinary catheter.
4. Transfuse packed cells if Anoushka becomes progressively anaemic.
5. Avoid loperamide (an antimotility agent), opioids and anticholinergics. In an acute episode of IBD, these agents can be associated with toxic megacolon.

Q: Three daily stool specimens were collected from Anoushka. Although they all demonstrate numerous white and red cells, they are negative for *Clostridium difficile* toxin and are culture-negative. Also, the pANCA and ASCA results return: the pANCA is elevated and the ASCA is negative. These blood results support your consultant's opinion that ulcerative colitis is the most likely diagnosis. Anoushka still remains very unwell. What treatment options are available for such a severe presentation of ulcerative colitis?

A: If this is ulcerative colitis with a severe presentation, the following approach is reasonable (Mowat *et al.*, 2011; Baumgart and Sandborn, 2007):

- IV corticosteroids (usually up to 5 days) in conjunction with corticosteroid enemas.
- If there is no response to IV corticosteroids, then other options are available, namely IV cyclosporine or IV infliximab.
- Transfuse to keep the haemoglobin >10 g/dL.

- Give subcutaneous heparin to reduce the risk of thromboembolic disease.

Q: Your consultant commences IV hydrocortisone 100 mg every 6 hours. Within 72 hours, Anoushka improves. Her fevers have stopped, her appetite is returning and she is having only 1–2 loose bowel motions per day. About one-third of these motions contain small amounts of blood.
What should be done now?

A: Anoushka should undergo a diagnostic endoscopic procedure such as a flexible sigmoidoscopy or colonoscopy to confirm that she does indeed have IBD.

Q: What are some of the other differences between Crohn disease and ulcerative colitis (apart from ulcerative colitis being more strongly associated with positive pANCA and Crohn being more strongly associated with ASCA)?

A:

Feature	Ulcerative colitis	Crohn disease
Clinical		
Perianal disease	Absent	Fairly common
Abdominal mass	Absent	Common
Site		
Colon	Always	2/3 cases
Ileum	Never	2/3 cases
Jejunum and proximal	Never	Infrequent
Distribution	Contiguous	Discontinuous ('skip lesions')
Transmural disease	No	Yes
Intestinal complications		
Stricture	Unknown	Common
Fistulae	Absent	Fairly common
Cancer	Common	Fairly common
Colonoscopic findings		
Aphthous and linear ulcers	Absent	Common
Cobblestone appearance	Absent	Common
Histology		
Granulomas	Absent	Fairly common

Source: Adapted from Friedman and Blumberg (2002).

Despite all these differences, about 10% of IBD cases will be classed as indeterminate.

Q: Anoushka has a colonoscopy on the following day. The endoscopic appearance is consistent with severe ulcerative colitis. Anoushka has macroscopic disease of the rectum and the sigmoid colon that is contiguous. The mucosa is haemorrhagic and oedematous with multiple ulcerated areas.

Biopsies are taken and demonstrate contiguous acute neutrophilic infiltration of the mucosa and submucosa. No granulomas are seen.

What do you conclude?

A: Anoushka's clinical presentation, raised pANCA, negative ASCA, endoscopic and histologic findings are all consistent with a diagnosis of ulcerative colitis.

Q: The patient is surprised. 'I lead such a healthy life and I still get this weird disease. I should have taken up smoking and binge drinking a long time ago', she jokes.

What is the unintentional irony in her remarks?

A: Smoking is protective against ulcerative colitis. Nevertheless, it is a risk factor for Crohn disease and may be associated with higher relapse rates in Crohn disease.

Q: Now that a diagnosis of ulcerative colitis has been made, your consultant asks you how you would grade the severity of Anoushka's attack. Although she has obviously been very sick, is there an objective way to assess severity?

A: Yes, there is. Ulcerative colitis can be graded as follows:

	Mild	Moderate	Severe
Number of stools	<4/day	4–6/day	>6/day
Blood in stool	Small	Moderate	Severe
Fever	None	<37.5 °C mean	>37.5 °C mean
Tachycardia	None	<90 mean	>90 mean
ESR	<30 mm/hour		>30 mm/hour
Endoscopic appearance	Erythema	Marked erythema	Spontaneous bleeding
	Fine granularity	Course granularity	Ulceration
	Reduced vascular markings	Absent vascular markings	

Source: Adapted from Friedman and Blumberg (2002).

As you may recall, Anoushka averaged 7 stools a day, half of which were bloody. She was febrile and tachycardic. Her ESR was less than 70 mm/hour and she had ulceration and haemorrhage visible on endoscopy. You can conclude that Anoushka had severe disease.

Q: Anoushka asks: 'Is there any treatment for this other than these steroids? My aunt takes steroids for asthma and she gets horrible side effects'.

A: Steroids have no role in long-term maintenance therapy in either Crohn disease or ulcerative colitis. Nevertheless, they can be used for acute exacerbations and should be weaned over a period of weeks to months.

The mainstay of treatment for ulcerative colitis has been the 5-aminosalicylic acid (5-ASA) group of medications, which are anti-inflammatory and act on a number of levels. Medications such as sulfasalazine, olsalazine, mesalazine and balsalazide belong to the 5-ASA family.

In patients with ulcerative proctitis or left-sided colitis, such as Anoushka, topical therapy with 5-ASA medications can be beneficial in the form of enemas or foam. For more extensive disease, oral 5-ASA therapy is recommended.

For those patients with ulcerative colitis and a poor response to 5-ASA medications, other maintenance options include azathioprine, mercaptopurine and infliximab.

Finally, patients whose disease is refractory to the above medications should be considered for elective bowel surgery (Mowat *et al.*, 2011; Baumgart and Sandborn, 2007).

Q: Does the maintenance therapy for Crohn disease differ from that of ulcerative colitis?

A: Yes, it does. Unlike ulcerative colitis, the 5-ASA drugs are not recommended for maintenance therapy. Instead, azathioprine, mercaptopurine, methotrexate and anti-TNF antibodies (such as infliximab, certolizumab and adalimumab) are primarily used. In the presence of perianal fistulae, the preceding agents can also be given; however, antibiotics such as metronidazole and ciprofloxacin are commonly used in clinical practice. But the evidence for use of these antibiotics is not strong (Mowat *et al.*, 2011; Baumgart and Sandborn, 2007).

Q: The gastroenterologist commences Anoushka on topical and oral mesalazine and begins weaning her steroid dose. He asks you, 'By the way, how were her liver function tests on admission?'

A: You show him the following results, which have not changed significantly since admission.

Albumin	33–48 g/L	30*
Bilirubin	0–25 μmol/L	20
ALP	38–126 U/L	250*
GGT	0–30 U/L	60*
AST	<45 U/L	56*
ALT	<45 U/L	61*

* Abnormal results.

Q: Your consultant reviews these results. He looks worried. What could he be concerned about?

A: Primary sclerosing cholangitis, which is one of the extraintestinal manifestations of IBD.

Q: What do you know about the extraintestinal manifestations of IBD?

A: There are numerous extraintestinal manifestations of IBD. The majority are most likely autoimmune in origin and can be divided into various systems:

System	Manifestations in IBD	Comments
Rheumatological	Peripheral arthropathy Axial arthropathy (sacroiliitis or spondylitis)	Responds to treating colitis No response to treating colitis
Musculoskeletal	Osteoporosis In CD even without steroids Osteopaenia Osteomalacia Osteonecrosis (avascular necrosis)	In UC with steroid treatment
Dermatological	Erythema nodosum Pyoderma gangrenosum Aphthous and angular stomatitis Psoriasis	
Ocular	Episcleritis Uveitis	
Hepatobiliary	Primary sclerosing cholangitis Cholangiocarcinoma Cholelithiasis Granulomatous or autoimmune hepatitis Cirrhosis Portal vein thrombosis	

System	Manifestations in IBD	Comments
Haematological	Anaemia Leukocytosis, Thrombocytosis	Multifactorial
	Hypercoagulabe state	DVT, PE
Urogenital	Nephrolithiasis Obstructive uropathy Fistula formation	Extrinsic compression
Cardiovascular	Pleuropericarditis	
Respiratory	Altered lung function tests Fibrosing alveolitis Vasculitis Bronchiectasis Apical fibrosis Tracheal stenosis	
Neurological	Peripheral neuropathy Myopathy Seizures Meningitis Vasculopathy	
Metastatic CD	Skin	Rare

UC—ulcerative colitis; CD—Crohn disease.
Source: Adapted from Su *et al.* (2002).

Q: Why does your consultant look so concerned about the possibility of primary sclerosing cholangitis (PSC) in Anoushka?

A: PSC is a progressive disease characterised by inflammation, fibrosis and destruction of the biliary duct system that results in cirrhosis. Patients are often asymptomatic at diagnosis and are picked up through abnormal liver function tests.

The best way to diagnose PSC is through cholangiography, usually during an ERCP. Once a diagnosis has been established, PSC can be staged by liver biopsy.

The concern is that there is very limited therapy for PSC. Ursodeoxycholic acid improves laboratory tests without reducing time to death, decompensated liver disease or time to transplantation. In addition, PSC is associated with an increased risk of cholangiocarcinoma and is likely to be associated with an increased risk of colorectal neoplasia (Mowat *et al.*, 2011).

The treatment of choice for end-stage PSC is orthotopic liver transplantation.

Q: Anoushka undergoes an ERCP. Thankfully, she does not have PSC. As luck would have it, the liver function tests return to normal over the next 2 days.

Is there any other long-term concern that Anoushka needs to know about regarding ulcerative colitis?

A: She needs to be warned about colon cancer. Patients with ulcerative colitis develop colorectal carcinoma at a younger age than the general population.

The risk is increased by:

- pancolonic disease (Anoushka has only left-sided disease but is still at risk)
- longer duration of disease
- early age at diagnosis (like Anoushka)
- coexisting PSC
- possibly a family history of colorectal cancer.

A reasonable approach would be to begin regular colonoscopies with multiple biopsies 8–10 years after symptoms began to look for cancer or dysplasia. Colectomy is recommended for colorectal cancer and certain types of dysplasia. The colonoscopies should be performed every 1–2 years initially but then annually after 20 years. Patients with concurrent PSC and ulcerative colitis should have annual colonoscopies as soon as PSC has been diagnosed.

Patients with Crohn disease and colonic involvement are also at risk of colorectal cancer and should undergo similar screening. Crohn disease patients are also at risk of small bowel cancers which typically involve the inflamed ileum (Baumgart and Sandborn, 2007).

Scenario

Anoushka is discharged with a plan for follow-up in the consultant's clinic in 2 weeks' time.

Three weeks later, you are called to the Emergency Department to see a patient. It is Anoushka, and she looks unwell. She tells you that she ceased her medications 10 days ago because she didn't want to feel like a patient all the time. She also forgot to see the gastroenterologist for her follow-up appointment.

About 3 days later, she again developed diarrhoea with increasing amounts of blood day by day. She now has chills and sweats and feels very weak. She is drinking fluids as much as possible to maintain her state of hydration, but feels she is losing the battle.

On examination, she has a regular tachycardia (125/minute) and a blood pressure of 95/60. Her temperature is 39 °C. She is clearly dehydrated.

Her abdominal examination reveals a distended abdomen with diffuse tenderness without peritonism. There are no masses. Bowel sounds are reduced. She is anaemic (110 g/L) with a neutrophilia (25 × 10⁹/L).

An abdominal X-ray is performed. It demonstrates marked colonic distension of 7 cm in diameter.

Q: What is your diagnosis? (A clue is that the diameter of the distended bowel is more than 6 cm.)

A: Anoushka has a toxic megacolon. This is colonic dilatation associated with systemic toxicity that is not due to obstruction.

Q: What are the causes of toxic megacolon?

A: Think of the 3 'I's:

1. IBD
2. ischaemic colitis
3. infective colitis

There are diagnostic criteria for toxic megacolon. You do not have to remember them, but it is worth being aware that they exist so you can refer to them when you suspect toxic megacolon.

The crucial thing to remember in diagnosing toxic megacolon is that the colonic dilatation on plain X-ray is more than 6 cm.

The diagnostic criteria for the condition are:

- radiographic evidence of colonic distension
- at least 3 of the following:
  - fever over 38 °C
  - heart rate over 120/minute
  - neutrophilic leucocytosis greater than 10.5×10^9/L
  - anaemia
- and at least 1 of the following:
  - dehydration
  - altered consciousness
  - electrolyte disturbances
  - hypotension.

Once again, do not try to memorise these criteria.

Q: Anoushka meets the criteria for toxic megacolon. How will you treat her?

A: About 50% of patients respond to medical therapy without the need for surgery.

Basic management for Anoushka's toxic megacolon would include:

- nil by mouth with IV fluids and nasogastric tube
- monitor in an intensive care unit
- at least daily plain abdominal X-rays and daily blood tests

- IV corticosteroids (hydrocortisone 100 mg every 6 hours)
- broad-spectrum IV antibiotics
- blood transfusion if necessary.

Indications for surgery include:

- persisting colonic dilatation after 48–72 hours
- free perforation
- haemorrhage
- increasing signs of toxicity
- increasing transfusion requirements.

Scenario

You are pleased to see Anoushka respond well to conservative therapy over the next few days. She repeatedly tells you how stupid she was not to take her medication in the first place and promises that she will never do this again.

When she is discharged 3 weeks later, she returns to the original regimen of oral and rectal mesalazine and a weaning dose of steroids.

Four months later, you have finished your gastroenterology term and moved on to the Emergency Department. Your first patient of the day is a young woman with diarrhoea—Anoushka! She is pleased to see you, and quickly asserts that she has been compliant with her medication: 'I don't know why I have diarrhoea this time. I've taken my medication religiously. I don't want to get that toxic megathing ever again. Maybe it has something to do with this infection I have'.

She tells you that she had been well until a week ago, when she developed dysuria. Her GP collected a urine specimen, which confirmed a urinary tract infection (UTI). The GP prescribed a 5-day course of cephalexin (a first-generation cephalosporin). Today is the final day of the course. Anoushka developed diarrhoea yesterday. Since recommencing treatment for ulcerative colitis, she has had only 1–2 bowel motions a day. Yesterday, however, she had 7 watery stools and a further 5 so far today. There has been no blood whatsoever. She has noticed some lower abdominal cramping and has experienced some chills. Her physical examination is unremarkable.

Q: What do you suspect has happened?

A: It is possible that this presentation represents an acute exacerbation of ulcerative colitis. However, given that Anoushka has been compliant with therapy, this is less likely. She has also been on immunosuppression in the last few months so cytomegalovirus (CMV) colitis must be considered. On the other hand, the diarrhoea and cramping began

3 days after commencing cephalexin. She may have antibiotic-related diarrhoea.

Q: What organism is classically associated with antibiotic-related diarrhoea?

A: Clostridium difficile accounts for approximately 25% of antibiotic-related diarrhoea. An organism is usually not identified in the other 75% of cases.

Q: Which antibiotics can cause *C. difficile* infection (CDI)?

A: All classes of antibiotics have been associated with CDI— even those used to treat the condition! However, the 3 most commonly associated with CDI are the penicillins, cephalosporins and clindamycin. And Anoushka is taking a cephalosporin.

Interestingly though, the epidemiology of this infection is changing. It previously targeted elderly and sick people institutionalised in nursing homes and hospitals. Nowadays, however, healthy young people with no history of antibiotic use or contact with the health care system are presenting with this infection. Even person-to-person transmission has been suggested in some cases (Kelly and LaMont, 2008). Furthermore, *C. difficile* has now been identified in the food chain and in animal products, thereby raising the possibility of food-borne transmission (Songer *et al.*, 2009).

Q: Apart from antibiotics, is there any other reason Anoushka may be at higher risk of CDI?

A: People with IBD are 3 times more likely than those without IBD to develop CDI. Also, Anoushka's glucocorticoid use in recent times is another risk factor (Czepiel *et al.*, 2014).

Q: What are the clinical manifestations of CDI?

A: These are highly variable, but include:
- diarrhoea
- colitis without pseudomembrane
- colitis with pseudomembrane
- fulminant colitis (including toxic megacolon).

Some strains of *C. difficile* can be more virulent (e.g. the NAP-1/027 strain that not only causes a marked increase in incidence of CDI, but also leads to more deaths and colectomies than other strains) (Kelly and LaMont, 2008).

Q: How would you investigate and manage Anoushka initially?

A: It would be reasonable to use the same approach as when Anoushka was first diagnosed with ulcerative colitis (see page 109). In addition, you should cease the cephalexin and repeat a midstream urine specimen to ensure that her UTI has resolved. Make sure you request *C. difficile* testing of the stool samples.

Q: How do laboratories test for *C. difficile*?

A: This will vary a little between hospitals, but a fairly common approach in Australia would be:

1. Initially use a combined enzyme immunoassay (EIA) for *C. difficile* glutamate dehydrogenase (GDH) and toxins.*
2. If the EIA is GDH+/toxin+, then a diagnosis of CDI is made.
3. If the EIA is GDH−/toxin−, then CDI is excluded.
4. If the EIA is GDH+/toxin−, a more sensitive toxin PCR will be performed to diagnose or exclude CDI.

Q: Anoushka's blood tests demonstrate a mild neutrophilia, but are otherwise unremarkable. The abdominal X-ray and non-contrast CT abdomen are normal.

The stool culture results are as follows:

White cells: numerous

Red cells: nil

Clostridium difficile GDH+/toxin+

Anoushka has CDI. How do you treat her?

A:

1. For mild disease: use oral metronidazole 400 mg q8h for 10 days. IV metronidazole can be used if the patient can't tolerate oral therapy (Antibiotic Expert Group, 2014).
2. For severe disease, use oral vancomycin 125 mg q6h for 10 days (Antibiotic Expert Group, 2014).

Q: What are signs of severe *C. difficile* disease?

A: Signs of severity of CDI include (Cheng *et al.*, 2011):
- clinical features (T > 38.5 degrees Celsius, haemodynamic instability, peritonitis, ileus or toxic megacolon)
- lab features (WCC >15 × 10^9/L and <20% neutrophils, elevated serum lactate, >50% rise in creatinine above baseline, albumin <25 mg/L)

---

*The EIA for GDH is a very sensitive test for the presence of *C. difficile* in the bowel; however, it doesn't tell you if the organism is producing toxin (i.e. even though it's there, it might not be causing diarrhoea). The EIA for toxin, on the other hand, is very specific for *C. difficile* as being the cause of diarrhoea; however, it isn't especially sensitive.

- other parameters (e.g. pseudomembranous colitis on colonoscopy, distended or thickened colon, fat stranding, unexplained ascites).

Q: You are confident that CDI is the cause of Anoushka's current illness. Since she doesn't have any signs of severe disease, you commence a course of oral metronidazole. However, you warn her that if she doesn't improve with the metronidazole, she will need a colonoscopy to ensure that acute ulcerative colitis or even CMV colitis isn't contributing to her illness.

Fortunately, after ceasing the cephalexin and commencing metronidazole, Anoushka improves quickly. Understandably, she wants to know if this will happen again. What do you tell her?

A: Unfortunately, up to 20% of individuals with CDI will relapse within 2 weeks of ceasing therapy.

Q: This relapse rate concerns Anoushka. She asks, 'What can be done if this keeps happening despite all the antibiotics?'

A: Although we have only discussed metronidazole and oral vancomycin, there are a number of other antibiotics that can be used for CDI—which you don't need to know. But for persistent cases or severe cases not responding to antibiotics, there are two non-pharmacological therapies:

1. **infusion of donor faeces into the GI tract** (van Nood *et al.*, 2013): the so-called 'faecal transplant'

2. **surgery**, typically a subtotal colectomy with end-ileostomy (Cheng *et al.*, 2011).

Q: One of the nurses in the Emergency Department asks you about CDI: 'Isn't yoghurt good for *C. difficile*?' Is he right?

A: The nurse is referring to the use of probiotics such as *Saccharomyces* and *Lactobacillus* organisms. One large study suggested that lactobacillus GG did not decrease the rate of *C. difficile* infection or the rate of diarrhoea. Another study found that *Saccharomyces boulardii* stimulated the secretion of intestinal IgA directed against *C. difficile* toxin A; however, probiotics aren't effective monotherapy for CDI and the evidence isn't compelling for their use in preventing CDI either (Kelly and LaMont, 2008). Similarly, a recent randomised controlled trial found that a multistrain preparation of lactobacilli and bifidobacteria wasn't effective in preventing either antibiotic-associated diarrhoea or CDI (Allen *et al.*, 2013).

Q: A few months later, you run into the gastroenterologist who looked after Anoushka with you. He is pleased to see you—after all, you were an excellent gastroenterology intern! You ask him about Anoushka's progress.

He reviewed Anoushka about 2 weeks ago. Her colitis is under control and she has returned to university. However, she has developed lower back pain and the specialist is concerned about an axial arthropathy (the disease activity of which, as shown in the table on page 111, is independent of the colitis).

What medications should Anoushka be cautious of in view of her lower back pain?

A: NSAIDs are effective for back pain, but can exacerbate IBD.

Achievements

You now:
- know causes of acute colitis
- know how to investigate acute colitis
- appreciate that multiple stool specimens and not 1 should be taken
- can institute basic management measures for acute colitis
- have a basic understanding of acute and long-term pharmacotherapy of IBD
- can recognise the differences between Crohn disease and ulcerative colitis
- can classify ulcerative colitis according to severity
- know the common extraintestinal manifestations of IBD
- realise that IBD is associated with a risk of colon cancer
- know how to diagnose and treat toxic megacolon
- know which antibiotics commonly cause CDI
- can diagnose and treat CDI.

References

Ahmad, J. and Slivka, A. (2002), 'Hepatobiliary disease in inflammatory bowel disease', *Gastroenterology Clinics of North America*, vol. 31, no. 1, pp. 329–345.

Alapati, S.V. and Mihas, A.A. (1999), 'When to suspect ischemic colitis. Why is this condition so often missed or misdiagnosed?', *Postgraduate Medicine*, vol. 105, no. 4, pp. 177–180, 183–184, 187.

Allen, S.J., Wareham, K., Wang, D., *et al.* (2013), 'Lactobacilli and bifidobacteria in the prevention of antibiotic-associated diarrhoea and Clostridium difficile diarrhoea in older inpatients (PLACIDE): a randomised, double-blind, placebo-controlled, multicentre trial', *Lancet*, vol. 382, no. 9900, pp. 1249–1257.

Antibiotic Expert Group (2014), *Therapeutic Guidelines: Antibiotic*, Version 15, Therapeutic Guidelines Ltd, Melbourne.

Baumgart, D.C. and Sandborn, W.J. (2007), 'Inflammatory bowel disease: Clinical aspects and established and evolving therapies', *Lancet*, vol. 369, no. 9573, pp. 1641–1657.

Cheng, A.C., Ferguson, J. K., Richards, M.J., *et al.* (2011), 'Australasian Society for Infectious Diseases guidelines for the diagnosis and treatment of Clostridium difficile infection', *Medical Journal of Australia*, vol. 194, no. 7, pp. 353–358.

Czepiel, J., Biesiada, G., Perucki, W., Mach, T. (2014), 'Clostridium difficile infection in patients with inflammatory bowel disease', *Przeglad Gastroenterologiczny*, vol. 9, no. 3, pp. 125–129.

Friedman, S. and Blumberg, R.S. (2002), 'Inflammatory bowel disease', in E. Braunwald, A.S. Fauci, D.L. Kasper, S.L. Hauser, D.L. Longo and J.L. Jameson (eds), *Harrison's Principles of Internal Medicine*, McGraw-Hill, New York, pp. 1679–1692.

Gastrointestinal Writing Group (2011), *Therapeutic Guidelines: Gastrointestinal*, Version 5, Therapeutic Guidelines Ltd, Melbourne.

Kelly, C.P. and LaMont, J.T. (2008), 'Clostridium difficile—more difficult than ever', *New England Journal of Medicine*, vol. 359, no. 18, pp. 1932–1940.

Mowat, C., Cole, A., Windsor, A., *et al.* (2011) 'Guidelines for the management of inflammatory bowel disease in adults', *Gut*, vol. 60, no. 5, pp. 571–607.

Mylonakis, E., Ryan, E.T. and Calderwood, S.B. (2001), 'Clostridium difficile-associated diarrhea: A review', *Archives of Internal Medicine*, vol. 161, no. 4, pp. 525–533.

Podolsky, D.K. (2002), 'Inflammatory bowel disease', *New England Journal of Medicine*, vol. 347, no. 6, pp. 417–429.

Sharan, R. and Schoen, R.E. (2002), 'Cancer in inflammatory bowel disease: An evidence-based analysis and guide for physicians and patients', *Gastroenterology Clinics of North America*, vol. 31, no. 1, pp. 237–254.

Sheth, S.G. and LaMont, J.T. (1998), 'Toxic megacolon', *Lancet*, vol. 351, no. 9101, pp. 509–513.

Songer, J.G., Trinh, H.T., Killgore, G.E., Thompson, A.D., McDonald, A.C. and Limbago, A.M. (2009), 'Clostridium difficile in retail meat products, USA, 2007', *Emerging Infectious Diseases*, vol. 15, no. 5, pp. 819–821.

Stoddart, B. and Wilcox, M.H. (2002), 'Clostridium difficile', *Current Opinion in Infectious Diseases*, vol. 15, no. 5, pp. 513–518.

Su, C.G., Judge, T.A. and Lichtenstein, G.R. (2002), 'Extraintestinal manifestations of inflammatory bowel disease', *Gastroenterology Clinics of North America*, vol. 31, no. 1, pp. 307–327.

van Nood, E., Vrieze, A., Nieuwdorp, M., *et al.* (2013), 'Duodenal infusion of donor feces for recurrent Clostridium difficile', *New England Journal of Medicine*, vol. 368, no. 5, pp. 407–415.

Chapter 11
A case of confusion in a man with cirrhosis

Scenario

You are the gastroenterology intern. It is Friday afternoon and you are looking forward to a quiet weekend away from work. You are just about to turn off your pager when it beeps. It is your consultant.

'I'm sending a patient from my rooms,' he tells you. 'He has alcoholic cirrhosis and became confused in the past 2 days. His wife is very concerned. Sort him out before the weekend.'

The patient and his wife arrive at the ward. The patient is a heavily jaundiced, cachectic man with a distended abdomen. He is obviously confused, so his wife tells you his medical history.

The patient is 58 years old and was diagnosed with alcoholic cirrhosis 7 months ago. He stopped drinking alcohol 3 months ago after a long history of heavy drinking. Six weeks ago, he required abdominal paracentesis for ascites.

Q: The patient's current medications include spironolactone and frusemide. He was told that these were for his liver. What role do these medications play in chronic liver disease?

A: Spironolactone and frusemide are both diuretics. In combination, they are first-line therapy for ascites, typically starting at 100 mg/d of spironolactone and 40 mg/d of frusemide (Runyon, 2013).

Q: What other basic management strategies can be used for ascites apart from oral diuretics (Liou, 2014; Runyon, 2013)?

A:

1. **Education regarding dietary salt restriction**. The main factor in the pathogenesis of ascites in chronic liver disease is sodium retention. Restricting dietary sodium to 40–60 mmol/day (1–1.5 g) should be the first measure used to control the condition. Unfortunately, compliance is a problem due to the deleterious effect this on the taste of food!
2. **Regular monitoring of weight and electrolytes**.

3. **Avoid drugs like ACE inhibitors and angiotensin receptor blockers (which can lead to hypotension and renal failure), propranolol and nonsteroidal anti-inflammatory drugs where possible.**
4. **Fluid restriction is rarely used (e.g. if the serum sodium is < 120).**

Q: What further options are available for the control of ascites that is refractory to these basic measures?

A: Further options would be (Runyon, 2013):
- serial therapeutic paracentesis
- peritoneovenous shunt
- transjugular intrahepatic portosystemic shunt (understandably shortened to TIPS!)[1]
- liver transplantation
- use of midrodine (not readily available in Australia at this time).

Q: On closer questioning, the patient's wife acknowledges that her husband is meant to be on a low sodium diet. However, he couldn't tolerate the bland taste and gave up.

But she is most concerned about her husband's confusion. She first noticed that he became irritable 2 days ago. Additionally, he has been sleeping during the day and staying awake at night. He has been increasingly forgetful. A few hours ago he went to get the mail from the postbox wearing only his underwear, which is completely out of character for him. He is usually mentally alert.

'Doctor, what is happening to my husband?'

A: In a man with chronic liver disease, the most likely cause of mental deterioration is hepatic encephalopathy.

The irritability, inverted sleep pattern, forgetfulness and loss of inhibition would support such a diagnosis, although other illnesses can manifest this way.

Q: What is hepatic encephalopathy?

A: This is a neuropsychiatric syndrome. It is clinically diverse, with very subtle abnormalities detectable only with neuropsychometric testing at one extreme and deep coma at the other. Some 50–70% of patients with cirrhosis may have hepatic encephalopathy.

---

[1] Peritoneovenous shunting and TIPS are rarely used because of the various side effects associated with these procedures. Nevertheless, they may still be used to buy the patient some time before a transplant can be performed.

Most of the clinical manifestations of hepatic encephalopathy are reversible with medical therapy. Nevertheless, some patients experience a progressive, chronic, debilitating syndrome.

Q: What is the pathogenesis of hepatic encephalopathy?

A: Although accumulation of ammonia due to impaired metabolism is the best-known factor, many other mechanisms have been proposed. These include manganese deposition in the basal ganglia, zinc deficiency and production of false neurotransmitters.

Q: Apart from hepatic encephalopathy, what are the other possible causes of confusion in a patient with chronic alcoholic liver disease?

A: Other possible causes would be:
- hypoglycaemia due to liver disease
- electrolyte imbalance due to liver disease and diuretic treatment
- hypoxia due to intrapulmonary shunting in liver disease
- AKI (acute kidney injury; hepatorenal syndrome)
- alcohol (he may have started drinking alcohol again)
- alcohol withdrawal
- subdural, intracerebral or subarachnoid haemorrhage contributed to by a coagulopathy from chronic liver disease
- other causes of delirium not specific to chronic liver disease (see Chapter 30).

Q: The patient's wife is sure that her husband has not drunk any alcohol for months. This makes an alcoholic encephalopathy or alcohol withdrawal unlikely.

What are the symptoms of alcohol withdrawal?

A: Most commonly, the signs and symptoms of alcohol withdrawal begin 5–10 hours after the last drink. They usually peak within 48 hours and can spontaneously resolve after 4–7 days.

Symptoms can temporally occur as follows.

1. **Autonomic hyperactivity** (onset typically 5–10 hours after cessation).

    Symptoms such as tremor, tachycardia, gastrointestinal problems and hypertension occur. These can progress to agitation, insomnia and hypervigilance.

    The autonomic symptoms often resolve within 5–7 days without requiring treatment.

2. **Withdrawal seizures** (typically 7–16 hours after the last drink).

    These are typically single, tonic-clonic grand mal seizures, and may be the only manifestation of alcohol withdrawal. About 10% of subjects who have withdrawal seizures proceed to delirium tremens. About 90% of these seizures occur within 48 hours.

3. **Sensory disturbances** (onset is typically within 24–48 hours). Sensory disturbances range from vivid dreams to illusions (where objects appear abnormal; e.g. the pattern on a carpet may appear to be moving) and hallucinations (seeing things that are not there; e.g. frightening animals such as snakes or crocodiles).

4. **Delirium tremens.** Delirium tremens is the label given to a constellation of signs characterised by confusion and agitation. In addition to being tremulous, patients experience fever, tachycardia and hypertension, and often also paranoid ideation, apprehension, hallucinations and disorientation. Delirium tremens is a medical emergency, as patients are at risk of harming themselves and others. It is most likely to occur when an alcohol-dependent person stops drinking abruptly in the setting of intercurrent medical illness, such as pneumonia or trauma.

Q: How do you treat alcohol withdrawal?

A: It is best to anticipate and prevent the development of major withdrawal rather than try to treat established delirium. To monitor for the beginnings of withdrawal, it can be helpful to use an alcohol withdrawal scale, which can be administered by nursing staff. A rising score on the scale points to the need for medical review and initiation of treatment.

In the management of alcohol withdrawal, supportive measures include a calm, quiet room with minimal lighting, little interpersonal contact and orienting the patient with reassurance. Nutritional support includes correcting dehydration and vitamin deficiencies.

Not all heavy drinkers develop withdrawal, but, where necessary, benzodiazepines are the drugs of choice. Diazepam, with its rapid oral absorption and long half-life, is probably the most commonly used medication for treating alcohol withdrawal in Australian hospitals. A loading dose of diazepam can prevent all manifestations of alcohol withdrawal. But benzodiazepines with an intermediate half-life, such as lorazepam, may be safer in those with concomitant liver disease.

There is a variety of adjuvant agents, which can have beneficial effects on various aspects of alcohol withdrawal such as hallucinations, confusion and autonomic dysfunction; however, they should only be used in conjunction with benzodiazepines.

With regard to alternatives to benzodiazepines, many studies have examined anticonvulsants (especially carbamazepine) (McKeon *et al.*, 2008; Kosten and O'Connor, 2003) although diazepam is still the most commonly used agent in Australia.

For delirium tremens, benzodiazepines remain the mainstay of therapy while haloperidol can be added if further control of agitation, disordered thought or perceptual disturbances is required. Despite all this, patients with delirium tremens may even need to be intubated in order to sedate them adequately (McKeon *et al.*, 2008).

It is also worth giving thiamine 100 mg daily to prevent Wernicke syndrome and 1 mg daily of folic acid replacement (Merrill and Duncan, 2014).

Q: What is the underlying pathophysiology of alcohol withdrawal?

A: It is thought that enhanced neurotransmission of glutamate (N-methyl-D-aspartate) pathways with a concomitant reduction in type A gamma-aminobutyric acid (GABA) pathway neurotransmission is responsible. Benzodiazepines act at the type A GABA receptor, which may partly explain their therapeutic role in alcohol withdrawal (Kosten and O'Connor, 2003). There is also enhanced dopaminergic transmission which may play a role in hallucinations. Early in alcohol withdrawal, there is an increase in noradrenergic activity which contributes to the heightened sympathetic activity (McKeon *et al.* 2008).

Q: You are sure that alcohol withdrawal is not the cause of confusion in this man. You are still concerned about hepatic encephalopathy. Will a physical examination help you diagnose this condition?

A: Possibly. Some patients with hepatic encephalopathy will have obvious signs, while others have very subtle features. Even the obvious signs can be non-specific and common to a number of conditions.

Nevertheless, the following signs will support a diagnosis of hepatic encephalopathy:

- disordered mentation (abnormal mini-mental test)
- hepatic fetor (unpleasant, musty odour of the breath due to mercaptans)
- asterixis (impaired proprioception best demonstrated by dorsiflexing the hands with the arms extended)
- constructional apraxia (inability to copy a shape such as the Star of David)
- hyperreflexia, or extensor plantar responses.

Stages and grades based on clinical features have been developed to assess the severity of hepatic encephalopathy. Although they are too difficult to remember, it may be worth referring to them in a textbook or on the hospital intranet whenever you encounter a possible case of hepatic encephalopathy. They are based on a combination of intellectual function, behaviour/personality, neuromuscular abnormalities and level of consciousness. The most severe stage or grade basically refers to a comatose person who is barely responsive (Munoz, 2008). Hepatic encephalopathy can be further divided into 'covert'/'minimal' (only detectable on neuropsychometric testing) or 'overt' where neurologic and psychiatric abnormalities are apparent on clinical bedside testing (Liou, 2014).

Q: The patient is deeply jaundiced and tachycardic. His blood pressure is 110/70. Oxygen saturation on room air is 97%. He is disoriented to time and place and demonstrates asterixis. He has constructional apraxia, but no other focal neurological signs. Apart from large amount of ascites and ankle oedema bilaterally, his gastrointestinal examination is normal. A rectal examination does not reveal faecal impaction (constipation is a cause of hepatic encephalopathy). The respiratory and cardiovascular systems are also unremarkable. You conclude that hepatic encephalopathy is still the most likely diagnosis.
What causes hepatic encephalopathy?

A: The most common precipitants of hepatic encephalopathy are:
- spontaneous bacterial peritonitis (SBP)
- gastrointestinal haemorrhage
- constipation
- hepatoma
- hypokalaemia
- alkalosis
- acute renal failure (ARF)
- portosystemic shunts (including TIPS and surgical shunts)
- anaemia

Q: What investigations would help you identify the causes of hepatic encephalopathy or other causes of confusion?
A:
1. **Full blood count**. Anaemia can precipitate hepatic encephalopathy.
2. **Electrolytes, urea, creatinine**. Hypokalaemia and ARF can precipitate hepatic encephalopathy. Hyponatraemia can cause confusion.
3. **Alpha fetoprotein**. This is a marker of hepatocellular carcinoma (also known as hepatoma).
4. **Blood cultures**.
5. **Chest and abdominal X-ray**. An abdominal X-ray may demonstrate constipation (faecal loading) as a precipitant of

hepatic encephalopathy. A chest X-ray may show pneumonia, which can cause confusion.

6. **Upper abdominal ultrasound**. This can identify a hepatoma.
7. **Electroencephalography (EEG)**. Hepatic encephalopathy can lead to triphasic waves (5 cycles a second) or delta waves.
8. **Diagnostic abdominal paracentesis**. This will identify SBP.
9. **Cerebral CT**. If there is any doubt about your diagnosis of hepatic encephalopathy, you must exclude a intracerebral haemorrhage, large stroke or other causes of space-occupying lesions with a CT brain scan.

And note ...

Although liver function tests and coagulation studies should be ordered for prognostic purposes, they will not help you sort out the cause of this man's confusion. Also, you must check his coagulation studies before performing invasive procedures, such as abdominal paracentesis, in order to prevent bleeding complications.

Q: A medical student watches on with interest and asks you, 'If ammonia accumulation causes hepatic encephalopathy, then wouldn't testing blood ammonia levels be a good idea?'

A: There previously were a number of issues related to blood ammonia levels, for example the inaccuracy of assays, venous versus arterial ammonia levels and how labile ammonia is. But now reliable assays for venous ammonia levels exist as long as the sample is correctly processed, for example using the right tube, putting it on ice and having the assay performed within 30 minutes. It would therefore be a good idea to speak to your pathology lab before taking the blood just to make sure that you do everything correctly.

As for the test itself, it seems to have a fairly good negative predictive value. In other words, a normal ammonia level in blood from a patient with severe mental abnormalities does not support a diagnosis of hepatic encephalopathy. Unfortunately, it is a non-specific test, so elevated levels in this type of patient can be due to other causes (Munoz, 2008).

Q: Your patient has thrombocytopaenia, abnormal liver function tests and a raised INR of 1.8, which are all consistent with chronic liver disease. The electrolytes, urea and creatinine are normal. The X-rays, upper abdominal ultrasound and cerebral CT are also all normal. The alpha fetoprotein result will be available in a few days. The EEG can only be performed tomorrow.

The gastroenterology registrar is concerned about SBP and suggests that you perform abdominal paracentesis. Do you need to give blood products before the procedure to reduce the bleeding complications?

A: This is an interesting question. Despite over 70% of these patients having an abnormal INR, only about 1% develop haemorrhagic complications following paracentesis (e.g. abdominal wall haematoma); so, abnormal coagulation tests in cirrhosis do not reflect bleeding risk. More serious bleeding complications, such as haemoperitoneum, occur in <1/1000 cases. In fact, despite the abnormal coagulation tests, cirrhotic patients often have overall normal coagulation activity due to both procoagulants and anticoagulants being deficient. Patients with marked thrombocytopaenia and INRs > 8 have undergone large volume paracentesis without haemorrhagic complications (Runyon, 2013).

Q: The gastroenterology registrar is happy to go ahead with the paracentesis without giving any vitamin K or blood products. You explain to the man's wife that the most important aspect of this investigation is to exclude SBP. She is surprised that you think her husband might have peritonitis, 'My aunt had peritonitis when her appendix burst. She had terrible abdominal pain and jumped off the bed when the doctor felt her tummy. My husband isn't complaining of pain and he didn't even wince when you felt his tummy. Does he really need this test?'

A: Although she has made a very good point, you explain to her that the only symptoms and signs of SBP may be the onset of hepatic encephalopathy. Fevers, abdominal pain and tenderness do not have to be present. Therefore, SBP must be excluded in any patient with hepatic encephalopathy and ascites.

Q: You easily remove straw-coloured but slightly cloudy ascitic fluid. What tests will you order on this?

A: You should ask for:
- cell count
- Gram stain
- culture
- albumin
- amylase
- cytology (malignancy)
- protein.

Q: The preliminary results are available.
- Gram stain is negative.

- There are 300×10^6/L polymorphonuclear cells.
- The albumin level in the ascites is 10 g/L.
- The ascitic protein is 29 g/L.

You explain to your patient's wife that bacteria could not be seen on Gram stain. You will therefore have to wait for the cultures to grow an organism in the next 48 hours before a diagnosis of SBP can be made. Is this correct?

A: Wrong! Although the figures vary, 40% of cases of SBP are culture-negative. As a result, the diagnosis can be made on the number of polymorphonuclear cells in the ascites. A level of 250×10^6/L is diagnostic for SBP.

Q: Your patient has 300×10^6/L polymorphonuclear cells in the ascites. You confidently inform his wife that he has SBP. Which bacteria are most likely to cause SBP?

A: Enteric gram-negative bacilli are by far the most likely culprits. Streptococci, including pneumococcus, are a less common cause.

Q: What antibiotic treatment will you commence in this patient?

A: The Therapeutic Guidelines: Antibiotic (Antibiotic Expert Group, 2014) recommends third-generation cephalosporins (such as cefotaxime or ceftriaxone). Broad-spectrum penicillins such as piperacillin-tazobactam as empiric therapy. A different antibiotic regimen may have to be used if the SBP occurred while the patient was already on antibiotic prophylaxis.

Q: Why did you order an albumin level on the ascitic fluid?

A: You wanted to know the serum to ascites albumin gradient (SAAG). Although the SAAG will not help you in diagnosing SBP, it will demonstrate that the patient's ascites is due to portal hypertension.

The SAAG involves a simple calculation: serum albumin minus ascites albumin.

In portal hypertension, the SAAG is greater than 11 g/L. In contrast, an SAAG of less than 11 g/L reflects normal portal pressures.

For example, your patient has a serum albumin level of 29 g/L and his ascitic albumin is 10 g/L. Therefore, the SAAG = 29 – 10 = 19 g/L. This is consistent with the raised portal pressures of portal hypertension.

Q: You have done well. There are 2 levels of treatment of hepatic encephalopathy, namely treatment of the precipitating cause and then treatment of the hepatic encephalopathy itself. You have initiated ceftriaxone to treat the SBP, so how do you treat the hepatic encephalopathy itself?

A: The use of lactulose (a nonabsorbable disaccharide) alone may be sufficient to cure the encephalopathy. An initial dose of 30 mL orally every 1–2 hours can be given until a laxative effect is reached. Then the dose can be reduced to 30 mL tds-qid (Gastrointestinal Writing Group, 2011).

Q: How does lactulose (a bowel aperient) cure something as serious as hepatic encephalopathy?

A: As discussed earlier, ammonia accumulation is thought to play an important role in the pathogenesis of this condition. One source of ammonia is the colon. Here urease-producing bacteria use gut epithelial cells that have been shed by the bowel wall as a substrate for ammonia production.

Lactulose acts at 2 levels. First, it promotes bowel catharsis and removes the shed gut epithelial cells from the bowel. Second, it lowers the colonic pH, which is unfavourable to the urease-producing bacteria. You should aim to induce a laxative effect with mild diarrhoea.

Q: If lactulose does not work, what other measures can be used?

A: An antibiotic such as rifaximin (550 mg bd) can be used; however, it is meant to be used as secondary prophylaxis against recurrent hepatic encephalopathy rather than being used for primary treatment.

Q: You add lactulose to the ceftriaxone and inform the specialist of your progress. He is pleased with your work and will review the patient over the weekend.

You return on Monday to find that the patient is doing well. His wife tells you that his confusion resolved within 24 hours of your treatment. The culture of the ascites has remained negative.

The patient wonders if he should be on antibiotics to stop getting the SBP again. What do you think?

A: Although he responded well to antibiotics, even a single episode of SBP has terrible prognostic implications. He has a 70% chance of recurrence at 1 year and only 30–50% of patients will survive if they haven't been on secondary prophylaxis. On the other hand, secondary prophylaxis reduces the recurrence rate of SBP from 68% to 20%. So it would be reasonable to put him on antibiotic prophylaxis (Liou, 2014).

Q: On the following day, your patient is ready to be discharged. Just as you are about to start writing his discharge summary, his nurse comes to the desk looking very worried and tells you that he has just had a haematemesis.

What is the likely cause?

A: The most common cause of upper gastrointestinal bleeding is peptic ulcer disease. However, in patients with chronic liver disease, the biggest concern is bleeding from gastro-oesophageal varices. The morbidity and mortality arising from variceal bleeding is higher than from other causes of upper gastrointestinal bleeding.

Q: What do you do?

A: You rush to the room. Your patient looks slightly pale and is holding a bowl filled with about 100 mL of blood.

He needs his haemodynamic status assessed, urgent IV access with IV fluids and blood taken for a number of tests, including an urgent cross-match and insertion of a urethral catheter (see Chapter 8 on upper gastrointestinal bleeding for a detailed approach to this initial part of resuscitation).

Q: Your patient is awake. His blood pressure is 110/60 and his heart rate is 100/minute. His oxygen saturation is 97% on room air. A physical examination reveals no new findings.

You already know his medical history and are aware that there is no known history of peptic ulcer disease, aspirin or non-steroidal anti-inflammatory drug use.

What further treatment would you institute?

A: Based on Liou, 2014; Toubia and Sanyal, 2008; and the Gastrointestinal Writing Group, 2011:

1. **Call the gastroenterology registrar.**
2. **General resuscitation measures** (insert 2 large-bore IV cannulae, consider intubation and ventilation, transfuse if haemoglobin is <7 g/dL).
3. **Octreotide infusion (50 microgram bolus, then an infusion of 25–50 microgram/hr for 2–5 days)**. Octreotide is a somatostatin analogue that can stop up to 80% of cases of variceal bleeding, possibly by reducing portal pressure. But this does not improve mortality.

    An alternative is 2–5 days of IV terlipressin (1.7 mg q6h), which is a vasopressin analogue. Terlipressin has a milder side effect profile to vasopressin, which can lead to such severe vasoconstriction that bowel necrosis can occur.
4. **Endoscopic therapy** can stop almost 90% of cases of oesophageal variceal bleeding. Ligation (banding) of oesophageal varices is preferred to sclerotherapy. A delay of >15 hours to endoscopic therapy is associated with increased mortality.

5. **Antibiotic prophylaxis (ceftriaxone 1 g daily)**. There is an increased risk of sepsis or SBP in patients with variceal bleeding, particularly when the cirrhosis is advanced.

Q: What techniques can be used for refractory variceal bleeding?

A: Possibilities include:

- Balloon tamponade, where a tube is inserted into the oesophagus and stomach and a balloon is inflated to compress the bleeding vessels. It is very effective in stopping the bleeding once the balloon is inflated; however, it is prone to complications and bleeding often recurs with deflation of the balloon.
- TIPS.
- Surgical portosystemic shunting—less commonly seen these days due to the availability of the above techniques and fewer experienced surgeons.

Q: Your patient's haemoglobin is 80 g/L. You immediately commence an octreotide infusion. An endoscopy is performed. This reveals oesophageal varices, which are treated by ligation. The patient has no further bleeding and recovers.

Should the patient have secondary prophylaxis for gastroesophageal haemorrhage?

A: Yes, because almost 70% of patients with variceal bleeding will suffer another bleed within the year (mainly within the first 6 weeks) which is associated with a 70% 1-year mortality (Toubia and Sanyal, 2008).

Q: What would you recommend for secondary prophylaxis of his oesophageal varices?

A: A combination of non-selective beta-blockers and regular endoscopic variceal ligation is first-line for secondary prophylaxis (Liou, 2014; Toubia and Sanyal, 2008).

- **Non-selective beta-blockers**. Beta-blockers reduce portal pressure, thus lessening the risk of recurrent bleeding and prolonging survival.
- **Endoscopic therapy**.[2] Ligation of oesophageal varices every 10–14 days until they are obliterated is also recommended with further endoscopic monitoring every 3–6 months after that.

---

[2]The treatment of gastric varices is not as straightforward as oesophageal varices with 'tissue glue' (N-butyl-2-cyanoacrylate) and sclerotherapy playing a greater role than with oesophageal varices.

Q: Your patient is commenced on a beta-blocker. He will return to hospital in 10 days to begin ligation of his oesophageal varices. Your medical student wonders what the prognosis is. Do you know any objective markers of severity for chronic liver disease?

A: There are two well-known prognostic scores: the Child–Pugh classification and the MELD (Model for End-stage Liver Disease) score.

The Child–Pugh classification is based on 2 clinical criteria and 3 laboratory criteria. Each factor is given a score out of 3: the higher the score, the worse the prognosis. Also, the worse the Child–Pugh grade, the higher the risk of variceal bleeding and difficulty controlling acute haemorrhage (Toubia and Sanyal, 2008).

It is worthwhile remembering what the 5 factors are, but you do not have to learn the exact scoring system. There will always be a book or computer nearby where you can look up the complete system.

Out of interest, though, the scoring system is as follows:

	1 point	2 points	3 points
Hepatic encephalopathy	None	Grade 1 or 2	Grade 3 or 4
Ascites	None	Mild	Moderate
Bilirubin (mmol/L)	<35	35–50	>50
Albumin	>35	28–35	<28
INR	<0.7	1.7–2.3	>2.3

Source: Adapted from Patel (1999) and Riley and Bhatti (2001).

- Child–Pugh A: 5–6 points (life expectancy 15–20 years, 10% perioperative mortality)
- Child–Pugh B: 7–9 points
- Child–Pugh C: 10–15 points (life expectancy 1 to 3 years, 80% perioperative mortality)

Your patient currently has no encephalopathy (1 point), gross ascites (3 points), albumin 29 g/L (2 points), bilirubin 60 mmol/L (3 points) and INR 1.4 (1 point). Therefore, he is Child–Pugh C classification, which is the worst prognostic group.

The MELD score has been used to prioritise the waiting lists for a liver transplant. It also has a number of other uses, including being a good marker of prognosis in a variety of complications of chronic liver disease, such as variceal bleeding, SBP and hepatorenal syndrome (Kim and Lee, 2013). The score consists of 3 components: bilirubin, creatinine and INR. However, the formula is complicated so you will have to use an app or online calculator to determine the score.

Q: You determine that your patient's MELD score is 20, which means he has around a 20% 3-month mortality. Your medical student hears his Child-Pugh and MELD scores and shakes her head, 'He's an alcoholic, so I guess they can't offer him a liver transplant'. What is your response?

A: You inform your student that alcoholic cirrhosis is in fact one of the indications for liver transplantation. However, there must be evidence that the patient has controlled their drinking.

The Australian National Liver Transplantation Unit (2013) reported that the most common causes for liver transplantation in adults were:
- hepatitis C (23%)
- alcoholic liver diseases (12%)
- malignancy (11%)
- primary sclerosing cholangitis (10%)
- fulminant hepatic failure (10%)
- hepatitis B (7%).

Achievements

You now:
- know the management principles of ascites
- know causes of confusion in a man with alcoholic liver disease
- can describe the temporal sequence of clinical features in alcohol withdrawal
- know how to treat alcohol withdrawal
- know the precipitants of hepatic encephalopathy
- can order appropriate investigations for hepatic encephalopathy
- know how to diagnose SBP using ascitic fluid
- know the appropriate treatment for SBP
- are aware of the use of the serum to ascites albumin gradient
- can institute treatment for hepatic encephalopathy
- know how to manage acute variceal bleeding
- are aware of the Child-Pugh classification and MELD scores for cirrhosis
- know the common causes for liver transplantation in Australia.

References

Antibiotic Expert Group (2014), *Therapeutic Guidelines: Antibiotic*, Version 15, Therapeutic Guidelines Ltd, Melbourne.

Australian National Liver Transplantation Unit (2013), 'Liver transplantation: Australian National Liver Transplantation Unit', The Australian National

Liver Transplantation Unit, at <www.sswahs.nsw.gov.au/gastro/livertransplant/RPAH2013/2013Report.pdf>, accessed 11 November 2014.

Chang, P.H. and Steinberg, M.B. (2001), 'Alcohol withdrawal', *Medical Clinics of North America*, vol. 85, no. 5, pp. 1191–1212.

Gastrointestinal Writing Group (2011), *Therapeutic Guidelines: Gastrointestinal*, Version 5, Therapeutic Guidelines Ltd, Melbourne.

Kim, H.J. and Lee, H.W. (2013), 'Important predictor of mortality in patients with end-stage liver disease', *Clinical and Molecular Hepatology*, vol. 19, no. 2, pp. 105–115.

Kosten, T.R. and O'Connor, P.G. (2003), 'Management of drug and alcohol withdrawal', *New England Journal of Medicine*, vol. 348, no. 18, pp. 1786–1795.

Krige, J.E. and Beckingham, I.J. (2001), 'ABC of diseases of liver, pancreas, and biliary system: Portal hypertension-2. Ascites, encephalopathy, and other conditions', *British Medical Journal*, vol. 322, no. 7283, pp. 416–418.

Liou, I.W. (2014), 'Management of end-stage liver disease', *Medical Clinics of North America*, vol. 98, no. 1, pp. 119–152.

McKeon, A., Frye, M.A. and Delanty, N. (2008), 'The alcohol withdrawal syndrome', *Journal of Neurology, Neurosurgery and Psychiatry*, vol. 79, no. 8, pp. 854–862.

Merrill, J.O. and Duncan, M.H. (2014), 'Addiction disorders', *Medical Clinics of North America*, vol. 98, no. 5, pp. 1097–1122.

Mowat, C. and Stanley, A.J. (2001), 'Spontaneous bacterial peritonitis—diagnosis, treatment and prevention', *Alimentary Pharmacology and Therapeutics*, vol. 15, no. 2, pp. 1851–1859.

Munoz, S.J. (2008), 'Hepatic encephalopathy', *Medical Clinics of North America*, vol. 92, no. 4, pp. 795–812.

Patel, T. (1999), 'Surgery in the patient with liver disease', *Mayo Clinic Proceedings*, vol. 74, no. 6, pp. 593–599.

Riley, T.R. 3rd and Bhatti, A.M. (2001), 'Preventive strategies in chronic liver disease: Part II. Cirrhosis', *American Family Physician*, vol. 64, no. 10, pp. 1735–1740.

Riordan, S.M. and Williams, R. (1997), 'Treatment of hepatic encephalopathy', *New England Journal of Medicine*, vol. 337, no. 7, pp. 473–479.

Runyon, B.A. (2013), 'Management of adult patients with ascites due to cirrhosis: Update 2012', American Association for the Study of Liver Diseases, at <www.aasld.org/publications/practice-guidelines>, accessed 10 November 2014.

Sharara, A.L. and Rockey, D.C. (2001), 'Gastroesophageal variceal hemorrhage', *New England Journal of Medicine*, vol. 345, no. 9, pp. 669–681.

Toubia, N. and Sanyal, A.J. (2008), 'Portal hypertension and variceal haemorrhage', *Medical Clinics of North America*, vol. 92, no. 3, pp. 551–574.

Chapter 12
Mr Perez presents with right-sided weakness

Scenario

A 63-year-old man presents to the Emergency Department with right-sided weakness. Mr Perez was at home with his wife when his right arm and leg suddenly became weak. Mrs Perez called an ambulance and she and her husband were quickly brought to the hospital. The weakness has neither worsened nor improved since it began about 30 minutes ago. Mr Perez takes simvastatin for high cholesterol and has smoked 10 cigarettes a day for 30 years.

Q: What are your concerns?

A: Mr Perez could be suffering from a stroke due to a thromboembolic infarct or an intracerebral haemorrhage.

Q: Your examination demonstrates a facial droop and 4/5 upper and lower limb weakness on the right. Mr Perez clinically is in sinus rhythm and has no carotid bruits. His blood pressure is 170/100.
What do you do now?

A: Your clinical assessment supports the diagnosis of a stroke. You now need to establish whether this is haemorrhagic or thromboembolic in origin, which can be quite difficult to differentiate clinically. Therefore, although you would normally order baseline blood tests, the most important and urgent investigation is a CT brain scan. A CT brain scan is a test that should be easily accessible at any hour in an Australian teaching hospital.

Q: The nurse is concerned about Mr Perez's blood pressure, which is 170/100. He asks if you want to reduce it now. How do you respond?

A: About 70% of acute stroke patients have elevated blood pressure. The concern in reducing it is that this could extend the stroke. The ischaemic penumbra loses autoregulation, which results in a direct relationship between blood pressure and cerebral blood flow through the ischaemic penumbra. Consequently, it is feared that lowering the blood pressure will lead to a reduction in blood flow to the ischaemic penumbra, causing another ischaemic stroke. Furthermore, the hypertension often settles with bed rest alone. Recent guidelines (National Stroke Foundation, 2010; Hill and ASMEWG, 2008) do support cautious reduction of blood pressure if extremely high (e.g. >220/120 mm Hg), but by no more than 10–20% and observing the patient carefully for signs of deterioration neurologically.

But as an intern, you do not have to make this decision alone. Do not lower a patient's blood pressure without first seeking the advice of a more senior staff member, such as the neurology registrar or on-call neurologist.

Q: You page the neurology registrar. She is comfortable with Mr Perez's blood pressure and does not advise lowering it. The nurse notes that his oxygen saturation on room air is 96%. 'Shall I give him some oxygen?'

A: In the setting of acute stroke, supplemental oxygen should only be given to patients with an oxygen saturation <95% (National Stroke Foundation, 2010). So you tell the nurse that supplemental oxygen is not necessary.

Q: What other investigations should be ordered in these early stages of Mr Perez's presentation?

A:

1. **An urgent CT brain**.
2. **Carotid artery doppler ultrasound**.
3. **Full blood count**. This provides baseline values that can be very useful if heparin-induced thrombocytopaenia (HIT) develops while on deep vein thrombosis (DVT) prophylaxis. Rarely, a full blood count might identify a myeloproliferative cause of stroke (e.g. polycythaemia or thrombocytosis).
4. **Coagulation studies**. These provide a baseline and will be needed if anticoagulation is being considered. Occasionally, an abnormality here might identify an uncommon cause of stroke (e.g. a raised APTT due to a lupus anticoagulant).
5. **Electrolytes, liver function tests and blood sugar**. Again, these provide baseline values. Occasionally, you will identify hypoglycaemia and hyponatraemia severe enough to cause focal neurological symptoms. In addition, hyperglycaemia may be identified (see page 140).
6. **ESR and CRP**. Rarely, this might identify a patient whose stroke is due to an underlying vasculitis (e.g. giant-cell arteritis).
7. **12-lead ECG**. This may identify an underlying cause of stroke such as:
   - atrial fibrillation (AF)

- old anterior MI (resulting in left ventricular thrombus)
- new MI (resulting in a hypotensive stroke).
8. **Fasting lipids.**
9. **In certain patients, other testing such as syphilis serology, a vasculitis screen, prothrombotic screen and catheter angiography may have to be performed.**

Q: Will a CT brain scan demonstrate a cerebral infarct?

A: A CT brain scan in this setting will demonstrate an intracerebral haemorrhage or another space-occupying lesion such as a tumour. However, unless the patient has suffered a massive cerebral infarct, you are unlikely to see an infarct on a CT in the first 48–72 hours after a stroke.

In the acute stroke setting, it appears that MRI of the brain is the imaging modality of choice compared to CT with a superior sensitivity (0.99 versus 0.39) but similar specificity (0.92 versus 1.00) (National Stroke Foundation, 2010; Chalela *et al.*, 2007); however, an MRI is a very difficult test to order at short notice in many Australian hospitals.

Q: A CT brain scan is performed within an hour of your request. It appears to be normal and certainly does not demonstrate an intracerebral haemorrhage.

Your medical student asks you if Mr Perez should be thrombolysed, given that this is a thromboembolic stroke. What do you tell him?

A: It is a good question. Thrombolysis is an important therapeutic intervention for acute ischaemic stroke. There is an increased risk of intracranial haemorrhage and early death from thrombolysis; however, once the risk period from early bleeding has ended, the long-term outcomes at 3 and 6 months following thrombolysis are good. This is contingent on the thrombolysis being given early in the course of acute stroke (Wardlaw *et al.*, 2014).

In Australia, recombinant tissue plasminogen activator (rt-PA) can be given for acute ischaemic stroke within 4.5 hours of stroke onset. This should only be done in a hospital that is set up with a multidisciplinary acute stroke team and ready access to radiology facilities. An intervention other than systemic thrombolysis is intra-arterial thrombolysis (e.g. with urokinase). Intra-arterial thrombolysis can be offered within 6 hours in select patients only (National Stroke Foundation, 2010).

Of course, there is also a large list of contraindications to thrombolysis, and these are not dissimilar to those for thrombolysis in acute myocardial infarction.

Q: Mr Perez has presented within 3 hours of the onset of his symptoms and had an immediate CT brain to exclude an intracranial haemorrhage; therefore, he meets the timeframe for thrombolysis. You call the neurology registrar who rapidly comes and assesses the patient. He agrees that Mr Perez should be thrombolysed with IV rt-PA. Should he get aspirin before the thrombolysis?

A: Once an intracranial haemorrhage has been excluded by imaging, aspirin should be given within 48 hours of stroke onset. This can be given orally or by nasogastric tube. The initial dose should be at least 150–300 mg, after which a smaller daily dose can be given such as 100 mg/day (National Stroke Foundation, 2010). A daily dose of aspirin started within 48 hours of an acute ischaemic stroke is beneficial in reducing incidence of recurrent stroke within 2 weeks and improving mortality and functional outcome (Sandercock *et al.*, 2008).

However, if a patient is going to be thrombolysed, delay the administration of aspirin for 24 hours, until progress imaging rules out significant haemorrhage (National Stroke Foundation, 2010).

Q: Mr Perez isn't given aspirin right now as he is going to be thrombolysed. He receives the thrombolysis and is transferred to the stroke unit. Your student also wonders if Mr Perez needs deep venous thrombosis (DVT) heparin prophylaxis. What do you tell him?

A: The third most common cause of deaths in stroke patients is pulmonary embolism; therefore, DVT and PE are important considerations in the management of an acute stroke patient. However, the use of low molecular weight heparin or unfractionated heparin is only recommended for select stroke patients at high risk of DVT or PE (e.g. those with a thrombophilic disorder or a past history of DVT/PE). Also, thigh-length antithrombotic stockings are not recommended in the post-stroke setting. Other important interventions to reduce the risk of DVT or PE in acute stroke patients include (National Stroke Foundation, 2010):

- early mobilisation
- maintaining adequate hydration.

However, since Mr Perez has just been thrombolysed, many neurologists would defer DVT prophylaxis for 24 hours.

Q: The on-call neurologist agrees that TED stockings should be given. Patients with acute stroke are potentially at risk of aspiration pneumonia due to factors such as reduced level of consciousness, reduced gag reflex and cough. If you have any such concerns about

Mr Perez, it would be reasonable to make him nil by mouth until he has been reviewed by a speech pathologist.

What ward is ideal for Mr Perez and why?

A: Not all hospitals have a stroke unit, but if there is one this is the ward to which patients such as Mr Perez should be admitted. In stroke units, a multidisciplinary team looks after stroke patients only. Care in a stroke unit increases the chances of stroke patients being alive, living at home and being independent 1 year after the stroke (Stroke Units Triallists' Collaboration, 2007).

Q: Before being moved to the stroke unit, you assess Mr Perez's blood tests. You discover that he has a blood sugar level of 9.8 mmol/L. Mrs Perez is surprised as she is certain that her husband's fasting blood sugar only 2 weeks ago was normal. Is this surprising?

A: Acute hyperglycaemia following stroke in non-diabetics is not uncommon. It does not have to mean that the patient is diabetic. Allport *et al.* (2008) found that 34% of non-diabetic patients with acute hemispheric ischaemic stroke were hyperglycaemic for part of the acute post-stroke period. Furthermore, the hyperglycaemia might lead to adverse outcomes following a stroke (Lindsberg and Roine, 2004; Parsons *et al.*, 2002). But the best way to deal with this is yet to be seen (National Stroke Foundation, 2010).

Q: Mr Perez is moved to the stroke unit. By the following day, his weakness has greatly resolved. The speech pathologist has assessed his swallowing and is happy to start him on a normal diet. He will have carotid dopplers later today. But should he also have a cardiac echo?

A: Echocardiography is not a routine diagnostic tool in acute stroke. But it may be useful in those with an abnormal ECG, pre-existing cardiac abnormalities or those in whom the cause of stroke is not apparent after routine tests (National Stroke Foundation, 2010).

Q: Which type of cardiac echocardiography—transoesophageal echocardiogram (TOE) or transthoracic echocardiogram (TTE)—is superior in evaluating a source of cardioembolic stroke?

A: Both procedures have their strengths and weaknesses. Ideally, they should be complementary procedures that are performed together. Many cardiology departments, however, will not perform a TOE until a TTE has been performed.

TTE is better than TOE at visualising left ventricular (LV) apex, LV thrombi and certain aspects of prosthetic valves. TOE is better at visualising the left atrial appendage, left atrium, left atrial thrombi, small valvular abnormalities and the interatrial septum.

The neurologist comes to see the patient and is pleased to see that you have ordered the carotid dopplers for tomorrow. She feels that a carotid source of the stroke is most likely so she is happy to defer echocardiography for now. She notices that Mr Perez is on aspirin and asks you if there is another agent you could add.

Q: You confidently tell the specialist that the long-term use of dipyridamole in combination with aspirin is more effective than aspirin alone in the secondary prevention of stroke (National Stroke Foundation, 2010; ESPRIT Study Group *et al.*, 2006). A commercial formulation of both aspirin and dipyridamole is available in Australia; however, it should not be used in patients with concomitant coronary artery disease. Clopidogrel, the antiplatelet agent, is an alternative to the aspirin-dipyridamole combination (National Stroke Foundation, 2010).

The specialist is impressed with your knowledge and ceases the aspirin. She commences the patient on combined dipyridamole/aspirin therapy.

The following day the TTE and TOE demonstrate no intra-cardiac source of embolus. However, the left internal carotid artery has a 75% narrowing on the Doppler study. Mr Perez wants to know what this means. What do you tell him?

A: In general, carotid endarterectomy (CEA) (National Stroke Foundation, 2010) is:
1. recommended for patients with a non-disabling stroke or TIA with ipsilateral 70–99% stenosis and should only be performed by surgeons with <6% perioperative morbidity and mortality rates
2. recommended for certain select patients with a symptomatic stenosis of 50–69% or asymptomatic stenosis of >60% being only performed by surgeons with <3% perioperative morbidity and mortality rates
3. recommended to be performed within 2 weeks of the stroke in appropriate patients (see criteria above)
4. not recommended in symptomatic stenosis <50% or asymptomatic stenosis of <60%.

Q: Your student says, 'Surely carotid artery stenting is a safer procedure than carotid endarterectomy?' What is your response?

A: Currently, carotid surgery is preferred to stenting, although studies continue on this topic (National Stroke Foundation, 2010; Hill and ASMEWG, 2008).

Q: The vascular surgeons agree that a CEA should be performed and arrange a time for early next week. Should Mr Perez be commenced on a statin for secondary prevention of stroke?

A: Yes. Although statins are indicated for all patients with a TIA or ischaemic stroke, they are not routinely recommended for haemorrhagic stroke (National Stroke Foundation, 2010).

Scenario

On your next overtime shift in the Emergency Department, you see 2 patients with acute neurological symptoms. The first patient you see is a 72-year-old man, Mr Barber, with profound right-sided hemiparesis and his first documented episode of atrial fibrillation. He is not using antiplatelet or anticoagulant agents. The CT brain scan excludes intracerebral haemorrhage. Your diligent medical student points out that the stroke most likely is cardioembolic secondary to the AF, and is keen to commence heparin immediately.

Q: What do you think?

A: The routine use of anticoagulation early in acute cardioembolic stroke is not recommended (National Stroke Foundation, 2010; Hill and ASMEWG, 2008); however, the patient will require long-term anticoagulation to prevent further strokes.

Q: The neurology registrar is on hand and starts seeing Mr Barber. You move on to the next patient. It is 72-year-old Mrs Jameson, with diabetes, who experienced transient right-sided weakness. It has never happened before. It only lasted for about 15 minutes but her husband was anxious for her to be reviewed in hospital. Her physical examination and ECG are unremarkable. She is fairly relaxed about the whole episode. 'It was nothing. Can't I just go home and see my GP next week?' What do you tell her?

A: It is likely that Mrs Jameson suffered from a transient ischaemic attack (TIA). The ABCD^2 tool can be used to assess risk of stroke after a TIA with a score >3 regarded as high risk (other high-risk factors include atrial fibrillation, carotid territory symptoms or crescendo TIA). The tool uses the following (National Stroke Foundation, 2010):

- Age 60 or over—1 point
- Blood pressure (systolic 140 mm Hg or more and/or diastolic 90 mm Hg or more)—1 point
- Clinical features: unilateral weakness—2 points; speech impairment without weakness—1 point
- Diabetes—1 point

Mrs Jameson has a score of 4, which puts her at high risk of stroke following her TIA. She should be admitted for urgent imaging of the brain and carotids, in addition to standard blood tests.

Achievements

You now:
- know which investigations to order in the initial assessment of a stroke patient
- know uses and limitations of a CT brain scan in early assessment of a stroke
- are aware of the role of thrombolysis in stroke
- realise that treatment of hypertension in acute stroke must be considered carefully
- realise that hyperglycaemia is common in the setting of acute stroke
- understand the importance of stroke units in the management of acute stroke
- realise that DVT is a common complication after acute stroke
- know the role of antiplatelet agents in early management of stroke
- can undertake investigations to find the source of stroke
- appreciate the indications of CEA in treating carotid stenosis
- are aware of the ABCD^2 tool for assessing stroke risk in TIA patients.

References

Adams, H.P. Jr, del Zoppo, G., Alberts, M.J. *et al.* (2007), 'Guidelines for the early management of adults with ischemic stroke: A guideline from the American Heart Association/American Stroke Association Stroke Council, Clinical Cardiology Council, Cardiovascular Radiology and Intervention Council, and the Atherosclerotic Peripheral Vascular Disease and Quality of Care Outcomes in Research Interdisciplinary Working Groups. The American Academy of Neurology affirms the value of this guideline as an educational tool for neurologists', *Stroke*, vol. 38, no. 5, pp. 1655–1711.

Albers, G.W. and Amarenco, P. (2001), 'Combination therapy with clopidogrel and aspirin: Can the CURE results be extrapolated to cerebrovascular patients?', *Stroke*, vol. 32, no. 12, pp. 2948–2949.

Allport, L., Baird, T., Butcher, K. *et al.* (2008), 'Frequency and temporal profile of poststroke hyperglycemia using continuous glucose monitoring', *Diabetes Care*, vol. 29, no. 8, pp. 1839–1848.

Amarenco, P., Bogousslavsky, J., Callahan, A. 3rd *et al.* (2006), 'High-dose atorvastatin after stroke or transient ischemic attack, *New England Journal of Medicine*, vol. 355, no. 6, pp. 549–559.

Brickner, M.E. (1996), 'Cardioembolic stroke', *American Journal of Medicine*, vol. 100, no. 4, pp. 465–474.

Broderick, J.P. and Hacke, W. (2002a), 'Treatment of acute ischemic stroke Part I: Recanalization strategies', *Circulation*, vol. 106, no. 12, pp. 1563–1569.

Broderick, J.P. and Hacke, W. (2002b), 'Treatment of acute ischemic stroke Part II: Neuroprotection and medical management', *Circulation*, vol. 106, no. 13, pp. 1736–1740.

Chalela, J.A., Kidwell, C.S., Nentwich, L.M. *et al.* (2007), 'Magnetic resonance imaging and computed tomography in emergency assessment of patients with suspected acute stroke: A prospective comparison', *Lancet*, vol. 369, no. 9558, pp. 293–298.

Donnan, G.A., Davis, S.M. and Thrift, A. (2003), 'The role of blood pressure lowering before and after stroke', *Current Opinion in Neurology*, vol. 16, no. 1, pp. 81–86.

ESPRIT Study Group *et al.* (Halkes, P.H., van Gijn, J., Kappelle, L.J., Koudstaal, P.J. and Algra, A.) (2006), 'Aspirin plus dipyridamole versus aspirin alone after cerebral ischaemia of arterial origin (ESPRIT): Randomised controlled trial', *Lancet*, vol. 367, no. 9523, pp. 1665–1673.

Gerraty, R.P. (2003), 'Stroke prevention: What's new?', *Internal Medicine Journal*, vol. 33, no. 4, pp. 177–181.

Hacke, W., Kaste, M., Bogousslavsky, J. *et al.* (2003), 'European Stroke Initiative Recommendations for Stroke Management—update 2003', *Cerebrovascular Disease*, vol. 16, no. 4, pp. 311–337.

Hacke, W., Donnan, G., Fieschi, C. *et al.* (2004), 'Association of outcome with early stroke treatment: Pooled analysis of ATLANTIS, ECASS, and NINDS rt-PA stroke trials', *Lancet*, vol. 363, no. 9411, pp. 768–774.

Hart, R.G., Palacio, S. and Pearce, L.A. (2002), 'Atrial fibrillation, stroke, and acute antithrombotic therapy: Analysis of randomized clinical trials', *Stroke*, vol. 33, no. 11, pp. 2722–2727.

Hill, K. and ASMEWG (Australian Stroke Management Expert Working Group) (2008), 'Australian clinical guidelines for acute stroke management 2007', *International Journal of Stroke*, vol. 3, no. 2, pp. 120–129.

Johnston, S.C. (2002), 'Clinical practice: Transient ischemic attack', *New England Journal of Medicine*, vol. 347, no. 21, pp. 1687–1692.

Lindsberg, P.J. and Roine, R.O. (2004), 'Hyperglycaemia in acute stroke', *Stroke*, vol. 35, no. 2, pp. 363–364.

McGovern, R. and Rudd, A. (2003), 'Management of stroke', *Postgraduate Medical Journal*, vol. 79, no. 928, pp. 87–92.

National Stroke Foundation (2010), 'Clinical guidelines for stroke managemen 2010', National Stroke Foundation, Melbourne, Australia, at <http://strokefoundation.com.au/site/media/clinical_guidelines_stroke_managment_2010_interactive.pdf>, accessed 11 November 2014.

O'Regan, C., Wu, P., Arora, P., Perri, D. and Mills, E.J. (2008), 'Statin therapy in stroke prevention: A meta-analysis involving 121,000 patients', *American Journal of Medicine*, vol. 121, no. 1, pp. 24–33.

Parsons, M.W., Barber, P.A., Desmond, P.M. *et al.* (2002), 'Acute hyperglycemia adversely affects stroke outcome: A magnetic resonance imaging and spectroscopy study', *Annals of Neurology*, vol. 52, no. 1, pp. 20–28.

Sandercock, P.A., Counsell, C., Gubitz, G.J. and Tseng, M.C. (2008), 'Antiplatelet therapy for acute ischaemic stroke', *Cochrane Database of Systematic Reviews*, 3: CD000029.

Stroke Unit Triallists' Collaboration (2007), 'Organised inpatient (stroke unit) care for strokes', *Cochrane Database of Systematic Reviews*, 4: CD000197.

Wahlgren, N., Ahmed, N., Davalos, A. *et al.* (2007), 'Thrombolysis with alteplase for acute ischaemic stroke in the Safe Implementation of Thrombolysis in Stroke-Monitoring Study (SITS-MOST): An observational study', *Lancet*, vol. 369, no. 9558, pp. 275–282.

Wardlaw, J.M., Murray, V., Berge, E. and del Zoppo, G.J. (2014) 'Thrombolysis for acute ischaemic stroke', *Cochrane Database of Systematic Reviews*, issue 7, art. no. CD000213, DOI: 10.1002/14651858.CD000213.pub3.

Chapter 13
Marwan presents with seizures

Scenario

It is midday in the Emergency Department. You have sorted out all the patients from the morning, and are hoping to grab a quick lunch. But just as you start to make your way towards the culinary delights of the hospital cafeteria, a nurse grabs you.

'Can you come to the Resus Room? A dental student who is doing an elective in the hospital collapsed and is having a generalised tonic–clonic seizure. He has never been responsive, but his observations are fine: heart rate 85/minute, blood pressure 130/70, temperature 36.9 °C, oxygen saturation 97% on room air. We haven't given him anything for the seizure. It's been going on for just over 3 minutes.'

Q: Is this a case of status epilepticus?
A: Technically, no. The definition of status epilepticus is:
- continuous seizure activity for more than 30 minutes OR
- 2 or more sequential seizures over this period without full recovery between seizures.

However, for practical purposes, people should begin treatment for status epilepticus after 5 minutes of continued seizures (Neurology Writing Group, 2011; Millikan *et al.*, 2009). So this young man currently doesn't meet the criteria for status epilepticus.

Q: What are the consequences of not ending status epilepticus promptly?
A: Think of the 4 Hs:
1. hypoxia (potentially resulting in chronic brain injury)
2. hyperthermia
3. pH (acidosis)
4. hypotension.

Status epilepticus is a serious condition—the 30-day mortality of people with status epilepticus is 19–27% (Millikan *et al.*, 2009).

Q: You are concerned about impending status epilepticus in this young man. What would you do if the seizure were to continue beyond 5 minutes and he required treatment for status epilepticus?

A:
1. **Assess the airway.** If the fitting is interfering with respiration, he may require intubation and assisted ventilation.
2. **Insert a large-bore IV cannula and commence IV fluids.**
3. **Collect blood for the following tests:**
   a. full blood count
   b. EUC, calcium, magnesium and phosphate
   c. blood sugar
   d. liver function tests
   e. anticonvulsant levels
   f. serum and urinary screen for recreational drugs
   g. arterial blood gas.
4. **Insert a second IV line for administration of anticonvulsants.**

And note ...

A pinprick blood glucose can be taken at this early stage. This can almost immediately identify individuals with seizures due to hypoglycaemia.

Q: What IV anticonvulsants would you use for a patient in status epilepticus?

A: Start with (Neurology Writing Group, 2011):
1. **Benzodiazepines**[1] (clonazepam 1mg IV or diazepam 10-20mg IV or midazolam 5–10 mg IM or IV, bucally or intranasally) AND
2. **Phenytoin IV or sodium valproate IV** (give phenytoin, 15–20 mg/kg (1000–2000 mg is the usual dose in adults).
   IV phenytoin must be given no faster than 50 mg/minute. Otherwise, there is a risk of hypotension, arrhythmias and central nervous system depression.
   Dilute phenytoin in saline, not dextrose, or else there is a risk of extravasation of phenytoin and tissue necrosis.
3. **If seizures continue, repeat the IV benzodiazepine dose in 15 minutes.**

---

[1] Although it is not mentioned in the Therapeutic Guidelines: Neurology (Neurology Writing Group, 2011), there are data supporting the use of another benzodiazepine, IV lorazepam, as the first-line agent for treating status epilepticus (Millikan *et al.*, 2009; Prasad *et al.*, 2005).

4. If seizures still persist, intensive care monitoring and a propofol or thiopentone infusion can be used.

Q: Are there any other medications that you would initially give in status epilepticus?

A: Thiamine 100 mg IVI. If the pinprick glucose demonstrates hypoglycaemia, he should receive IV 50% dextrose.

Q: Why would you administer thiamine?

A: Wernicke's encephalopathy is due to thiamine deficiency. It is commonly associated with chronic alcohol abuse. It is classically associated with a triad of ataxia, ophthalmoplegia and confusion, which can progress to seizures, coma and death. It is therefore always worth giving thiamine to an individual in status epilepticus in case of a thiamine deficiency. Make sure that the thiamine is given before the glucose infusion.

Q: Thankfully, the young man stops fitting after 4 minutes. He is awake but looks groggy. He tells you his name is Marwan, but does not respond to any other questions for the moment. You attribute this behaviour to postictal confusion and proceed to examine him.

He has been incontinent of urine, which is common during a seizure. He is still afebrile. His blood pressure and heart rate are normal. There is no neck stiffness to suggest meningitis. You note 4/5 weakness of the right upper limb. There is a superficial laceration of the tongue. The remainder of the examination is unremarkable.

What do you make of the weakness in the right arm?

A: It could be Todd's paresis, which is a focal neurological deficit after a seizure that spontaneously resolves within minutes to hours.

Q: Within 15 minutes, Marwan is fully alert but looks exhausted after his ordeal. His right upper limb weakness has resolved, confirming that it resulted from Todd's paresis.

Marwan tells you that he is a 23-year-old dentistry student who began his elective in the hospital earlier this week. He has 'never been sick in his life' until today. He recalls looking at some X-rays in the Emergency Department. He then felt 'a bit odd', and has no further recollection of events until now.

Marwan takes no medications and has no known allergies. He drinks 10 grams of alcohol a week, and denies recreational drug use.

The consultant neurologist comes down to see Marwan but gets the history from you first. You confidently tell the neurologist that this is Marwan's first seizure. The neurologist asks, 'How do you know that? Where are the relevant negatives?'

What 'relevant negatives' in the history is the neurologist referring to?

A: Around 50% of patients presenting with their 'first' seizure have evidence of seizures in the past; however, it is important to take a directed history to tease out this information since patients may not appreciate its significance and not volunteer it. It is therefore important to ask about the following (Angus-Leppan, 2014):
- bed wetting
- tongue biting
- blood on pillows
- early morning headache
- hangover without alcohol.

The presence of these features suggest recurrent seizures and a diagnosis of epilepsy.

Q: You admit to the neurologist that you didn't ask Marwan about those specific points. The neurologist is forgiving, however, and takes a history from Marwan, who does not give any evidence of previous seizures. The consultant neurologist decides to admit him to the neurology ward. How are you going to investigate Marwan?

A: You check the results of the blood tests you took earlier. They are all normal—there are no electrolyte abnormalities to account for Marwan's seizures.

The serum and urinary drug screen won't be available for some time. Although Marwan denies using recreational drugs, many individuals are initially reluctant to disclose such information.

Marwan needs a CT brain scan with contrast to identify a space-occupying lesion that served as an epileptogenic focus. You should order an EEG to look for an epileptogenic focus. A 12-lead ECG is also important to exclude a cardiac cause resulting in a hypoxic seizure.

Q: The ECG shows sinus rhythm and is otherwise unremarkable. The EEG is also normal. Does a normal EEG following a seizure surprise you?

A: No. Interictal EEGs (EEGs between seizures) are not very sensitive, identifying abnormalities in only 8–50% of cases. Therefore, you should not dismiss a diagnosis of epilepsy on the basis of a normal EEG.

However, a positive result is most likely in the first 24 hours after the seizure and certain techniques (e.g. hyperventilation and photic stimulation) can increase the sensitivity (Angus-Leppan, 2014). So it was an appropriate test to order.

Q: Marwan's CT brain scan is normal. Does he need further imaging or are you satisfied with the contrast CT scan?

A: Given the normal EEG, it would be reasonable to order a MRI brain for Marwan at some stage. The MRI will pick up 10% of abnormalities after a first seizure and is more sensitive than a CT scan (Angus-Leppan, 2014). It does not have to be performed immediately; however, Marwan can come in later as an outpatient.

Q: But you are lucky and an MRI is arranged soon after admission. The MRI is normal, as are the urinary and serum drug screens.
Should Marwan commence regular anticonvulsants for his epilepsy?

A: Generally, the risk of another seizure is only about 50% (range 6–82%) so it would be reasonable to NOT prescribe antiepileptic medications following a first seizure (Angus-Leppan, 2014; Neurology Writing Group, 2011). Neurologists might be more inclined to initiate anticonvulsants if an individual has risk factors for recurrence. These would include (Angus-Leppan, 2014):
- MRI brain abnormality
- abnormal EEG
- neurological deficit
- individual factors (e.g. needing to drive immediately, social isolation or risk of injury).

Q: Marwan has none of these risk factors so he is not prescribed antiepileptic medications. Although he is pleased to go, he wants to know if he can drive. What do you tell him?

A: You tell him that unfortunately, he will need to be seizure-free for 6 months before he can return to driving (Tan, 2014).

Q: A month passes and you find yourself working nights in the Emergency Department. As you arrive at work, you pass through the acute section and are surprised to see Marwan. He greets you before letting you know that he had another witnessed tonic–clonic seizure that resolved within 2 minutes. The neurologist has already seen him and commenced him on anticonvulsants. What anticonvulsant would he normally start on?

A: The first-line drug for generalised seizures is sodium valproate; for partial seizures it is carbamazepine (Neurology Writing Group, 2011).

Q: Marwan has been started on sodium valproate for generalised seizures. He looks a bit depressed and asks you, 'Am I going to be on these tablets for the rest of my life?'

A: Not at all. If a patient is seizure-free for 3–5 years, neurologists will often cease the anticonvulsant.

Q: Marwan looks relieved to hear this. 'So apart from taking these pills, I can do whatever I like?'

A: Unfortunately, there will be restrictions on certain activities where the onset of a seizure could be disastrous:
- no driving (discussed above)
- no climbing (e.g. ladders)
- no operating heavy machinery
- no swimming in deep water and no swimming alone.

The duration of these restrictions is variable. The restrictions on the other activities may remain for much longer. Nevertheless, it would be reasonable to revise the restrictions when Marwan ceases anticonvulsants if he has been free of seizures for 3–5 years.

Q: Marwan also wants to know what else he can do to avoid having further seizures.

A: Avoid:
- sleep deprivation
- excess alcohol
- stress
- non-compliance with anticonvulsants.

Q: Your medical student is busily scribbling down every word you say. He looks up and says, 'What do you do for patients whose seizures are refractory to all anticonvulsants?'

A: Unfortunately, this scenario does occur. Medical therapy is thought to have failed when 3 appropriate anticonvulsants have not succeeded in controlling a patient's seizures.

In this case, patients may be evaluated for surgery. If surgery is not feasible, then consider implantation of a vagus nerve stimulator.

1. **Surgery.** A thorough preoperative evaluation is required to pinpoint the epileptogenic focus and ensure there are not multiple foci.

   Neuropsychological testing, structural tests (MRI), electrophysiological tests (EEG), functional tests (SPECT and PET scans[2]) and tests of cortical function (Wada scan[3]) may all be used in the preoperative evaluation.

   Surgery can be successful. For example, of those who undergo a temporal lobectomy, 68% become seizure-free and 23%

---

[2]SPECT and PET scans are studies of perfusion and metabolism, respectively. It is thought that between seizures, both perfusion and metabolism are reduced in the area of the brain serving as the epileptogenic focus.

[3]Wada tests involve injecting sodium amytal into the internal carotid artery. This allows assessment of the lateralisation of memory and language.

improve, while 9% show no improvement. This is in contrast to a callosotomy, where only 8% become seizure-free, 61% improve and 31% fail to improve.

2. **Vagus nerve stimulation**. This is similar to a cardiac pacemaker. It involves insertion of a generator in the left chest region, with a lead going up to the neck. The system is programmed to deliver regular stimulation to the vagus nerve. In addition, the patient or a carer can terminate an anticipated seizure by creating more stimulation with a magnet (Mapstone, 2008).

Adverse effects from implantation of the device include (Mapstone, 2008):

- infection (5–7%)
- vocal cord paralysis (1%)
- transient mild effects (cough, dyspnoea, hoarse voice, nausea, obstructive sleep apnoea).

Q: About 6 weeks later you review a young woman, Elaine, in the Emergency Department. She was discharged from hospital a few weeks ago following a traumatic brain injury complicated by seizures. She was sent home on phenytoin. Although she remains seizure-free, her presenting complaint is unsteadiness on her feet for the past 3 days. Your examination demonstrates nystagmus and ataxia.

What do you think has happened?

A: Although there are a number of possibilities, the most likely cause of nystagmus and ataxia in Elaine would be phenytoin toxicity.

Q: Is there a definitive test to demonstrate phenytoin toxicity?

A: Well, almost. Phenytoin plasma levels can be measured and can be very useful. A concentration of 40–80 mmol/L will usually suppress seizures without causing toxicity. Toxicity usually occurs above 80 mmol/L. Nevertheless, there are situations where individuals will have toxicity in the presence of a therapeutic plasma level.

Q: Elaine's plasma phenytoin level returns at 120 mmol/L, which is clearly too high. She has phenytoin toxicity. What are the most likely causes?

A: The most common causes are:

- acute alcohol ingestion
- drug interactions (drugs that inhibit the metabolism of phenytoin include amiodarone, allopurinol, erythromycin, cimetidine, metronidazole, omeprazole and sulfonamides, to name a few)
- phenytoin overdose.

Q: Elaine only drinks 10 grams of alcohol a day. She has taken 300 mg of phenytoin a day as she was told to. But she did commence erythromycin 5 days ago for a chest infection. You realise that the erythromycin inhibited the metabolism of phenytoin, which resulted in toxicity. You assure Elaine that she will be fine once she stops taking the antibiotic. You mention Elaine's story to another intern during a coffee break. Your colleague's ears prick up with interest as he has seen another patient earlier this week with a similar story. This particular patient had nystagmus and ataxia and also was taking phenytoin. She had a background of chronic renal failure with nephrotic syndrome. But the phenytoin level was 60 mmol/L.

'The phenytoin level was normal. So I initially thought she couldn't have phenytoin toxicity. But the ED registrar explained it all to me.' What was the ED registrar's explanation?

A: As noted earlier, there are situations where the plasma levels are normal but phenytoin toxicity is present. This is because the plasma phenytoin level represents both protein-bound and unbound phenytoin. It is the unbound portion that is responsible for its effects. Normally, about 90% of plasma phenytoin is bound to plasma. In situations where there is more unbound phenytoin in the blood than protein-bound phenytoin, toxicity can arise even though the total phenytoin level is therapeutic.

Hypoalbuminaemia, arising from chronic liver disease, nephrotic syndrome, nutritional deficiency, malabsorption or pregnancy, is one such situation. In hypoalbuminaemia, there is less protein to bind the phenytoin. Therefore, a higher proportion of the drug will be unbound. But the plasma levels, representing both the bound and the unbound drug, may still be normal.

Furthermore, chronic renal failure itself is associated with reduced affinity of albumin for phenytoin. Therefore your colleague's patient probably still has phenytoin toxicity despite the therapeutic level.

Q: Do you know any other side effects of phenytoin?

A: The side effects include:
- acne
- hirsutism
- folate deficiency
- coarsened facial features
- gingival hyperplasia
- lymphadenopathy (benign or lymphomatous).

Because of these side effects, it is now relatively uncommon to commence newly diagnosed patients with epilepsy on phenytoin.

Q: While on a relief term, you spend a week in the neurology unit and attend an outpatient clinic. You present a patient you have just seen to your consultant. It is a 45-year-old Chinese woman with partial seizures. In an attempt to impress the consultant neurologist, you state that the patient should be started on carbamazepine, as it is first-line treatment for partial seizures.

'Shouldn't we do something first before starting it in this woman?'

You are surprised to be asked a question instead of having praise lavished upon you for your detailed knowledge of antiepileptic drugs. What is the neurologist on about?

A: Many antiepileptic drugs can cause a life-threatening cutaneous reaction called Stevens–Johnson syndrome (SJS). Phenytoin, lamotrigine, phenobarbitone and carbamazepine have all been implicated. With regard to carbamazepine and SJS, the presence of the HLA-B*1502 allele predicts a higher risk in people of Han Chinese and South-East Asian ethnic backgrounds. People of these ethnicities should be tested for HLA-B*1502 prior to commencing carbamazepine.

Achievements

You now:
- can treat status epilepticus
- know to give IV phenytoin in saline, not dextrose
- know to give thiamine before IV glucose in status epilepticus
- know how to investigate and treat (or not treat) a patient experiencing a seizure for the first time
- realise that a diagnosis of epilepsy does not have to mean lifelong anticonvulsants
- know available management strategies for patients who fail anticonvulsant therapy
- can recognise and identify causes for phenytoin toxicity
- know the importance of HLA testing in certain ethnic groups prior to commencing carbamazepine.

References

American Epilepsy Society (1999), Medical Education Program Residents Version, at <www.aesnet.org/pdf/C21-30.pdf> and <www.aesnet.org/pdf/C41-50.pdf>.

Angus-Leppan, H. (2014), 'First seizures in adults', *British Medical Journal*, vol. 348, no. g2470, doi: 10.1136/bmj.g2470.

Aronson, J.K., Hardman, M. and Reynolds, D.J. (1992), 'ABC of monitoring drug therapy: Phenytoin', *British Medical Journal*, vol. 305, no. 6863, pp. 1215–1218.

Austroads (n.d.), 'Assessing fitness to drive: For commercial and private vehicle drivers', at <www.austroads.com.au/downloads/ AFTD_2003.pdf>.

Berkovic, S.F. (2005), 'Treatment with anti-epileptic drugs', *Australian Family Physician*, vol. 34, no. 12, pp. 1017–1020.

Mapstone, T.B. (2008), 'Vagus nerve stimulation: Current concepts', *Neurosurgical Focus*, vol. 25, no. 3, E9.

Millikan, D., Rice, B. and Silbergleit, R. (2009), 'Emergency treatment of status epilepticus: Current thinking', *Emergency Medicine Clinics of North America*, vol. 27, no. 1, pp. 101–113.

Neurology Writing Group (2011), *Therapeutic Guidelines: Neurology*, Version 4, Therapeutic Guidelines Ltd, Melbourne.

Prasad, K., Al-Roomi, K., Krishnan, P.R. and Sequeira, R. (2005), 'Anticonvulsant therapy for status epilepticus', *Cochrane Database of Systematic Reviews*, 4: CD003723.

Sperling, M.R., Bucurescu, G. and Kim, B. (1997), 'Epilepsy management: Issues in medical and surgical treatment', *Postgraduate Medicine*, vol. 102, no. 1, pp. 102–104, 109–112, 115–118 passim.

Tan, M. (2014), 'Epilepsy in adults', *Australian Family Physician*, vol. 43, no. 3, pp. 100–104.

Chapter 14
Mrs Flint presents with lower limb weakness

Scenario

It is the final day of your 10-week term in the Emergency Department. Mrs Flint is a 45-year-old woman who is complaining of difficulty walking in the past 48 hours. Several days before this, she noticed tingling in her feet and ankles and back pain.

She is otherwise healthy, takes no regular medications and has no allergies. The only thing of note is an upper respiratory tract infection she had 3 weeks ago. However, this resolved within a week without antibiotics.

Q: Does the combination of weakness and a recent upper respiratory tract illness suggest any particular syndrome?

A: It raises the possibility of Guillain–Barré syndrome.

Q: What is Guillain–Barré syndrome?

A: This is an autoimmune neurological disorder that can manifest with a wide variety of motor and sensory symptoms.

Q: Mrs Flint tells you that she first developed pins and needles in the feet and lower back pain that radiated down her legs. After a couple of days, she became progressively weak. On examination, she has a heart rate of 110/minute and blood pressure of 140/90. Her neurological examination reveals symmetrical 3–4/5 weakness of the lower limbs with absent reflexes. The sensory exam is unremarkable, as is the remainder of the physical examination.

Are her clinical features consistent with Guillain–Barré syndrome?

A: Yes. The flaccid paralysis is typical. About 90% of individuals with Guillain–Barré syndrome have pain that can be severe. It is common for symptoms to begin with pins and needles in the extremities (but a normal sensory exam). The tachycardia and hypertension could represent autonomic dysfunction, which is seen in two-thirds of cases.

Q: What other observations do you need to make to find out if this is Guillain–Barré syndrome? Why?

A: It is vital to check oxygen saturation and spirometry. Up to 30% of people with Guillain–Barré syndrome develop respiratory muscle failure from respiratory muscle paralysis. The most common cause of death, however, is cardiac arrest from autonomic dysfunction.

Q: Mrs Flint's oxygen saturation and spirometry are normal. She can't understand how she could have developed such an illness. She asks, 'Did my cold have anything to do with this?'

A: It probably did. Two-thirds of patients with Guillain–Barré syndrome experience an infection in the preceding month. About 40% report a respiratory tract illness, while 20% report a gastrointestinal illness.

Q: What organisms have been identified?

A:
- *Campylobacter jejuni* (the most common)
- *Cytomegalovirus*
- Epstein–Barr virus
- human immunodeficiency virus (HIV)
- herpes simplex virus
- *Mycoplasma pneumoniae*

Q: 'A simple infection could cause this?' Mrs Flint asks with wonder. 'Are you sure this isn't cancer?'

A: Occasionally, anti-Hu antibodies in patients with malignancy have been associated with a Guillain–Barré-like syndrome, but this is very uncommon (Pritchard, 2008).

Q: What are the other possibilities?

A: There is a broad range of differential diagnoses including (Pritchard, 2008):
- viral encephalomyelitis
- botulism
- porphyria
- diphtheria (very uncommon in Australia due to our immunisation program)
- paraneoplastic syndrome and lymphoma
- toxic neuropathies.

Q: What investigations will support your diagnosis?

A:
1. **Lumbar puncture**. This demonstrates elevated protein and very few mononuclear cells ($\leq 10/\mu L$) in about 90% of cases. The term for these lumbar puncture findings is 'albuminocytologic

dissociation'. Using it is sure to impress neurologists and registrars! In the first week of illness, however, the protein may not yet have risen in up to 50% of cases.

2. **Electromyography/nerve conduction studies (EMG/NCS).** There are electrophysiological features particular to each clinicopathologic type.

3. **Magnetic resonance imaging.** Gadolinium enhancement of the spinal nerve root is a non-specific finding. Enhancement of the cauda equina roots and anterior root can be very suggestive of Guillain–Barré syndrome.

4. **Antiganglioside antibodies.** Molecular mimicry is proposed as one of the mechanisms of Guillain–Barré syndrome, particularly when Campylobacter and possibly cytomegalovirus are involved. Antibodies formed against epitopes on the infective agent cross-react with ganglioside molecules in the nervous system, causing damage to the nerves. Some of these antibodies can be detected and, in fact, different antiganglioside antibodies are associated with certain forms of Guillain–Barré syndrome (see below). Examples include anti-GM1 antibodies in acute inflammatory demyelinating polyneuropathy and anti-GQ1b antibodies in the Miller–Fisher variant.

   But there are 2 limitations with antiganglioside antibodies in the clinical setting. First, the results may take some time to return; therefore, it isn't a useful diagnostic test in the acute setting. Also, the sensitivity is variable; for example, in the UK only 25% of people with acute demyelinating polyneuropathy have anti-GM1 antibodies (Pritchard, 2008). In other words, you can't rule out Guillain–Barré syndrome because of a negative test.

5. **Look for an infective cause:**
   a. 3 stool cultures for Campylobacter over 3 days
   b. HIV, EBV, CMV, HSV, Mycoplasma serology (check serology for Lyme disease if there has been travel to a Lyme-endemic area).

6. **12-lead ECG.** Arrhythmias can occur with autonomic disturbances.

7. **Blood tests.**
   a. Hypokalaemia and elevated creatine kinase (myopathy) are alternative causes of weakness.
   b. Liver function tests and ESR can be abnormal due to Guillain–Barré syndrome.

    c. Serum immunoglobulins and serum electrophoresis (IgA deficiency increases the risk of anaphylaxis to IV immunoglobulin treatment of Guillain–Barré syndrome; therefore, it is worth looking for at this early stage).

    d. Serum angiotensin converting enzyme (to evaluate for sarcoidosis).

  8. Chest X-ray. To exclude malignancy or sarcoidosis.

Q: What are the clinicopathologic types of Guillain–Barré syndrome?

A: Guillain–Barré syndrome can be broken down into the following clinicopathologic types:

- acute inflammatory demyelinating polyneuropathy (the most common type)
- acute motor axonal neuropathy
- acute motor sensory axonal neuropathy
- Miller–Fisher syndrome (a triad of ophthalmoplegia, ataxia and areflexia)
- pure sensory syndrome, pure dysautonomic, paraplegic.

Q: You perform a lumbar puncture on Mrs Flint. The cerebrospinal fluid is clear with no cells and elevated protein of 1.2 g/L (normal range 0.15–0.45 g/L). This is consistent with Guillain–Barré syndrome.

The EMG/NCS testing is done urgently. It is consistent with acute inflammatory demyelinating polyneuropathy (AIDP) and demonstrates reduced conduction velocity, prolonged terminal latency, absent F-waves and abnormal temporal dispersion. The on-call neurologist is confident of his diagnosis of Guillain–Barré syndrome. Mrs Flint and her family want to know her outlook. What do you tell them?

A: She is likely to get worse but start recovering after 4 weeks. Eighty per cent of people will have recovered by day 200 although many continue to have minor residual complaints. The mortality rate is about 5% (Dimachkie and Barohn, 2013).

Q: The neurologist wants to commence treatment. What do you suggest?

A: Therapy should be as follows (Pritchard, 2008):

- Careful monitoring of respiratory/cardiovascular function and commencement of supportive therapy if either is badly affected.
- Directed therapy against Guillain–Barré syndrome with either IV immunoglobulin or plasma exchange. They are thought to be equally efficacious in non-ambulant patients in the first 2 weeks of symptoms.

IV steroids have no benefit in acute management.

Q: Mrs Flint receives IV immunoglobulin treatment for 5 days and after 7 days is almost back to normal. Her serology is consistent with acute cytomegalovirus infection. Although relieved to be well, Mrs Flint is still clearly troubled by these recent events. 'Could this happen again, Doctor?' What do you tell her?

A: In a small proportion of cases, relapse can occur. About 10% of patients have an early relapse 1–2 weeks post-therapy while 3% will have a relapse years later (Pritchard, 2008); therefore, although the chances of relapse are low, it is important to make her aware of the possibility so she can seek urgent treatment as soon as she relapses.

Achievements

You now:

- know the clinical features of Guillain–Barré syndrome (GBS)
- appreciate the life-threatening respiratory and cardiovascular complications of GBS
- realise that infection often precedes cases of GBS
- know which organisms are most commonly identified in association with GBS
- know how to investigate patients with suspected GBS
- can treat patients with GBS.

References

Dimachkie, M.M. and Barohn, R.J. (2013), 'Guillain–Barré syndrome and variants', *Neurology Clinics*, vol. 31, no. 2, pp. 491–510.

Pritchard, J. (2008), 'What's new in Guillain–Barré syndrome?', *Postgraduate Medical Journal*, vol. 84, no. 996, pp. 532–538.

Seneviratne, U. (2000), 'Guillain–Barré syndrome', *Postgraduate Medical Journal*, vol. 76, no. 902, pp. 774–777.

Chapter 15
Mr Quixote presents with headache

Scenario

You pick up the next patient card in the Emergency Department. This will be the last patient you see in a 15-hour shift before 4 blissful days off work. You hope this will be a nice, easy case—cellulitis or an uncomplicated laceration, for instance. You read the triage notes: it is a 50-year-old man with a headache. Oh well, so much for a quick case.

Mr Quixote looks very uncomfortable. He is staying still, but is grimacing in pain. He tells you that he is an accountant with mild hypertension, for which he takes an ACE inhibitor. He was fine this morning and has been working in the garden all day. But about 2 hours ago, while digging in the garden, he was overwhelmed by a headache that came on over a minute. It is the worst headache he has ever had. He recalls dropping his spade, holding his head in his hands and falling to his knees. A few minutes later he started vomiting. The headache has not improved. It is still 10/10 in severity. He denies any neck pain or focal neurological symptoms.

Q: 'What do you think this could be, Doc?'
A: Mr Quixote has suffered a 'thunderclap headache', which is a headache of severe intensity that reaches its maximum intensity in less than a minute. One of the most serious possibilities is subarachnoid haemorrhage (SAH), which has a mortality rate of about 50% (Schwedt, 2013). One study evaluated the cause of a sudden-onset and thunderclap-type headache in a series of patients. They found that SAH was responsible for the headache in only 11% of cases (Landtblom *et al.*, 2002). Nevertheless, SAH is such a serious diagnosis that it should be excluded in this type of patient. It has a mortality of 32–67% with up to 30% of those surviving being left with serious sequelae (Ferro *et al.*, 2008). Other causes of a thunderclap headache include cervical artery dissection, cerebral venous thrombosis, intracerebral haemorrhage, unruptured intracranial aneurysm and spontaneous intracranial hypotension (Schwedt, 2013).

Q: What is SAH?

A: This is bleeding into the subarachnoid space. A ruptured saccular (berry) aneurysm around the base of the brain is responsible for approximately 85% of cases.

Q: Is Mr Quixote's history typical for SAH?

A: The classical history for SAH is a headache that develops instantaneously and is the worst headache the patient has ever had. Mr Quixote's headache is consistent with the classical history of SAH.

It is important to realise that not all patients with SAH will have the classical presentation. In fact, 20% of patients with SAH are missed on their first presentation (Ferro *et al.*, 2008). So always consider SAH for a headache that a patient considers significant enough to go to hospital (as Mr Quixote has done).

Vomiting occurs in 70% of individuals with rupture of an aneurysm. However, this is a non-specific finding that occurs in other headache syndromes and other intracranial disorders.

Q: Mr Quixote's headache occurred while he was exerting himself in the garden. Again, the pain of SAH often occurs during exertion, but can also occur during sleep.

What risk factors for SAH will you look for in the history?

A: The most common risk factors are:
- first-degree relative with SAH
- hypertension
- smoking
- heavy alcohol consumption
- previous SAH.

Less common associations include:
- autosomal dominant polycystic kidney disease
- Ehlers–Danlos IV
- neurofibromatosis type I.

Mr Quixote smokes half a packet of cigarettes a day. As mentioned, he has hypertension. He has 2 risk factors for SAH.

Q: In individuals whose SAH is not due to a ruptured saccular aneurysm, what are other possible causes?

A: Other possible causes include:
- non-aneurysmal perimesencephalic haemorrhage (10%)
- arterial dissection
- arteriovenous malformations
- cardiac myxoma
- septic aneurysms

- pituitary apoplexy
- cocaine abuse
- anticoagulants
- sickle cell disease
- superficial central nervous system siderosis (iron overload).

Q: You proceed to examine Mr Quixote. He is alert and oriented. His temperature is 38.1 °C, his blood pressure is 140/90 and his heart rate is 80/minute. He has no neck stiffness. The temporal arteries are not prominent and there are no focal neurological deficits. The remainder of the examination is normal. Fundoscopy is normal.

Are you surprised that Mr Quixote doesn't have neck stiffness?

A: Neck stiffness is a common feature of SAH, occurring in up to 70% of cases. But it may take hours to develop. Mr Quixote has presented to hospital promptly, so it may be too early for him to experience neck stiffness.

Q: But surely the fever of 38.1 °C makes SAH an unlikely diagnosis?

A: Not at all. Fever can be seen in SAH. In fact, refractory fever after SAH is associated with a higher mortality and worse prognosis; however, it isn't clear if correcting a fever reduces that risk (Caplan et al., 2013).

Q: Why did you examine Mr Quixote's fundi?

A: In patients with SAH, subhyaloid, retinal or vitreous haemorrhages (Terson's syndrome) may be visible on fundoscopy (Ferro et al., 2008). However, much depends on the expertise of the operator of the ophthalmoscope even if they are present.

Q: You tell Mr Quixote that SAH is a possibility. How are you going to investigate him?

A: A CT brain scan without contrast is a very good test for detecting blood in the subarachnoid spaces. The CT scan in this case does in fact demonstrate a small SAH.

Q: What are the limitations of a CT scan for SAH?

A: It is important to realise that patients with SAH and minimal symptoms may have normal scans. Also, the sensitivity of CT scanning diminishes with time, as the following table demonstrates:

Time of CT scan after SAH	Sensitivity
12 hours	98%
3 days	85%
7 days	50%

Source: Adapted from Edlow (2003).

Therefore, do not dismiss a diagnosis of SAH if the CT scan is normal in a patient with a history consistent with SAH. An MRI is an alternative to a CT but in most Australian hospitals, a CT will be far more readily accessible.

Q: In Mr Quixote's case, however, you have the luxury of a positive CT scan.

What would have been the next step if your patient's CT scan had been inconclusive or normal, given that you have a strong clinical suspicion of SAH?

A: A lumbar puncture would be the next investigation of choice (Steiner *et al.*, 2013).

Q: What is the classical finding of a lumbar puncture in SAH?

A: Xanthochromia, which is a yellow discolouration of the CSF due to formation of bilirubin and oxyhaemoglobin after red cell lysis. It used to be identified by the naked eye of the lab scientist; however, many labs now have formal spectrophotometry to detect xanthochromia. It takes a variable time (2–12 hours) after the SAH for xanthochromia to appear, after which it will remain for 2 weeks. Xanthochromia can be used to distinguish SAH from a 'traumatic tap' (Ferro *et al.*, 2008).

Q: What will you do now that you have diagnosed SAH in Mr Quixote?

A: It is time to call the neurosurgical registrar.

Q: Just as you are about to call the neurosurgical registrar, an alarmed ED nurse shows you a routine ECG performed on Mr Quixote. It shows widespread T-wave changes. 'Could he be having an acute coronary syndrome at the same time as having a SAH?' the nurse asks you.

A: It is possible. Up to 75% of SAH patients will have a variety of ECG abnormalities. Some will even have abnormal cardiac wall motion on echocardiography, elevated cardiac enzymes or even develop pulmonary oedema. In fact, in the acute setting of SAH, sudden death from cardiac arrest can occur. These cardiac abnormalities are thought to reflect the impact of a SAH on the sympathetic and parasympathetic system of the heart (Ferro *et al.*, 2008). It will therefore be important to monitor Mr Quixote's cardiac status very closely over the next few hours.

Q: Despite the pain, Mr Quixote is anxious to learn more. 'Doctor, is there any chance that this will happen again?'

A: Is there ever! Rebleeding is a common, life-threatening complication of SAH.

Time after onset of SAH	Risk of rebleeding without intervention
First few hours	15%
1 day to 4 weeks	35–40%
Long term	3% per year

Source: Adapted from Edlow (2003).

Q: You tell Mr Quixote as much as you know about SAH. Instead of reassuring him, you are shocked to find that he starts crying, saying how miserable he is. His wife is upset and surprised. 'My husband is always such a stoic man. He never complains and he never cries like this. What is wrong with him? Did this bleed in the brain do this to him?'

A: She may be right. SAH can present with psychiatric manifestations ranging from depression to apathy to delirium (Ferro *et al.*, 2008).

Q: Given that Mr Quixote is going to be immobile, should he receive prophylaxis for deep venous thrombosis (DVT)?

A: At this stage, only prescribe compression stockings or pneumatic devices for DVT prophylaxis. Only once an aneurysm has been treated can low-molecular-weight heparin be considered (Steiner *et al.*, 2013).

Q: The neurosurgical registrar manages to calm Mr Quixote down somewhat and tells him that he will need to undergo angiography to visualise the culprit aneurysm. Angiographic techniques include intra-arterial, CT or MRI angiography of which intra-arterial angiography is the most common technique for detecting aneurysms (Ferro *et al.*, 2008). Once the aneurysm has been identified, it will need to be obliterated.

How can an aneurysm be obliterated?

A:
1. intraoperative clipping of the aneurysm OR
2. endovascular treatment using detachable coils.

The decision on whether to coil or clip is a complex one; however, when both options are equally effective, coiling is preferred (Steiner *et al.*, 2013).

Q: 'Does my husband have a good prognosis?' asks Mrs Quixote as her husband is being wheeled away for the angiogram. What do you tell her?

A: There are various ways to grade the severity of SAH, for example, World Federation of Neurological Surgeons (WFNS) system and the Prognosis on Admission of Aneurysmal Subarachnoid Haemorrhage (PAASH) scale, both of which are based on the Glasgow Coma Scale (GCS). Although it is unrealistic for an intern to memorise them, it is worth knowing that they exist. Mr Quixote is completely alert with no neck stiffness and no focal neurological deficits (apart from possibly being depressed following the SAH). This would make him Grade I for both WFNS and PAASH scales with a 14.8% chance of a poor outcome (compared to around a 93% chance of a poor outcome with a GCS of 3) (Steiner *et al.*, 2013).

Q: You explain to them that although SAH is very serious, he is at the less dangerous extreme of the scale. Mrs Quixote then says, 'Looking back on it, my husband had a less severe headache about 2 weeks ago. It lasted for a couple of days and then left. We didn't bother seeing the doctor. Could that have had something to do with this problem?'

A: Up to about 40% of SAH patients recall a milder headache preceding the SAH by 2–8 weeks. It is due to a minor haemorrhage (a 'warning leak' or 'sentinel bleed'). The presence of such a sentinel headache means that a person has a 10-fold higher odds of early rebleeding (Steiner *et al.*, 2013).

Q: Mr Quixote is given analgesia for his headache. He then undergoes a CT angiogram, which fails to identify an aneurysm; therefore, digital subtraction angiography (DSA) is performed. The DSA demonstrates a middle cerebral artery aneurysm (see Fig. 15.1 below).

Unfortunately, there is nobody at your hospital with the expertise to coil this aneurysm; therefore, the neurosurgeons operate on Mr Quixote 24 hours later and clip the aneurysm. Is he finally out of danger?

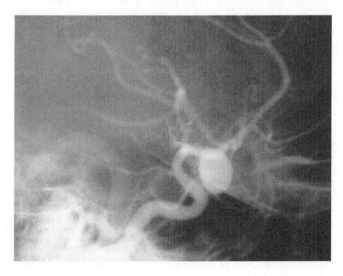

Figure 15.1 A cerebral angiogram demonstrating a middle cerebral artery aneurysm

A: Unfortunately, no. Another serious cause of morbidity and mortality after SAH is delayed cerebral ischaemia secondary to vasospasm. This occurs in about one-third of cases, typically in the first 2 weeks after the haemorrhage.

Q: How can this be detected?

A: Any clinical deterioration should alert you to the possibility of delayed cerebral ischaemia.

Transcranial Doppler studies of the arteries of the brain can be helpful in detecting and excluding vasospasm although the evidence for the accuracy of transcranial Doppler studies is limited to the anterior and middle cerebral arteries (Ferro *et al.*, 2008). A CT brain scan can exclude other causes of clinical deterioration, for example hydrocephalus, rebleeding, etc. In other words, often a combination of clinical and radiological factors may point to delayed cerebral ischaemia (Caplan *et al.*, 2013).

Q: What treatment will you use to prevent secondary cerebral ischaemia in Mr Quixote?

A: The main way to prevent vasospasm is to give nimodipine, a calcium antagonist, at a dose of 60 mg every 4 hours for 3 weeks (Steiner *et al.*, 2013).

Q: Mr Quixote is placed on nimodipine to prevent vasospasm. What can be done if vasospasm develops despite the nimodipine?

A: The treatment options for established vasospasm include (Caplan *et al.*, 2013; Ferro *et al.*, 2008):

1. triple H therapy (hypertension, hypervolaemia and haemodilution)
2. endovascular intervention (balloon angioplasty or injection of intra-arterial vasodilators such as papaverine).

Q: What complication, other than rebleeding and cerebral ischaemia, can cause severe neurological deterioration after SAH?

A: Hydrocephalus, which can be diagnosed on CT scanning.

Q: One of the nurses asks, 'Given the irritation to his brain from the SAH, won't he need antiepileptic medication to prevent seizures?'

A: No. Prophylactic use of antiepileptic drugs is not recommended in SAH patients (Steiner *et al.*, 2013).

Mr Quixote, however, has no such difficulties. He receives nimodipine and IV normal saline and improves quite quickly before being discharged. Even his initially depressed mood seems to resolve.

Q: Although he did not experience any of the acute major complications of SAH, is he likely to experience any long-term difficulties from the SAH?

A: Possibly. These include (Ferro *et al.*, 2008):
- neuropsychological disturbances of memory and executive function
- disturbed sleep–wake cycle
- pituitary deficiency
- epilepsy.

Achievements

You now:
- know that SAH does not always present with the classical clinical picture
- know risk factors for SAH
- know the roles and limitations of CT and lumbar puncture in diagnosing SAH
- understand the principles of managing SAH
- are aware of the risks of vasospasm, rebleeding and hydrocephalus after SAH.

References

Caplan, J.M., Colby, G.P., Coon, A.L., Huang, J. and Tamargo, R.J. (2013), 'Managing subarachnoid hemorrhage in the neurocritical care unit', *Neurosurgery Clinics of North America*, vol. 24, no. 3, pp. 321–337.

Edlow, J.A. (2003), 'Diagnosis of subarachnoid hemorrhage in the emergency department', *Emergency Medicine Clinics of North America*, vol. 21, no. 1, pp. 73–87.

Ferro, J.M., Canhao, P. and Peralta, R. (2008), 'Update on subarachnoid haemorrhage', *Journal of Neurology*, vol. 255, no. 4, pp. 465–479.

Landtblom, A.M., Fridriksson, S., Boivie, J., Hillman, J., Johansson, G. and Johansson, I. (2002), 'Sudden onset headache: A prospective study of features, incidence and causes', *Cephalalgia*, vol. 22, no. 5, pp. 354–360.

Schwedt, T.J. (2013), 'Thunderclap headaches: A focus on etiology and diagnostic evaluation', *Headache*, vol. 53, no. 3, pp 563–569.

Steiner, T., Juvela, S., Unterberg, A., Jung, C., Forsting, M. and Rinkel, G. (2013), 'European Stroke Organization guidelines for the management of intracranial aneurysms and subarachnoid haemorrhage', *Cerebrovascular Diseases*, vol. 35, no. 2, pp. 93–112.

Van Gijn, J. and Rinkel, G.J. (2001), 'Subarachnoid haemorrhage: Diagnosis, causes and management', *Brain*, vol. 124, Pt 2, pp. 249–278.

Chapter 16
A case of elevated potassium in a man of non-English-speaking background

Scenario

You have just started an 8-hour shift in the Emergency Department. The ambulances are lined up outside, patients are yelling, staff are running around—another typical day!

Your first patient was handed over to you by one of the night residents and presents something of a challenge. He is an 84-year-old man who cannot speak English, and he doesn't look at all well.

It turns out that he lives alone in an apartment building. His neighbour noticed that he hadn't been collecting his morning newspapers, which had piled up outside his door. She became worried and called the police, who forced their way inside. They found the man lying in his bed, conscious, but very lethargic. His Medicare card revealed that he is Albert Fung.

The resident told you that Mr Fung looked a bit 'dry' (dehydrated) so she inserted an IV cannula, put up a bag of normal saline and took some baseline bloods. Mr Fung's baseline observations revealed a heart rate of 100/minute, blood pressure of 90/50, no fever, oxygen saturations of 97% on room air and a pinprick glucose of 6 mmol/L. However, the resident had no time to assess him further before the handover ward round.

Mr Fung looks very weak. He can't speak any English, but keeps pointing at his throat. You and the nurse are baffled by this, but are obviously keen to understand what he is trying to tell you.

Q: What are your options?

A: As an intern working in Australia, you will inevitably encounter migrants who cannot speak English very well. Given that taking a history is a vital part of assessing any patient, not being able to do so will immediately put you at a disadvantage.

However, there are usually 3 sources of interpretation available to you:
1. a family member (but not in the case of Mr Fung)
2. a bilingual health professional
3. an interpreter service.

Q: Which is the recommended source?

A: New South Wales Health Policy Directive PD2006_053 (2006), 'Interpreters—standard procedures for working with health care interpreters', recommends using an interpreter from the Health Care Interpreter Service. The service is available 24 hours a day, 7 days a week. In certain circumstances, telephone interviews with an interpreter can be performed.

Health care interpreters (HCIs) must receive accreditation prior to employment with the Health Care Interpreter Service. They then receive training in health-specific interpretation. As a result, they are very well qualified for their role. They should be used before bilingual health professionals or family members.

The New South Wales Health circular identifies various problems with using non-professional interpreters, including:
- uncertainty about the quality of the community language
- uncertainty about the accuracy of the translation
- distorted, suppressed or normalised information (especially with a family member interpreting)
- compromising of confidentiality (imagine a daughter telling her aged father that his blood tests reveal syphilis!)
- lack of knowledge of interpreting skills, medical concepts and ethics
- an invalid consent to a procedure.

The New South Wales Health circular also recommends that HCIs be present in the following situations:
- admission
- consent for operations, procedures, treatment and research
- counselling
- death of a patient and bereavement counselling
- discharge procedures and referrals
- explanation of medication
- health education and promotion programs
- medical instructions
- medical histories, assessments and treatment plans
- mental health review tribunals and magistrates' inquiries
- preoperative and postoperative instructions
- psychiatric assessment and treatment
- psychological assessment
- sexual assault, physical and emotional abuse
- speech therapy
- procedures relating to organ or tissue donation.

The nurse calls the Health Care Interpreter Service. An interpreter will be available in 45 minutes.

Q: Then the laboratory calls with an urgent message: Mr Fung has a plasma potassium of 7.2 mmol/L.

Boris, your medical student, hears the message and becomes very excited: 'High potassium! High potassium! We have to do something now!'

Is Boris's sense of urgency justified?

A: It is, because the usual range of potassium in the plasma is 3.5–5.0 mmol/L (depending on which hospital you work in). The major concern is cardiac toxicity resulting in ventricular arrhythmias and death, especially when the plasma potassium is more than 6.7 mmol/L. Therefore, it is recommended to urgently reduce plasma potassium whenever (Weisberg, 2008):

1. the plasma potassium is >6.5 mmol/L
2. there are ECG changes of hyperkalaemia, irrespective of the plasma potassium.

(Nevertheless, as Boris runs down the corridor shouting, 'Emergency! Emergency! Stat! Stat!', you make a mental note to tell him to watch less *Grey's Anatomy*.)

Q: What are your management aims?

A: Short term: prevent a cardiac arrest and reduce the plasma potassium level.

Intermediate term: identify the underlying cause of the hyperkalaemia.

Q: You arrange the following very quickly:

- Order a 12-lead ECG to look for any of the changes of hyperkalaemia.
- Keep the cardiac arrest trolley next to Mr Fung in case he suffers an arrhythmia.
- Tell the medical registrar or emergency registrar/physician.

Q: What are the ECG changes of hyperkalaemia?

A: You must be able to recognise the sequence of ECG changes of hyperkalaemia. This will not only save Mr Fung's life, but will also help you in your final year examinations! An inability to recognise these ECG changes may be grounds for failure:

1. peaking of T-waves
2. prolongation of PR and QRS intervals
3. loss of P-waves
4. occurrence of sine waves when the T-waves are incorporated into the widening QRS complex
5. asystole or ventricular fibrillation.

Q: A 12-lead ECG is performed (see Fig. 16.1 opposite). What does it show?

A: The ECG shows tall peaked T-waves, grossly widened QRS complexes, flattened P-waves that are barely visible, and sinus bradycardia with first-degree atrioventricular block. This ECG is definitely consistent with hyperkalaemia. Mr Fung may be moments away from a cardiac arrest!

Q: You must act immediately! What will you do?

A: The order and principles of treating hyperkalaemia acutely are as follows (Maxwell *et al.*, 2013; Weisberg, 2008; Endocrinology Expert Group, 2014):

1. Antagonise the excitatory effect of potassium on cell membranes.
2. Move potassium into the intracellular compartment.
3. Enhance removal of potassium from the body.

1. **Antagonise the excitatory effect of potassium on cell membranes.**
   a. **Give IV calcium gluconate (think of the rule of '10s'—10 mL of 10% given over 2–3 minutes).**
      - It should work within 3 minutes and last for 30–60 minutes which will allow you time to lower the plasma potassium by other means.
      - If the ECG hasn't improved or has worsened 5 minutes after giving it, then repeat the dose.
      - Hypercalcaemia is a complication of its use.
   b. **Give hypertonic saline (3%) ONLY IF THE PATIENT IS HYPONATRAEMIC (not often used in practice).**
2. **Move potassium into the intracellular compartment.**
   a. **Give 10 units of IV rapid-acting insulin (e.g. Actrapid) in conjunction with 50 mL of 50% glucose.**
      It should start working after 20 minutes and last for 4–6 hours.
      - After the initial bolus of dextrose, commence a dextrose infusion.
      - Continually check the blood glucose level for up to 6 hours after the insulin has been given.
   b. **Give salbutamol IV or as a 10 mg nebule in adults.**
   c. **Give IV sodium bicarbonate 8.4% (1 mmol/mL) 50 mL over 5–10 minutes under ECG control with a repeat dose 1–2 hours later.**[1]

---

[1]In practical terms, sodium bicarbonate is not often given in the ward setting. Most patients only receive insulin/dextrose and the salbutamol nebule.

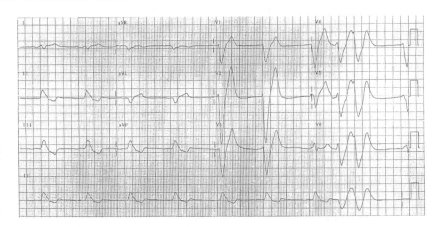

Figure 16.1 Mr Fung's 12-lead ECG

3. **Enhance removal of potassium from the body.**
   a. **Give sodium polystyrene sulfonate resins (e.g. Resonium).**
      - This is a cation exchange resin that exchanges sodium for potassium in the gut. It can be given orally or rectally. A reasonable oral dose would be 30 g stat (pending further serum potassium levels).
      - It works after 2 hours and lasts for 4–6 hours.
      - Toxicity includes fluid overload from increased sodium uptake, hypokalaemia and intestinal necrosis.
   b. **Perform dialysis (haemodialysis is more effective than peritoneal dialysis).**
      - This is a very effective means of removing potassium from the body.
      - Continuous ECG monitoring is required as there are concerns that there is an increased risk of ventricular arrhythmias in people receiving dialysis for severe hyperkalaemia.
      - It's usually reserved for patients who don't respond to the above measures.

And note ...

Flush the IV cannula with some of the 50% glucose before giving any of the IV insulin, because 50% glucose is a thick, syrupy liquid. This will tell you if the cannula is good enough to tolerate the thick glucose solution. You do not want to be in the situation of giving your patient IV insulin only to find that you can't administer glucose through the cannula! The result will be profound hypoglycaemia, which you definitely want to avoid.

Q: You end up administering calcium gluconate, actrapid, glucose and resonium to Mr Fung. You sit by the patient's bedside with the cardiac arrest trolley. After 5 uneventful minutes, a repeat ECG is performed—thankfully, it is now normal. You repeat the plasma potassium level after 45 minutes and find that it has come down to 5.9 mM. What else would you do?

A: It is important to ensure that the plasma potassium level does not rise again. Therefore, regular blood tests—perhaps every 1–3 hours—should be performed for the next 12 hours or so.

It would be reasonable to keep him under continuous cardiac monitoring in the Emergency Department, coronary care unit or intensive care unit until you are satisfied that the hyperkalaemia is under control.

Q: Apart from the cardiac effects, what else can hyperkalaemia cause?

A: It can also affect the neuromuscular and metabolic systems as follows (Weisberg, 2008):

1. neuromuscular—acute flaccid paralysis that spares the diaphragm and can be associated with paraesthesias
2. metabolic—hyperchloraemic metabolic acidosis.

Q: Now you must identify and correct the underlying cause of the hyperkalaemia. What are the most common causes of hyperkalaemia you will encounter in the hospital system?

A: The most common causes are:

- acute kidney injury (AKI) or chronic renal failure
- medications (angiotensin converting enzyme inhibitors [ACEI], NSAIDs, angiotensin II receptor antagonists and potassium-sparing diuretics are the most common groups involved)
- excessive potassium replacement
- rhabdomyovlysis.

Scenario

At this opportune time, the interpreter from the Health Care Interpreter Service arrives. Mr Fung relates his story to her.

Mr Fung has lived in Australia for 2 years, after migrating from Hong Kong. He does not take any regular medications and is normally independent. His only medical problem was an oesophageal web, for which he had an endoscopy in Hong Kong 5 years ago. He had had no recurrence until 2 months ago, when he developed difficulty in swallowing solids. In the past week, he has been unable to swallow liquids.

Normally he would tell his niece who lives nearby, but she had to return to Hong Kong a few months ago. Because of his lack of English, he felt helpless and alone. He has hardly eaten or drunk anything in the past week. He feels desperately weak and has been lying in bed for long periods. On examination, he is clearly dehydrated. He has a blood pressure of 90/60 with a postural drop of 25/10. He is tachycardic and has a dry tongue mucosa. His examination is otherwise normal.

Q: What do you think is the cause of hyperkalaemia in Mr Fung?

A: The most likely scenario is that Mr Fung's poor oral intake due to recurrence of his oesophageal web resulted in dehydration, AKI and hyperkalaemia. The prolonged immobility he describes may have resulted in rhabdomyolysis, also leading to hyperkalaemia and AKI.

Q: You examine Mr Fung's current results:

Test	Normal range	Result
Haemoglobin	130–180 g/L	170
Mean cell volume	80–100 Fl	82
White cell count	3.5–11 × 10^9/L	10
Platelet count	150–450 × 10^9/L	182
Sodium	135–145 mmol/L	137
Potassium	3.6–5.1 mmol/L	5.3*
Chloride	95–107 mmol/L	98
Bicarbonate	22–32 mmol/L	18*
Urea	2.9–7.1 mmol/L	15*
Creatinine	60–110 μmol/L	200*
Calcium	2.25–2.58 mmol/L	2.25
Troponin	0–0.1 μg/L	<0.1
Creatine kinase	<175 U/L	1600*
Albumin	33–48 g/L	35
Bilirubin	0–25 μmol/L	20
ALP	38–126 U/L	110
Test	**Normal range**	**Result**
GGT	0–30 U/L	25
AST	<45 U/L	40
ALT	<45 U/L	34

* Abnormal results.

Mr Fung's renal function on arrival (when his potassium was 7.2 mmol/L) is unchanged. (You also note that his creatinine from 2 months earlier, at the time of his endoscopy, was 70 mmol/L.)

The current elevated urea and creatinine, compared with levels 2 months ago, confirm AKI. What is the definition of AKI?

A: AKI can be defined and staged according to serum creatinine and urine output. The criteria for AKI are met if there is (KDIGO, 2012):

- an increase in serum creatinine above baseline* by 26 umol/L within 48 hours OR
- an increase in serum creatinine by 1.5–1.9 times above baseline creatinine* OR
- <0.5 mL/kg/hr urine output for >6 hours.

Q: Mr Fung meets the criteria for Stage 2 AKI. How do you further classify AKI?

A:

1. **Prerenal**. This can be due to any condition leading to reduced renal perfusion. Common causes include reduced intravascular volume secondary to dehydration (as with Mr Fung), compromised cardiac output, relative hypotension and hepatorenal syndrome (in the setting of liver failure).

2. **Intrarenal**. The most common cause of intrarenal AKI is acute tubular necrosis (ATN), which is secondary to toxin damage (haemoglobin, myoglobin), ischaemia or sepsis.

   As you may have realised, ischaemic ATN and prerenal AKI can both occur due to reduced renal perfusion. As a result, both conditions are often found simultaneously in patients with AKI. Although 'acute tubular necrosis' sounds horrendous, it is generally reversible once the underlying cause is identified and corrected.

   Injury to glomeruli (glomerulonephritis), vessels, nephrotoxins, infiltrative diseases (e.g. multiple myeloma) and interstitium (interstitial nephritis) can also lead to intrarenal AKI, however.

3. **Postrenal**. This refers to obstruction anywhere in the renal tract.

Q: How does medication-induced AKI fit into the above criteria?

A: It depends on the medication. ACEI and NSAIDs lead to renal hypoperfusion (prerenal AKI). Aminoglycosides (e.g. gentamicin), IV contrast, amphotericin B and cisplatin cause tubular damage (intrarenal AKI).

---

*Baseline creatinine is a reading ideally within a week of the current one. If not available within that timeframe, the lowest serum creatinine within 3 months can be used (KDIGO, 2012).

Q: Boris is excited by the elevated CK. He asks, 'Do you think he has rhabdo?' What is Boris referring to?

A: Rhabdomyolysis refers to a phenomenon where muscle injury results in the release of urate, potassium, phosphate, magnesium, calcium and myoglobin into the circulation.

Q: What are some of the causes of rhabdomyolysis?

A: These include:

- muscle compression (e.g. Mr Fung's prolonged immobility leading to prolonged muscle compression)
- severe muscle overexertion
- prescribed or illicit drug use[2]
- electric shock injury
- crush injury
- heat stroke
- polymyositis or dermatomyositis.

Q: How do you diagnose rhabdomyolysis?

A: The presence of an elevated CK indicates muscle damage. The combination of an elevated CK and a compatible history will support a diagnosis of rhabdomyolysis.

Mr Fung does have an elevated CK of 1600 U/L. Although there is a possibility that this reflects damage to myocardial muscle, this seems unlikely given the normal troponin. A CKMB fraction will confirm whether the CK has arisen from cardiac muscle. Also, Mr Fung's history of prolonged immobilisation supports a diagnosis of rhabdomyolysis from muscle compression.

Q: What are the complications of rhabdomyolysis?

A: Early complications include:

- hyperkalaemia
- AKI
- cardiac arrhythmia and arrest
- hypocalcaemia (secondary to deposition of calcium and phosphate product into tissues)
- elevated liver enzymes (transaminases secondary to muscle destruction).

Late complications include:

- disseminated intravascular coagulation.

---

[2]Prescription medications that can cause rhabdomyolysis include statins (hydroxy-methylglutaryl-coenzyme A reductase inhibitors), erythromycin, itraconazole, colchicine, cyclosporin, zidovudine and corticosteroids. All except statins are very rare causes.

Early or late complications include:
• compartment syndrome.

Q: Could rhabdomyolysis be contributing to Mr Fung's renal failure?

A: It is a possibility. The mechanism of AKI is mainly due to:
• obstruction of renal tubules by myoglobin
• hypovolaemia
• damage to the tubules by iron.

Two indications that rhabdomyolysis may be contributing to AKI are the level of CK and the presence of myoglobin in the urine (myoglobinuria). Although not a hard and fast rule, CK levels of more than 16 000 U/L are more likely to be associated with AKI. However, also consider that the CK may have peaked before Mr Fung presented and is now on the way down.

Q: How do you detect myoglobinuria?

A: Myoglobinuria is likely to be present if:
• dipstick urinalysis is positive for blood
• but urine microscopy does not reveal red cells
• serum sample is a normal colour (if the serum sample is brown or red, haemoglobinuria is the likely cause of the urinary abnormalities).

Q: Boris frantically writes down everything you say about rhabdomyolysis. 'Well then, I guess if his CK is only 1600, AKI from rhabdomyolysis is unlikely. Mr Fung has prerenal AKI with or without ATN because he is dehydrated. I guess there's no point in getting a urine sample.'

Is Boris right, or will examination of the urine help to determine the cause of AKI?

A: A urine specimen should be examined. But Boris's comments do have some truth to them. A CK of only 1600 U/L is unlikely to cause myoglobinuria and AKI. Also, in many cases of AKI, a thorough history and examination should point to the cause. For example:
• A history and examination demonstrating dehydration (as with Mr Fung) support a prerenal cause of AKI and/or ATN.
• A recent coronary angiogram might point to an intrarenal cause from IV contrast toxicity.
• The presence of a distended palpable bladder on examination points to a postrenal component of AKI.

Nevertheless, examination of the urine will be helpful. The following tests should be performed:
1. presence of blood on dipstick urinalysis (a negative result will make myoglobinuria very unlikely)

2. protein (rough estimate given on the dipstick urinalysis such as 1+ , 2+)
3. culture and sensitivity (in case of an underlying UTI, use a midstream urine specimen)
4. microscopy for cells and casts
5. urinary sodium, osmolality and creatinine.

After a dipstick urinalysis is performed, send the specimen to the lab and write on the form, 'MSU for M/C/S, casts, sodium, creatinine, osmolality'.

These results should also help you distinguish between ATN and prerenal AKI, as shown in the table below:

	Hypovolaemia	ATN
Sediment	Bland	Broad, brownish granular casts
Protein	None or low	None or low
Urine sodium, mEq/L	<20	>30
FENA %	<1	>1

FENA—Fractional excretion of sodium (this is the urine to plasma ratio of sodium (U/P) divided by the U/P of creatinine × 100). In order to calculate the FENA correctly you must collect both the serum and midstream urine samples at the same time.
Source: Adapted from Singri *et al.* (2003).

The dipstick urinalysis has 1+ protein, but is otherwise normal. Further examination reveals multiple granular casts, but no cells. The urinary sodium is 40 mEq/L. You calculate the FENA to be 5%. These results are consistent with ATN.

Q: Mr Fung commences IV rehydration. What fluids would you give him?
A: If there are hypovolaemic patients with hyperkalaemia, rhabdomyolysis or oliguric AKI, IV normal saline (0.9%) should be given. Initially, this can be prescribed as 500 mL boluses (250 mL if there is underlying heart failure or in the elderly). In other cases of hypovolaemia, solutions such as Hartmann's can be used (Anathanam and Lewington, 2013). It is important for the patient's fluid status to be regularly assessed during this process, otherwise complications such as pulmonary oedema can ensue.

Q: Mr Fung is given IV normal saline (0.9% NaCl). A urinary catheter is inserted to monitor his hourly urine output. He spends the night in the coronary care unit, where his plasma potassium level is closely monitored. He is sent to the ward the following day, when it is apparent that his plasma potassium level is stable.

He has been oliguric for the past 24 hours (defined as less than 400 mL of urine a day), but the treating renal physician is confident that he will recover (ATN often takes 2–4 weeks to start to resolve). Boris wonders if the addition of diuretics for Mr Fung's oliguria will help resolve the renal failure. What do you think?

A: Diuretics may make it easier to look after Mr Fung's fluid management only if he is now well hydrated. Diuretics will not change his outcome in terms of renal recovery or mortality, however.

Q: In ATN, is there any potential danger to consider in the recovery phase?

A: Sometimes a post-ATN diuresis can occur in the recovery phase. Patients may end up passing so much urine that they can become dehydrated and hypokalaemic! Therefore, monitor Mr Fung's urine output carefully, even though he is getting better. He may even require potassium replacement at this stage.

Scenario

After leaving Mr Fung, you are asked to admit a patient who has been sent to hospital to investigate an abdominal mass. The letter from his general physician states that the patient has chronic kidney disease and will require contrast for the CT study. The letter ends most helpfully with, 'Please do what is required'.

Q: What is required in this case?

A: If there are any doubts, speak to the general medicine registrar or the consultant. However, it sounds like the physician is worried about contrast-induced AKI. This is non-oliguric AKI occurring up to 72 hours after the administration of iodinated contrast. Some risk factors for this include chronic kidney disease, renal transplant, heart failure, age 75 years or over, and hypovolaemia. One recommendation to reduce the risk of contrast-induced AKI is the use of IV normal saline at a rate of 1 mL/kg/hour for 12 hours before and after the procedure. Although N-acetyl cysteine has been used to prevent contrast-induced AKI, the evidence doesn't really support it (Anathhanam and Lewington, 2013).

Achievements

You now:
- know the importance of HCIs for non-English-speaking patients
- realise the danger of hyperkalaemia and the urgency of correcting it

- can recognise the ECG changes of hyperkalaemia
- know how to correct hyperkalaemia
- are aware of the common causes of hyperkalaemia
- can classify AKI
- know what rhabdomyolysis is
- know the complications of rhabdomyolysis
- can diagnose myoglobinuria
- know the role of urine examination in determining the cause of AKI
- are aware of the potential danger of post-ATN diuresis in the recovery phase
- know about contrast-induced AKI.

References

Anathhanam, S. and Lewington, A.J.P. (2013), 'Acute kidney injury', *Journal of the Royal College of Physicians of Edinburgh*, vol. 43, no. 4, pp. 323–329.

Endocrinology Expert Group (2014), *Therapeutic Guidelines: Endocrinology*, Version 5, Therapeutic Guidelines Ltd, Melbourne.

Kidney Disease: Improving Global Outcomes (KDIGO) Acute Kidney Injury Work Group (2012), 'KDIGO clinical practice guideline for acute kidney injury', *Kidney International Supplement*, vol. 2, pp. 1–138.

Mandal, A.K. (1997), 'Hypokalemia and hyperkalemia', *Medical Clinics of North America*, vol. 81, no. 3, pp. 611–639.

Maxwell, A.P., Linden, O'Donnell, S., Hamilton, P.K. and McVeigh, G.E. (2013), 'Management of hyperkalaemia', *Journal of the Royal College of Physicians of Edinburgh*, vol. 43, no. 3, pp. 246–251.

NSW Health (2006), 'Interpreters—standard procedures for working with health care interpreters', PD2006_053, Sydney.

Sauret, J.M., Marinides, G. and Wang, G.K. (2002), 'Rhabdomyolysis', *American Family Physician*, vol. 65, no. 5, pp. 907–912.

Singri, N., Ahya, S.N. and Levin, M.L. (2003), 'Acute renal failure', *Journal of the American Medical Association*, vol. 289, no. 6, pp. 747–751.

Weisberg, L.S. (2008), 'Management of severe hyperkalemia', *Critical Care Medicine*, vol. 36, no. 12, pp. 3246–3251.

Chapter 17
Sasha presents with metabolic acidosis

Scenario

It is the morning handover round in the Emergency Department. You are just starting a 16-hour shift. Chandi, one of the night interns, tells you about a patient who arrived only an hour ago.

'This guy is an 18-year-old Year 12 student. He has been feeling generally unwell for the past 3 days. I haven't had a chance to take a history and examine him, but I did take some basic blood tests: full blood count, electrolytes, blood sugar and liver function tests. I also did an arterial blood gas because he was breathing quite quickly. Hopefully, the results are available now. Good luck! See you in 16 hours.'

You decide to see if the blood results are available before you see the patient, Sasha. They are, and they demonstrate the following:

Test	Normal range	Result
Haemoglobin	130–180 g/L	140
Mean cell volume	80–100 Fl	82
White cell count	3.5–11 × 10^9/L	20*
Platelet count	150–450 × 10^9/L	182
Sodium	135–145 mmol/L	137
Potassium	3.6–5.1 mmol/L	4.1
Chloride	95–107 mmol/L	102
Bicarbonate	22–32 mmol/L	14*
Urea	2.9–7.1 mmol/L	4
Test	Normal range	Result
Creatinine	60–110 µmol/L	105
Blood sugar		Pending
Albumin	33–48 g/L	30*

Bilirubin	0–25 μmol/L	20
ALP	38–126 U/L	100
GGT	0–30 U/L	26
AST	< 45 U/L	30
Lactate (tested on the arterial blood gas)	0.5–1.5 mmol/L	1.2
pH	7.35–7.45	7.25
PaCO$_2$		32
PaO$_2$		93

* Abnormal results.

Q: How do you interpret this?

A: He has a leukocytosis (which turns out to be a predominant neutrophilia) and hypoalbuminaemia. The low pH is consistent with acidosis.

Q: Is this a metabolic acidosis or respiratory acidosis?

A: In respiratory acidosis, the PaCO$_2$ is elevated. In metabolic acidosis, the bicarbonate level is low. Therefore, Sasha's results are consistent with metabolic acidosis.

As an intern and resident, you will definitely see patients with metabolic acidosis. It is worth having a basic understanding of the common causes and classification of this condition.

Q: How do you further classify Sasha's metabolic acidosis?

A: Metabolic acidosis can either be high-anion-gap or non-high-anion-gap acidosis.

Q: How do you calculate the anion gap?

A: The anion gap calculated as follows:
sodium – (bicarbonate + chloride)
The normal anion gap is approximately 12.
Sasha's anion gap is 137 – (14 + 102) = 21
Therefore, Sasha has a high-anion-gap acidosis.

(Try to remember this formula as it is fairly simple and is likely to assist you in assessing acidotic patients.)

Q: What could be the cause of Sasha's high-anion-gap acidosis?

A: There is a well-known mnemonic, among others, for the possible causes of high-anion-gap metabolic acidosis: KUSMAL.
Ketoacidosis (diabetes, starvation).
Uraemia (renal failure).

Salicylates (aspirin).
Methanol.
Alcohol, antifreeze (ethylene glycol).
Lactic acidosis (multiple causes).

Q: What commonly causes a non-high-anion-gap acidosis?

A: A common cause of the condition is loss of bicarbonate. This often occurs through gastrointestinal (diarrhoea) and renal (renal tubular acidosis) losses.

Scenario

You go and see Sasha. His worried mother is with him. Sasha was previously well. As a Year 12 student, his main concern this year is the Higher School Certificate. He feels that he is on top of his work, however, and certainly doesn't appear to be upset about it. He plays cricket for the school's second XI.

In the past 5 days, he has been feeling increasingly tired and nauseated. His appetite is well below normal. He has been passing urine far more than usual, getting up 2–3 times a night. Sasha attributes this to the large amount of fluid he has been drinking. He also has some upper abdominal pain, but this is extremely mild and hasn't required even simple analgesia. He denies using aspirin, is adamant that he does not consume ethylene glycol or methanol and, as far as he knows, he is not diabetic. He has no focal symptoms of infection or fevers (diabetic ketoacidosis may be precipitated by an infection).

On examination, Sasha does not look well. He is tachycardic (120/minute), with a blood pressure of 110/70. He is clearly dehydrated, with reduced tissue turgor and dry tongue mucosa. Despite an oxygen saturation on room air of 98%, he is taking deep breaths at a rate of 16/minute. The remainder of his physical examination is normal.

Q: To what do you attribute his unusual breathing?

A: This is Kussmaul respiration, which is a response to metabolic acidosis. (This is one reason why the KUSMAL mnemonic is so memorable!)

Q: The nurse taps you on the shoulder. The lab has phoned through a blood sugar result of 24 mmol/L. What diagnosis is looking more and more likely?

A: Diabetic ketoacidosis (DKA).

Q: You ask a passing medical student how to confirm the diagnosis of DKA. He says that a urinary dipstick positive for ketones is diagnostic. Is he correct?

A: Not always. Ketones can be present in the urine for reasons other than DKA, for example, starvation; therefore, if the urine dipstick is only weakly positive for ketones, you can't be certain that it is due to DKA.

Q: The nurse listening into your conversation says, 'Isn't a bedside blood ketone level the way to go?' Is the nurse right?

A: Yes. Many of the glucometers with which patients check their blood sugar levels every day at home now come with strips to test the blood for ketones. This provides an instantaneous estimate of serum ketones and can be performed at the bedside! Most Emergency Departments and wards would keep these machines and strips. In general, a reading greater than 3 mmol/L is regarded as high. In fact, if the reading is extremely elevated, the machine may just say 'HI' (as in 'high' rather than 'hello').

Q: Sasha's bedside ketone blood test comes back at 5.0 mmol/L, which is very high. This result, in combination with the polydipsia, polyuria, raised blood sugar and high-anion-gap acidosis, are all consistent with DKA.
What is the underlying pathogenesis of DKA?

A: Low insulin levels contribute to the breakdown of triglycerides with the release of free fatty acids. The free fatty acids are converted into ketone bodies in the liver. The 2 ketone acids responsible for DKA are beta-hydroxybutyric acid and acetoacetic acid.

Q: What are the common precipitants of DKA?

A: In the USA, omission of insulin is the most common cause (Gosmanov *et al.*, 2014).
    Other important causes include:
- infection (although Sasha's leukocytosis could represent infection, ketoacidosis alone can generate leukocytosis)
- acute coronary syndrome
- stroke
- mesenteric ischaemia
- acute pancreatitis
- acute gastrointestinal bleeding
- medications (thiazide diuretics, corticosteroids, calcium-channel blockers, propranolol, phenytoin, antipsychotics)
- surgery
- trauma.

DKA is idiopathic in 2–10% of cases.

Q: What additional investigations will you order to identify the source of DKA?

A:
1. **Midstream urine specimen.** Microscopy and culture are used to test for a urinary tract infection (UTI) (as a possible precipitant for DKA).
2. **Blood cultures.** These can also help identify an infection as a possible precipitant of DKA.
3. **12-lead ECG/serum and urinary drug screen/serial serum troponins.** Myocardial ischaemia can precipitate DKA. Although 18-year-old Sasha is extremely unlikely to have significant atherosclerosis, recreational drugs such as cocaine can precipitate MI. Sasha is unlikely to admit to using drugs in front of his mother.
4. **Serum amylase and lipase.** Sasha has mild upper abdominal pain. It is therefore worth excluding acute pancreatitis as a precipitant for his DKA.

   Although DKA can lead to a raised amylase, this is usually due to an extra-pancreatic source of amylase (e.g. from the salivary glands). A normal lipase will confirm that this is the case.

   The acidosis itself can generate abdominal pain. This is the most likely explanation. In fact, the pain from metabolic acidosis can be so severe that it is treated as an acute surgical abdomen!
5. **Chest X-ray.** This may reveal a precipitant for DKA, such as pneumonia.

Q: The preliminary examination of the midstream urine demonstrates more than 3+ organisms and numerous white cells in the absence of epithelial cells. Sasha appears to have a UTI. Dipstick analysis of the urine specimen reveals moderate to large ketones.

You are now confident that a UTI has precipitated an episode of DKA. What are the principles in managing DKA?

A: This is a fairly complex area and more senior medical staff will be involved in Sasha's management. Nevertheless, it is worth understanding the basic principles of managing DKA.
1. **Intensive care monitoring.** This involves regular monitoring of urine output (Sasha may need a urinary catheter), vital signs, pH, electrolyte and blood glucose levels.
2. **Treat any underlying precipitants.** In Sasha's case, this involves treating his UTI.
3. **Fluid therapy.** This involves expanding the extracellular (intravascular and extravascular) compartments.

   Often, initial fluid management involves using sodium chloride solutions of different strengths (0.9%, 0.45%, etc.), depending on the situation. However, once the blood glucose has been reduced to 12–14 mmol/L, the IV fluids should contain 5% dextrose.

In the initial stages of managing DKA, large amounts of fluid may need to be given as fluid losses average about 6–9 litres. The total volume of fluid loss should be replaced within 24–36 hours, with 50% of it given in the first 8–12 hours (Gosmanov *et al.*, 2014).

4. **Insulin therapy (insulin infusion).** Insulin is used to reverse the ketoacidosis, not just to reduce the hyperglycaemia. Therefore, do not cease the infusion when the plasma glucose is normal if the acidosis is still present (i.e. if the serum bicarbonate is still low). When the blood sugar level starts to fall, either decrease the rate of insulin infusion or increase the rate of the glucose infusion.

   Initially, insulin should be administered via a continuous IV infusion. Although protocols vary between hospitals, a reasonable regimen would be 50 units of a rapid-acting insulin in 50 mL of normal saline commencing at 0.5 units/hour and adjusted as per protocol. Aim for a 3–4 mmol/L fall in plasma glucose every hour. Once the plasma glucose reaches 12–14 mmol/L, the insulin infusion dose can be halved and IV 5% dextrose commenced.

5. **Potassium therapy.** For a variety of reasons, plasma potassium levels can become dangerously low during DKA. One of the most important contributors here is insulin therapy, which sends potassium into cells. For this reason, potassium replacement in IV fluids and careful monitoring of plasma potassium levels are essential in the management of DKA.

   You should begin to replace potassium when the patient begins to have a diuresis with fluid replacement. On the wards, IV potassium replacement should not exceed 10 mmol/hour. In an intensive care unit, where there is continuous cardiac monitoring, rates of 10 mmol/hour or higher can be used.

6. **Bicarbonate therapy.** This type of therapy is still somewhat controversial, and so will not be discussed here.

   More detailed management of DKA can be found in Therapeutic Guidelines: Endocrinology (Endocrinology Expert Group, 2014).

Q: What are the dangers of Sasha having low plasma potassium?
A:
- Muscular weakness can develop, with the lower limbs tending to be affected more than the upper limbs.
- Paralytic ileus can occur.

- Rhabdomyolysis and myoglobinuria, with resulting AKI, can occur.
- Severe hypokalaemia can cause respiratory muscle paralysis.
- ECG changes can occur, with more severe hypokalaemia leading to ventricular arrhythmias.

Some of the ECG changes of hypokalaemia include:
- flattened or inverted T-waves
- prominent U-waves
- ST-segment depression
- atrial tachycardia with or without block
- atrioventricular dissociation
- ventricular tachycardia
- ventricular fibrillation.

Q: What are some other causes of hypokalaemia?

A: Common causes include:
- diuretics
- alcoholism
- antibiotics (penicillin, carbenicillin, aminoglycoside, amphotericin)
- primary or secondary hyperaldosteronism
- magnesium depletion (it is always worth checking plasma magnesium levels in hypokalaemic patients you see on the wards)
- gastrointestinal disorders
- trauma
- type I and II renal tubular acidosis
- Bartter's syndrome
- drugs other than diuretics (e.g. beta-2-agonists, theophylline).

Q: In the setting of Sasha's DKA, IV potassium replacement should be used. But in a patient in a ward with mild hypokalaemia, how would you replace potassium?

A: Oral potassium replacement can be given. The dose will depend on the severity of the condition, but, in general, doses of 16–48 mmol a day should be adequate (Endocrinology Expert Group, 2014).

In Australia, commonly used oral potassium supplements include:

Tablet	Potassium content (mmol/tablet)
Span-K	8
Slow-K	8
Chlorvescent	14

For example, 3 slow-K/day equals 24 mmol of potassium while 2 Chlorvescent/day equals 28 mmol of potassium.

Q: Sasha responds well to treatment. The DKA resolves, as does the UTI.

Sasha's mother, alarmed at her son's new diagnosis of diabetes mellitus, wants to be tested for diabetes too. You explain that Sasha is likely to have type 1 diabetes and that he will be tested for antibodies known to be associated with this form of the disease. Although it is unlikely that his mother will also develop type 1 diabetes, Sasha's siblings are at increased risk.

What are the diagnostic criteria for diabetes mellitus?

A: Sasha's mother should demonstrate positive findings from any one of the following (Endocrinology Expert Group, 2014):

- symptoms of diabetes and a random venous glucose concentration ≥11.1 mmol/L
- symptoms of diabetes and a fasting venous glucose ≥7 mmol/L
- symptoms of diabetes and a HbA1C ≥6.5% (48 mmol/mol)*
- in the absence of symptoms, there should be 2 abnormal tests on separate days (ideally, the same test).

Q: What about an oral glucose tolerance test (OGTT)?

A: An OGTT is consistent with diabetes when there is a fasting venous glucose ≥7 mmol/L and a 2-hour post-glucose venous glucose ≥11.1 mmol/L. An OGTT only need be performed if 2 of the above tests are equivocal (Endocrinology Expert Group, 2014).

Q: Sasha's mother has an OGTT and tests negative for diabetes. She recalls that her uncle (Sasha's granduncle) was diagnosed with diabetes in his sixties. A few years later, he became extremely dehydrated with high sugars, went into a coma and died. This is one reason why she is extremely worried about Sasha's diagnosis of diabetes mellitus.

What syndrome could Sasha's granduncle have suffered from?

A: It is difficult to be sure, but it sounds as if he may have died from a hyperglycaemic hyperosmolar state (HHS), which is also known as hyperosmolar non-ketotic syndrome (HONK).

---

*The HbA1C can be affected by haemoglobinopathies and conditions with high cell turnover (e.g. malaria, haemolysis and large blood loss) (International Expert Committee, 2009). Also, a HbA1C < 6.5% does not eliminate a diagnosis of diabetes based on venous glucose levels (Endocrinology Expert Group, 2014).

Q: What is HHS?

A: DKA and HHS are different ends of the spectrum of acute metabolic decompensation in diabetes mellitus.

In HHS, insulin deficiency, among other factors, results in increased hepatic production of glucose. This, combined with reduced peripheral uptake of glucose, results in glycosuria, osmotic diuresis, dehydration, coma and eventually death.

Some of the similarities and differences are set out in the table below.

	DKA	**HHS**
Type	Usually type 1	Usually type 2
Age	Usually young lean individuals	Usually older obese individuals
	DKA	HHS
Precipitants	Similar to HHS*	Similar to DKA*
Kussmaul respiration	Often present	Absent
Polyuria	Often present	Often present
Polydipsia	Often present	Sometimes present
Plasma glucose	≥14 mmol/L	≥34 mmol/L
Arterial pH	≤7.30	>7.30
Serum bicarbonate	≤15 mmol/L	>15 mmol/L
Serum osmolality	≤320 mmol/kg	>320 mmol/kg
Anion gap	>12	Variable
Urinary ketones	Moderate to high	None or trace
Treatment	Similar to HHS	Similar to DKA but more gradual**

* Although the precipitants for both conditions are similar, older patients with HHS are more likely to have vascular precipitants than young patients with DKA.
** Correction of hyperglycaemia should be performed more slowly in HHS compared to DKA as rapid correction can be harmful to patients (Endocrinology Expert Group, 2014).
Source: Adapted from Chiasson *et al.* (2003).

Q: Is DKA exclusive to type 1 diabetes?

A: No. It can occur in type 2 diabetes, although this is very uncommon (Sherry and Levitsky, 2008).

Sasha commences a subcutaneous insulin regimen and is able to return to school to prepare for the Higher School Certificate.

Achievements

You now:

- can differentiate between respiratory and metabolic acidosis
- can calculate the anion gap
- know the causes of high-anion-gap acidosis
- understand the basic pathogenesis of DKA
- know the precipitants of DKA
- can diagnose DKA
- realise that there is a simple bedside test to determine serum ketone levels
- understand the basic management principles of DKA
- know the consequences of hypokalaemia
- know the causes of hypokalaemia
- know how to replace potassium, both orally and intravenously
- can diagnose diabetes mellitus
- understand the differences and similarities between DKA and HHS.

References

Chiasson, J.L. *et al.* (2003), 'Diagnosis and treatment of diabetic ketoacidosis and the hyperglycemic hyperosmolar state', *Canadian Medical Association Journal*, vol. 168, no. 7, pp. 859–866.

Colagiuri, S. (2002), 'When is diabetes really diabetes?', *Medical Journal of Australia*, vol. 176, no. 3, pp. 97–98.

Endocrinology Expert Group (2014), *Therapeutic Guidelines: Endocrinology*, Version 5, Therapeutic Guidelines Ltd, Melbourne.

Gosmanov, A.R., Gosmanova, E.O. and Dillar-Canon, E. (2014), 'Management of adult diabetic ketoacidosis', *Diabetes, Metabolic Syndrome and Obesity: Targets and Therapy*, vol. 7, pp. 255–264.

International Expert Committee (2009), 'International Expert Committee report on the role of the A1C assay in the diagnosis of diabetes', *Diabetes Care*, vol. 32, no. 7, pp. 1327–1334.

Mandal, A.K. (1997), 'Hypokalemia and hyperkalemia', *Medical Clinics of North America*, vol. 81, no. 3, pp. 611–639.

Sherry, N.A. and Levitsky, L.L. (2008), 'Management of diabetic ketoacidosis in children and adolescents', *Pediatric Drugs*, vol. 10, no. 4, pp. 209–215.

Chapter 18
A case of an acutely painful knee

Scenario

A 40-year-old man, Bill, presents to the Emergency Department with a 2-day history of a painful and swollen knee.

Q: What are the likely causes?

A: There is an extensive list of causes of acute monoarthritis but the most likely causes of acute knee pain are (Maury and Flores, 2006):

- septic arthritis
- crystal-induced arthritis
- trauma-related arthritis
- systemic inflammatory arthritis.

Q: What are the most common causes of septic arthritis in Australia?

A: Morgan *et al.* (1996) examined 18 years of cases of septic arthritis in tropical Australia. Their results showed that the most common causes (in order) are:

- *Staphylococcus aureus*
- streptococci (most commonly Group A streptococci)
- *Neisseria gonorrhoea*
- Gram-negative bacilli.

Q: What is the most common site of infection in non-gonococcal septic arthritis?

A: The knee is involved in 50% of cases.

Q: What questions might help provide a diagnosis?

A:

1. **Septic arthritis.** As with any infection, a history of constitutional symptoms such as rigors, sweats, fevers, anorexia and lethargy could point to an infective process.

    Neisseria gonorrhoea is the most common cause of septic arthritis in sexually active young adults. *Staphylococcus aureus* is the most common cause of non-gonococcal septic arthritis in adults. In both cases, haematogenous seeding of the joint is the mechanism of the septic arthritis.

Where gonococcal arthritis is suspected, you should take a detailed sexual history. It is also important to ask about other features of gonococcal disease such as urethral discharge, pharyngitis (after unprotected oral sex), maculopapular or vesicular rash and migratory arthralgias.

Often a cause of *S. aureus* septic arthritis is not found. This organism is a skin commensal, so any breach in the skin, no matter how small, can lead to a bacteraemia. It is worth asking if the patient has had any recent skin infections, surgery or IV lines, which could all allow *S. aureus* into the bloodstream. Do not rule out this organism if you don't elicit any of these risk factors.

2. **Crystal-induced arthritis** (Maury and Flores, 2006). The most common causes here are gout and pseudogout. The crystals that tend to cause an acute monoarthritis are:
   - monosodium urate (gout)
   - calcium pyrophosphate dihydrate (pseudogout)
   - hydroxyapatite (basic calcium phosphate)
   - calcium oxalate.

   A history of repeated attacks of monoarthritis that settled spontaneously can also point towards a crystal-induced arthritis.

   a. **Gout**. A previous history of gout can be helpful. Nevertheless, gout is a very common disease and its presence should not immediately dismiss the possibility of sepsis or another cause of arthritis.

   Try and identify precipitating factors for acute gout:
   - acute alcohol ingestion
   - ingestion of shellfish
   - diuretics
   - dehydration
   - trauma
   - severe illness
   - ceasing or starting medications to lower uric acid levels.

   b. **Pseudogout**. There are metabolic conditions associated with pseudogout. These include:
   - hyperparathyroidism
   - sarcoidosis
   - acromegaly
   - haemochromatosis.

It is worth asking about these when taking the history. Similarly, if the patient turns out to have pseudogout, it may be reasonable to look for some of these underlying diseases. As with gout, pre-existing pseudogout does not mean that the monoarthritis is due to superimposed sepsis.

c. **Basic calcium phosphate (BCP)**. BCP deposition is most commonly associated with patients on long-term dialysis. It is thought that periarticular deposits of BCP rupture into the joint or surrounding soft tissue, leading to the acute monoarthritis. The shoulder is most commonly involved.

3. **Systemic inflammatory arthritis**. For reactive arthritis, there may be a history of an infection (usually urogenital or gastrointestinal) 1–4 weeks prior to the onset of the monoarthritis. The presence of urethritis and/or conjunctivitis could support a diagnosis of Reiter's syndrome.

   A history of psoriasis, ankylosing spondylitis or inflammatory bowel disease would support a non-infective inflammatory cause of the monoarthritis.

4. **Trauma**. Tears of the menisci or ligaments are usually responsible. With meniscal tears, there may be no history of severe trauma. The precipitant may have been as subtle as jumping, decelerating suddenly or changing direction. The effusion often develops over several hours but may be more sudden if there is haemarthrosis.

Scenario

You find out that Bill felt generally unwell the day before the onset of the monoarthritis, with a reduction in appetite and reduced energy. Today he has been experiencing chills and sweats. He does have a 5-year history of gout, which caused acute swelling of his right ankle at the time of diagnosis. He has been taking 300 mg/day allopurinol since then, with no further episodes. He has been married for 15 years and has had no sexual encounters outside this relationship. He has no reason to doubt his wife's fidelity. There has been no history of acute trauma.

Q: What is your next step?

A: Physical examination may not be particularly helpful in this case. Both septic and crystal-induced arthritis can lead to extremely painful, joint-limiting movement.

Even if you found evidence of gouty tophi elsewhere in the body, this still wouldn't exclude any of the other causes of an acute monoarthritis.

Although physical examination may not give you an answer, it is worth looking for the following:

1. **Septic arthritis:**
   - purulent urethral discharge or a papular/pustular rash of mainly the extremities (gonorrhoea)
   - stigmata of endocarditis.
2. **Gout:**
   - the presence of gouty tophi.
3. **Pseudogout:**
   - look for other features of metabolic disorders associated with calcium pyrophosphate dihydrate crystals (discussed earlier).
4. **Systemic inflammatory arthritis** (Maury and Flores, 2006):
   - psoriatic rash
   - circinate balanitis (erythematous rash over the glans penis)
   - keratoderma blenorrhagicum (maculopapular rash which eventually forms pseudovesicles and hyperkeratotic plaques in Reiter's syndrome; it typically occurs over the soles and hands but can be more diffuse)
   - digital and nail changes of psoriasis
   - enthesitis (inflammation where a tendon inserts into the bone—classically involves the Achilles tendon).

Q: Where are gouty tophi usually found?

A: Deposits of tophaceous gout are most commonly found in the helix of the ear, the Achilles tendon and the elbow; however, a variety of joints can be involved (Maury and Flores, 2006).

Q: Bill is in a lot of pain. He has a low-grade fever of 38.1 °C and is tachycardic. His right knee is swollen, red and extremely tender, and pain almost completely restricts movement. He has no peripheral stigmata of bacterial endocarditis and the remainder of the physical examination is unremarkable. He has a fever, which means that this cannot be his gout. Bill must have septic arthritis.

Is this true?

A: No. Patients with acute gouty arthritis can have a fever. As in most cases of acute monoarthritis, the history and examination in this case have not provided a definitive diagnosis.

Q: What is the best way of making a diagnosis?

A: You should perform a joint aspirate.

Q: A nurse asks you whether a plain X-ray of the knee would be of any use.

A: Possibly. While the 'money' is with the joint aspirate, a plain X-ray might provide some useful information. Furthermore, it can be quickly performed. A plain X-ray of the knee might show (Maury and Flores, 2006):
- periarticular erosions with recurrent gout
- chondrocalcinosis with pseudogout (linear calcification of the cartilage of the knee menisci)
- calcific deposits in periarticular tissue with BCP.

Q: You aspirate 5 mL of turbid yellowish fluid. What tests would you request for the joint fluid?

A:

1. **Gram stain.** This test is positive in 50% of cases of non-gonococcal bacterial arthritis and in 25% of cases of gonococcal arthritis.
2. **White cell count and differential.**
3. **Culture.** This is positive in 90% of cases of non-gonococcal bacterial arthritis and in 50% of cases of gonococcal arthritis.
4. **Crystal analysis.**[1]

Q: Is the cell count useful?

A: Crystal arthritis tends to have a cell count of $5-50 \times 10^9$ white cells/L with a neutrophil predominance. Synovial fluid in acute bacterial septic arthritis often has $50-150 \times 10^9$ white cells/L, also with a neutrophil predominance.

However, these are not hard-and-fast rules and considerable variation can occur. In other words, do not dismiss or make a diagnosis of septic or crystal arthritis on the basis of the cell count alone.

Q: How is the synovial fluid examined for crystals?

A: Polarised light can be used. Under this, monosodium urate (gout) crystals are strongly negatively birefringent and needle-shaped, while calcium pyrophosphate (pseudogout) crystals tend to be weakly positively birefringent and rod-shaped. (Try to remember the 2 Ps: 'pyrophosphate positive birefrigence'. Therefore, gout crystals have to be negatively birefringent.)

Q: What blood tests would you order?

A:

1. **Blood cultures (2 sets from different sites).** Septic arthritis tends to occur in the setting of a bacteraemia. About 50% of

---

[1]Gram stain, a white cell count and differential and crystal analysis can be requested urgently. You should write 'URGENT' on the pathology form and ask the lab to contact you with the results as soon as they are available.

cases of acute non-gonococcal septic arthritis have positive blood cultures. This figure is lower in gonococcal arthritis, at 20%.

2. **Serum uric acid (for gout).**

3. **Full blood count, ESR, CRP.** These tests should be performed as a baseline to monitor the course of the disease and therapy. They are unlikely to have any diagnostic benefit.

   Bill may have a leukocytosis and neutrophilia. These are non-specific, however, as they can be found in both septic arthritis and acute crystal arthropathies. Similarly, an elevated CRP or ESR would be non-specific.

4. **Electrolytes, urea, creatinine and liver function tests.** These will provide a baseline result.

Q: Is it true that if Bill's serum uric acid level were normal, he could not be suffering from acute gout?

A: Not at all. It certainly is true that the risk of gout increases with increasing serum uric acid levels (the 5-year prevalence of gout is 30% in those with serum uric acid over 0.60 mmol/L, compared with 0.6% if the level is under 0.42 mmol/L).

However, acute gouty arthritis often arises from an acute change in serum uric acid levels (up or down). As a result, a normal serum uric acid may be associated with acute gout if there has been a rapid increase or decline in levels. Indeed, patients commencing allopurinol to treat gout may initially suffer an acute exacerbation due to the sudden decrease in serum uric acid levels from the medication! Furthermore, most people with hyperuricaemia do not have gout.

Q: Should you do any other diagnostic tests?

A: This patient's history suggests he is low risk for gonococcal infection. If it were suspected, however, polymerase chain reaction and culture for N. gonorrhoea should be performed on a urinary specimen and throat and rectal swabs. Remember that some patients are reluctant to disclose information about their sexual activity, particularly if someone else is present.

Q: The Gram stain is negative and monosodium urate crystals are seen in the joint aspirate. What else do you need to clarify about this result and does it exclude infection?

A: Gout is more likely to be the cause of the monoarthritis if the crystals are seen intracellularly as well as in the synovial fluid. You can ask the laboratory if intracellular crystals were seen. (Some labs in Australia will automatically report this on the computer. If not, you will have to call.)

Again, however, even the presence of crystals intracellularly does not completely exclude infection. And remember that this patient has already had 3 doses of cephalexin, which might mask a septic arthritis. It would therefore be reasonable to treat him with IV antibiotics for 48 hours to give the synovial fluid culture time to grow.

Q: What empirical therapy would you commence?

A: *Staphylococcus aureus* is the most likely cause of Bill's septic arthritis. Consequently, you should direct empirical therapy towards this organism.

Flucloxacillin 2 g every 6 hours intravenously (IV) is recommended by the Therapeutic Guidelines: Antibiotic (Antibiotic Expert Group, 2014) if he is not allergic to penicillin. If you feel that Bill has been at risk for gonococcal arthritis, a third-generation cephalosporin (such as ceftriaxone 1 g daily IV) should be added. If methicillin-resistant *S. aureus* (MRSA) is likely, empirical therapy with vancomycin would be appropriate.

Q: Who else would you involve at this early stage and why?

A: Although the cause of Bill's monoarthritis is still uncertain, septic arthritis has not been excluded.

The orthopaedic team should be urgently consulted about the need for surgical drainage of the joint. This is an important part of management in non-gonococcal septic arthritis. For infections in general, while antibiotic therapy is always an important part of the management, don't underestimate the role of 'scalpelmycin' in clearing an infection!

Having said that, remember that patients with gonococcal monoarthritis often do not require surgical drainage.

Q: What other treatment measures should you institute at this point?

A:

1. Analgesia
2. DVT prophylaxis.

Q: The orthopaedic registrar reviews Bill and agrees that septic arthritis is a strong possibility. He books him in for theatre later that day.

Twenty-four hours after admission, the microbiology laboratory calls you to say that both the synovial fluid and blood cultures are growing Gram-positive cocci in clusters consistent with *S. aureus*. You are relieved that you started antibiotic therapy and arranged the orthopaedic consultation.

How long will you treat Bill for?

A: In adults with *S. aureus* septic arthritis, 4 weeks' total therapy (at least 2 weeks IV and the remainder oral) should be adequate, although after 4 weeks of treatment, Bill needs to be reviewed in case longer treatment is required.

In gonococcal arthritis, 7 days of IV ceftriaxone is recommended.

Q: Given that Bill has a *S. aureus* bacteraemia resulting in septic arthritis, what other investigation should you undertake?

A: A transthoracic or transoesophageal echocardiogram should be undertaken to exclude bacterial endocarditis (see Chapter 21).

Q: Not surprisingly, Bill is feeling quite scared about all these developments. He asks, 'Doc, I will be fine, won't I? I mean, this is just an infected knee, nothing more?' Is he right?

A: Hopefully he will be fine, but septic arthritis is a serious condition. *S. aureus* bacteraemia in Australia has a 20.6% mortality at 30 days (Turnidge *et al.*, 2009) and permanent joint damage occurs in 50% of cases of acute monoarthritis.

Q: If Bill's acute monoarthritis had been clearly due to gout, what treatment options would have been available?

A: (Khanna and Khanna *et al.*, 2012; Maury and Flores, 2006; Rheumatology Writing Group, 2010):

1. **NSAIDs.** As a first-line therapy, all NSAIDs appear to be equally efficacious. Nevertheless, they should be used cautiously or avoided in people with heart failure, renal failure or factors for gastrointestinal haemorrhage. Unfortunately, these conditions are found in a large number of elderly patients with gout. Use the maximal dose for the first 2–3 days, then use a reduced dose until the attack has resolved.

2. **Colchicine.** Colchicine disrupts phagocytosis and chemotaxis by inflammatory cells. It is effective for acute gout, but limited by adverse reactions, mainly diarrhoea. For that reason, in acute gout, don't give more than 6 g in 4 days—a typical dose is 0.5 mg tds, which is adjusted according to renal function. (The American College of Rheumatology recommends a 1.2 mg bolus of colchicine followed by 0.6 mg 1 hour later and then 0.6 mg bd or daily if required. But this dosing regimen isn't widely used in Australia.)

3. **Corticosteroids.** Corticosteroids are an effective alternative in people who cannot have NSAIDs and can be administered through different routes and in different forms.

     a. Intra-articular. A very effective and safe treatment once sepsis has been excluded.

     b. Oral prednisolone. The American College of Rheumatology recommends a dose of 0.5 mg/kg/day for 5–10 days, then ceasing. Alternatively, give 2–5 days at a full dose with weaning over 7–10 days.

  4. Combination therapy. This can be considered when pain from an acute attack is extremely severe, especially with multiple large joints involved or with polyarticular gout. Combinations such as colchicine and NSAIDs, or colchicine and prednisolone, or intra-articular corticosteroids and an oral medication can all be considered.

  5. Remove any precipitants. Avoid or limit the use of food and beverages high in purines (e.g. fructose corn-syrup-containing drinks, alcohol, shellfish, sardines, beef, lamb, pork, sweetbreads, liver, kidney). If safely possible, cease medications that can increase urate levels (e.g. loop and thiazide diuretics and calcineurin inhibitors).

     (The pharmacotherapy for acute pseudogout is the same as for acute gout.)

Q: Six months later you are working as the orthopaedic intern in the preadmission clinic. You are surprised to find that your next patient is Bill. He is pleased to see you. You are glad to hear that his knee is fine, but he is about to have a total hip replacement because of osteoarthritis.

Bill still has nightmares about the septic arthritis of his knee. He asks you if his prosthetic hip can also become infected. What do you tell him?

A: Unfortunately prosthetic joint infections can occur. The rate of infection for knee and hip replacements is 0.5–2.0% (5–10% for a revision arthroplasty).

Q: Bill asks you if that 'wretched golden Staph' (i.e. *S. aureus*) is ever involved. What do you say?

A: Definitely. Prosthetic joint infections can be classified as:

- early (within the first 3 months of implantation)
- delayed (3 months to 2 years)
- late (more than 2 years).

(Early and delayed infections are usually related to implantation of the prosthesis whereas late infections are due to haematogenous spread.)

Staphylococcus aureus and *Staphylococcus epidermidis* account for 65% of total prosthetic joint infections, especially with early and late infections (Esposito and Leone, 2008).

Q: 'But Doc, if this artificial joint becomes infected, I can just have the antibiotics again, can't I?' Is this true?

A: Unfortunately, it is very difficult to treat prosthetic joint infections without removing the prosthesis and replacing it in a one-stage or two-stage exchange procedure. The latter procedure involves removal of the infected prosthesis, insertion of a spacer that contains antibiotic beads, 6 weeks of postoperative antibiotics and then insertion of a new prosthesis. The main difficulty in treating prosthetic joint infections without removing the prosthesis is the development of a biofilm. Bacteria, which attach to the prosthesis, can generate this biofilm (an exopolysaccharide), which protects them from phagocytes and antibiotics. However, if the prosthetic infection is early onset (less than 4 weeks postoperatively), the prosthesis is not loose and surgical debridement is prompt, then a successful cure without removing the prosthesis is more likely (Esposito and Leone, 2008). This 'debridement and implant retention approach' has a lower success rate (50–70%) than the 2-stage exchange but means that the whole prosthesis doesn't have to be removed (Antibiotic Expert Group, 2014). Irrespective of whether the prosthesis is removed or kept, adjunctive antibiotic therapy is always necessary.

Scenario

As orthopaedic intern, you meet Mr Sritala, a 52-year-old Thai man who was admitted with a painful first metatarsophalangeal (MTP) of the left foot. Although infection was initially considered, it turns out to be his first episode of gout. His serum uric acid is quite elevated. He is otherwise healthy and responds quickly to NSAID therapy. The rheumatology doctors see him and decide to start him on urate-lowering therapy with allopurinol, a xanthine oxidase inhibitor. But they want a special blood test performed before commencing allopurinol. What is the blood test likely to be for?

A: Allopurinol can be associated with a severe hypersensitivity reaction. The risk is increased in certain ethnic groups (e.g. Han Chinese, Thai people and Koreans with advanced chronic renal impairment) who are HLA-B*5801 polymerase chain reaction (PCR) positive. Mr Sritala is Thai and should be offered the HLA-B*5801 PCR assay (Khanna and Fitzgerald et al., 2012).

Q: Mr Sritala tests negative for HLA-B*5801 and is commenced on 50 mg/day of allopurinol. Despite the negative assay result, the rheumatologist will monitor him closely as an outpatient for any signs of hypersensitivity. Is there any other medication worth adding to the allopurinol?

A: Allopurinol might lead to further acute episodes of gout. It would therefore be reasonable to add either colchicine 0.5 mg bd or a NSAID to allopurinol to serve as prophylaxis until the target serum urate level is reached (e.g. 300 umol/L or less). The prophylactic colchicine or NSAID may be required for 6 months or more (Rheumatology Writing Group, 2010).

Achievements

You now:
- can list the common differential diagnoses of acute monoarthritis
- know the most common causes of septic arthritis
- are aware that gout can cause fever
- know what tests to order on synovial fluid
- know the appearance of different crystals under polarised light
- understand the limitations of serum uric acid in diagnosing acute gout
- know an appropriate empirical antibiotic regimen for septic arthritis
- realise the importance of surgical drainage of the joint in septic arthritis and know the duration of treatment in septic arthritis
- are aware of the different therapies available for acute gout
- know about the risk of prosthetic joint infection, can classify prosthetic joint infections and know which organisms are responsible
- understand how a biofilm may hinder successful treatment of prosthetic joint infections
- know the role of HLA testing to assess the risk of hypersensitivity from allopurinol.

References

Antibiotic Expert Group (2014), *Therapeutic Guidelines: Antibiotic*, Version 15, Therapeutic Guidelines Ltd, Melbourne.

Cibere, Y. (2000), 'Rheumatology 4: Acute monoarthritis', *Canadian Medical Association Journal*, vol. 162, no. 11, pp. 1577–1584.

Esposito, S. and Leone, S. (2008), 'Prosthetic joint infections: Microbiology, diagnosis, management and prevention', *International Journal of Antimicrobial Agents*, vol. 32, no. 4, pp. 287–293.

Goldenberg, D.L. (1998), 'Septic arthritis', *Lancet*, vol. 351, no. 9097, pp. 197–202.

Gottlieb, T., Atkins, B.L. and Shaw, D.R. (2002), '7: Soft tissue, bone and joint infections', *Medical Journal of Australia*, vol. 176, no. 12, pp. 609–615.

Khanna, D., Fitzgerald, J.D., Khanna, P.P., *et al.* (2012), '2012 American College of Rheumatology guidelines for management of gout. Part 1: Systematic nonpharmacologic and pharmacologic therapeutic approaches to hyperuricemia', *Arthritis Care & Research*, vol. 64, no. 10, pp. 1431–1446.

Khanna D., Khanna, P.P., Fitzgerald, J.D., *et al.* (2012), '2012 American College of Rheumatology guidelines for management of gout. Part 2: Therapy and antinflammatory prophylaxis of acute gouty arthritis', *Arthritis Care & Research*, vol. 64, no. 10, pp. 1447–1461.

Maury, E.E. and Flores, R.H. (2006), 'Acute monoarthritis: Diagnosis and management', *Primary Care*, vol. 33, no. 3, pp. 779–793.

Morgan, D.S. *et al.* (1996), 'An 18 year clinical review of septic arthritis from tropical Australia', *Epidemiology and Infection*, vol. 117, no. 3, pp. 423–428.

Rheumatology Writing Group (2010), *Therapeutic Guidelines: Rheumatology*, Version 2, Therapeutic Guidelines Ltd, Melbourne.

Rott, K.T. and Agudelo, C.A. (2003), 'Gout', *Journal of the American Medical Association*, vol. 289, no. 21, pp. 2857–2860.

Turnidge, J.D., Kotasanas, D., Munckhof, W., *et al.* (2009), 'Staphylococcus aureus bacteraemia: a major cause of mortality in Australian and New Zealand', *Medical Journal of Australia*, vol. 191, no. 7, pp. 368–373.

Chapter 19
Mrs Panetta has a painful jaw

Scenario

You are the colorectal intern. Your final task for the day is to change the IV cannula in Mr Panetta, a 61-year-old man who is day 4 after a right hemicolectomy. His wife is currently visiting him. She is sitting at his bedside eating an apple. They both greet you warmly as you enter the room.

While changing the cannula, you notice that Mrs Panetta stops eating her apple and starts rubbing her jaw. You ask her if there is a problem. She replies, 'Oh, it's nothing. These days, I find that after eating for a while, my jaw starts hurting. It disappears in a minute and I start eating again. Just a sign of old age. Nothing as serious as my husband's operation'.

Q: Your ears prick up at this revelation! What symptom has your patient's wife just described and what serious condition is it associated with?

A: This is jaw claudication, which may be seen in temporal (giant-cell) arteritis. Giant-cell arteritis is a vasculitis of medium-sized and large vessels.

Q: If Mrs Panetta does indeed have giant-cell arteritis, it is a matter of urgency to make a diagnosis and commence treatment. Why is this?

A: Blindness in one or both eyes occurs in up to 20% of individuals with giant-cell arteritis, and is often an early manifestation of the disease. This is why early diagnosis and treatment are extremely important.

Q: You tell Mr and Mrs Panetta that you would like to assess Mrs Panetta further immediately. They both agree to this.
What clinical features would support a diagnosis of temporal arteritis?

A:

1. **Age of onset over 50 years**.
2. **Headache** is the most frequent symptom, affecting up to two-thirds of individuals. Although it is typically occipital or temporal in location, consider giant-cell arteritis in any patient older than 50 years with a new headache.

3. **Jaw claudication** occurs in almost 50% of patients.
4. **Visual loss.** This occurs in 10–15% of patients (Weyand and Goronzy, 2014). Blindness is preceded by amaurosis fugax in nearly half of cases. Amaurosis fugax is transient monocular blindness classically described as a curtain being slowly drawn over the eye. Diplopia and visual hallucinations can also occur.
5. **Scalp tenderness over the temporal or occipital arteries.**
6. **Thickened, tender or nodular temporal arteries with reduced or absent pulses.** You may have noted the use of the term 'giant-cell arteritis', rather than 'temporal arteritis'. This is to reinforce the fact that this is a systemic process that is not restricted only to the head and neck. The following clinical features will demonstrate this.
7. **Polymyalgia rheumatica.** About 40% of patients experience polymyalgia rheumatica.
8. **Neurological findings.** These occur in about 30% of cases and include peripheral neuropathies and mononeuropathies of the arms and legs. Transient ischaemic attacks and strokes may also be seen.
9. **Peripheral arthritis and oedema of the hands and feet.** Peripheral arthritis and oedema of the hands and feet are seen in 25% of cases.
10. **Fever.** A review of fever (or pyrexia of unknown origin) (Mourad *et al.*, 2003) found that giant-cell arteritis in the elderly accounted for 17% of pyrexia of unknown origin.
    Therefore, you should always keep giant-cell arteritis in your possible diagnoses of pyrexia of unknown origin.
11. **Cough and sore throat** occur in 10% of cases.
12. **Ischaemia** may occur due to involvement of the branches of the aorta.
13. **Increased risk of thoracic aortic aneurysm.**

Q: What is polymyalgia rheumatica?
A: This is a condition characterised by aches or pains in the neck, shoulder and pelvic girdles for more than a month. The underlying process is a synovitis. Polymyalgia rheumatica is associated with an ESR of more than 40 mm/hour.

Scenario

You discover that Mrs Panetta is a previously well 57-year-old. She has suffered from episodic temporal headaches for the past month. The jaw claudication began soon after the onset of the headaches. Last week she had transient loss of vision in her right eye, which she attributed to anxiety over her husband's operation. She also recalls occasions where she felt unusually hot, but never thought of checking her temperature. Her examination reveals that she is afebrile. Her temporal arteries are prominent and slightly tender. You conclude that she may have giant-cell arteritis.

Q: You quickly call your consultant and express your concerns about his patient's wife. He is impressed with your resourcefulness and urges you to investigate Mrs Panetta.
What laboratory investigations support the diagnosis of giant-cell arteritis?

A:

1. **Elevated CRP.*** Studies have shown that this is an even more sensitive marker of diagnosis and disease activity than the ESR.
2. **Elevated ESR.*** The ESR is usually higher than 40–50 mm/hour. Even so, up to 20% of individuals with giant-cell arteritis do not have an elevated ESR. Therefore, you should not discount this diagnosis in the presence of normal ESR.
3. **Elevated liver function tests.** Salvarani *et al.* (2002) note that one-third of patients with giant-cell arteritis have abnormal liver function tests.
4. **Anaemia of chronic disease.** This is typically a normochromic and normocytic anaemia of chronic disease.
5. **Thrombocytosis.** Just under 50% of patients with giant-cell arteritis will have thrombocytosis. In patients where the clinical likelihood of giant-cell arteritis is high and the ESR is elevated, then a thrombocytosis $> 400 \times 10^9$/L is highly predictive of the condition (Kawasaki and Purvin, 2009).
6. **Elevated interleukin-6.** Although this may be a useful test, it is not freely available in all hospitals.

Q: Mr and Mrs Panetta are also impressed with your concern, and Mrs Panetta is happy for you to take blood from her. You do this and tell her the results should be available within an hour.

---

*At the time of diagnosis, only 4% of patients with confirmed giant-cell arteritis have a normal ESR and CRP; therefore, this combination has a good negative predictive value (Weyand and Goronzy, 2014).

Haemoglobin (120–150 g/L)	110*
Mean cell volume (80–100 fL)	85
White cell count (3.5–11 × 10^9/L)	6
Platelets (150–450 × 10^9/L)	520*
Electrolytes	Normal
Urea, creatinine	Normal
Liver function tests	Normal
ESR (<20 mm/hour)	75*
CRP (<10 mg/L)	70*

* Abnormal results.

Q: How do you interpret these results?

A: Mrs Panetta has a normochromic normocytic anaemia consistent with anaemia of chronic disease. Her CRP, platelet count and ESR are elevated. These findings are consistent with giant-cell arteritis.

Q: Are you sure that Mrs Panetta's ESR is not normal for her age?

A: It is true that the ESR increases with age, even in healthy people. Consequently, it is worth knowing how to calculate the approximate ESR for different age groups. Miller *et al.* (1983) describe one simple method:

For men: age/2   For women: (age + 10)/2

Using this method, 57-year-old Mrs Panetta's ESR should be $(57 + 10)/2 = 67/2 = 33.5$ mm/hour or less. Mrs Panetta's ESR of 75 mm/hour is definitely elevated for her age.

Q: Is there a more specific investigation that should be performed?

A: Absolutely. Mrs Panetta needs a temporal artery biopsy (1.5–2 cm in length) as soon as possible. A biopsy will be positive in 85–95% of cases and can distinguish vasculitis due to giant-cell arteritis from other causes (Weyand and Goronzy, 2014; Kawasaki and Purvin, 2009).

Q: Is there a role for imaging in giant-cell arteritis?

A: A quarter of those with giant-cell arteritis will have large vessel involvement (e.g. the aortic arch and its major branches). Therefore, magnetic resonance angiography (MRA) or CT angiography (CTA) is useful to determine the extent of vasculitis in those with confirmed giant-cell arteritis and to monitor response to treatment. Alternatively, it can aid diagnosis in those with suspected but unconfirmed giant-cell arteritis (e.g. if there is a negative biopsy) (Weyand and Goronzy, 2014).

Q: You speak to the on-call rheumatologist. She can see the patient tomorrow. But because Mrs Panetta has already experienced visual symptoms, the rheumatologist suggests that you commence treatment straight away. What is the best treatment to commence her on?

A: Corticosteroid therapy is the best therapy; however, there is some uncertainty about which route (IV versus oral), dose and duration of treatment are best. An oral dose of prednisone 1 mg/kg/day is often used but IV pulsed methylprednisolone may be offered if vision is threatened (Weyand and Goronzy, 2014).

Q: Mrs Panetta weights 61 kg so the rheumatologist recommends prednisolone 60 mg/day. You call the ophthalmology registrar and arrange for a temporal artery biopsy in 2 days. Mrs Panetta will have been on steroids for 48 hours by the time she has the biopsy. Will this affect the result of this procedure?

A: No. Biopsy results remain positive for 4–6 weeks after commencing corticosteroid therapy (Kawasaki and Purvin, 2009). Furthermore, the most important predictor for permanent loss of vision is how quickly treatment is started. If therapy is begun within 24 hours of the onset of visual symptoms, then 57% of patients experience visual improvement compared to only 6% if they receive their initial therapy after 24 hours (Kawasaki and Purvin, 2009). Therefore, don't delay the corticosteroids!

Q: You inform Mr and Mrs Panetta of the decision to use prednisolone immediately. Mrs Panetta wants to know if it has any side effects. What do you tell her?

A: Prednisolone is a very effective anti-inflammatory agent, but it does have a number of serious side effects, including:
- easy bruising
- thin skin that easily tears
- moon face and fat redistribution
- unmasking or aggravating diabetes mellitus
- osteoporosis
- proximal myopathy
- hypertension
- increased susceptibility to infections
- raised intraocular pressure
- cataracts
- hypokalaemia
- aseptic necrosis of the head of the femur
- peptic ulcer disease
- pancreatitis.

Q: Mrs Panetta raises her eyebrows at the long list of side effects you mention and asks whether any alternative agents can be used. Is there a role for steroid-sparing agents in giant-cell arteritis?

A: There aren't enough data to support the use of steroid-sparing agents in place of corticosteroids in giant-cell arteritis. Many agents have been studied either as monotherapy or in combination with corticosteroids but without clear benefit. These include agents such as methotrexate, azathioprine, cyclosporin, dapsone, aspirin, infliximab and tocilizumab (an anti-IL-6 monoclonal antibody) which might play a role in the future as more data become available (Weyand and Goronzy, 2014; Kawasaki and Purvin, 2009).

Mrs Panetta realises that corticosteroid therapy is best and also appreciates that the severity of uncontrolled giant-cell arteritis will outweigh the drug's side effects. They are therefore happy for you to commence treatment.

Q: Presumably without treatment, the giant-cell arteritis will progressively affect her until she dies. Is this true?

A: Surprisingly no. Due to giant-cell arteritis being treated as soon as it is recognised, we uncommonly see its natural history (and quite rightly so!). But it appears that it is a relapsing–remitting disease with eventual spontaneous recovery—although previous damage such as visual loss won't resolve. This is worth remembering in undiagnosed people who had an earlier episode that spontaneously resolved (Kawasaki and Purvin, 2009).

Q: A month passes and you receive a letter from the rheumatologist. It concerns Mrs Panetta's progress. Her temporal artery biopsy was indeed consistent with giant-cell arteritis. She has responded well to the prednisolone but the dose will have to be weaned over a period of months.
Is the disease likely to recur once it has resolved?

A: Unfortunately 30–50% of individuals with giant-cell arteritis will suffer exacerbations of the disease regardless of the steroid regimen used.

Q: The rheumatologist also noted that Mrs Panetta was very concerned about corticosteroid-induced osteoporosis and asked to be tested for it. How do you diagnose osteoporosis?

A: On the basis of a 't score' being $\leq$ –2.5 (i.e. 2.5 standard deviations below the mean); the t score compares an individual's bone mineral density (BMD) with the young normal mean. The most common ways of measuring BMD are dual-energy X-ray absorptiometry (DEXA) and quantitative ultrasound.

Q: What is the danger of osteoporosis?

A: Osteoporosis leads to an increased risk of hip and vertebral fractures. About 8% of men and 3% of women over 50 years of age die while in hospital for their hip fractures. The 1-year mortality rate after a hip fracture for men and women is 36% and 21%, respectively. The long-term morbidity from hip fractures is significant, with a large proportion of individuals who were independent prior to the fracture becoming partially dependent afterwards.

Vertebral fractures can lead to chronic pain and disability, resulting in a loss of independence and self-esteem, and even depression. Osteoporosis is definitely a disease that should be avoided.

Q: What are the major risk factors for osteoporosis?

A: The major risk factors are:
- in women, being postmenopausal (or prematurely menopausal)
- in men, being more than 50 years of age
- smoking
- lack of exercise or immobilisation
- family history of osteoporosis
- low body weight (body mass index less than 18)
- low trauma fracture
- low dietary intake of calcium.

Q: What are some causes of secondary osteoporosis?

A: There is a long list of secondary causes that includes (Sweet *et al.*, 2009):
- endocrine and metabolic disorders (hypogonadism, hyperthyroidism, hyperparathyroidism, diabetes mellitus, Cushing's syndrome, haemochromatosis)
- alcoholism (>2 drinks/day)
- medications (corticosteroids [relevant to our patient], anti-convulsants, immunosuppressants [cyclosporin, tacrolimus])
- hyperthyroidism
- malignancy (skeletal metastases, multiple myeloma)
- chronic inflammatory diseases (rheumatoid arthritis, inflammatory bowel disease, systemic lupus erythematosus, ankylosing spondylitis)
- chronic degenerative diseases (severe liver disease, chronic renal failure, chronic obstructive pulmonary disease)
- malabsorption
- HIV.

There are no clear guidelines for when to assess for secondary osteoporosis (as opposed to primary osteoporosis). In postmenopausal women, the prevalence of secondary osteoporosis is not thought to be high; but conversely, around 50% of perimenopausal and premeno-pausal women with osteoporosis have a secondary cause (Sweet *et al.*, 2009).

Q: What is the 'Z score' and how is it relevant to secondary osteoporosis?

A: The Z score, like the t score, is calculated from the DEXA scan. The Z score gives a measure of bone density relative to age-matched controls, whereas the t score gives bone density relative to the younger mean.

In patients with a low Z score (i.e. bone density below that expected for people of their age) you should be more suspicious of a secondary cause of osteoporosis.

Q: What blood tests would you order to look for secondary causes of osteoporosis and why?

A:

1. **Full blood count**. The finding of anaemia may support a number of causes of secondary osteoporosis, such as malignancy and malabsorption. The presence of a macrocytosis (mean cell volume) would support the presence of alcoholism and malabsorption.

2. **ESR**. This measure is elevated in some malignancies.

3. **Biochemistry (EUC, LFTs, 25-OH Vit D, Ca^{2+} Mg^{2+} PO_4^{3-}).** Hypercalcaemia and an elevated ALP can be associated with a number of causes of secondary osteoporosis. An elevated GGT can be associated with alcoholism. An elevated blood sugar might unmask diabetes mellitus. These tests should also identify chronic renal and liver impairment.

4. **Thyroid function tests**. Hyperthyroidism can cause secondary osteoporosis.

5. **Urine and serum immunoelectrophoresis**. In multiple myeloma, these tests may demonstrate the presence of a paraprotein.

6. **Sex hormones (for hypogonadism)**. Abnormalities with the following are associated with hypogonadism:
   a. testosterone
   b. sex hormone binding globulin
   c. luteinising hormone
   d. follicle stimulating hormone (in men).

7. **Prostate specific antigen** (looking for skeletal metastases from prostate cancer).

8. **HIV test** (if the patient has been at risk).

9. **Autoimmune markers** (this includes ANA, ENA, dsDNA, ANCA, rheumatoid factor, anti-CCP).

Q: Mrs Panetta is at risk of secondary osteoporosis from corticosteroid use. Even so, isn't it true that corticosteroid-induced osteoporosis will occur only after years of high-dose prednisolone therapy?

A: Wrong! Actually, bone loss tends to occur after the first 3–6 months of treatment. A dose as small as 7.5 mg/day is sufficient to cause bone loss.

Because Mrs Panetta will most likely use prednisolone at a dose and duration sufficient for bone loss, she should have a baseline DEXA scan to assess her BMD. In fact, the rheumatologist mentions in her letter that she has organised a DEXA scan for next week. (Medicare will even provide a rebate for BMD testing of individuals who take more than 7.5 mg of prednisolone a day for more than 4 months.)

Q: Two weeks later, you run into the rheumatologist on the wards. She greets you and gives an update on Mrs Panetta. A blood sugar and BMD were performed. The blood sugar was normal, but the BMD testing revealed a t score of –2.0. What do you do about this?

A: Although Mrs Panetta doesn't meet the criteria for osteoporosis (t less than –2.5), bone loss and fractures in individuals on corticosteroids can occur at higher BMDs. An important step in minimising damage from secondary causes of osteoporosis is to treat or remove the underlying precipitant.

Q: Unfortunately, in Mrs Panetta's case the steroids are vital to treating the giant-cell arteritis and cannot be ceased. Her rheumatologist wants to commence treatment to reduce further bone loss and osteoporosis. In general, what strategies are available for the treatment or prevention of osteoporosis?

A: There are a number of strategies (Honig *et al.*, 2013; Bell *et al.*, 2012; Sweet *et al.*, 2009).

1. **Non-pharmacologic.** This includes ceasing medications that can predispose to falls, addressing medical conditions that predispose to falls and optimising the home environment to minimise the likelihood of falls and damage from falls.

2. **Calcium and vitamin D supplementation**. This combination should be used if dietary calcium is below the recommended daily intake of 1200–1300 mg. It seems to reduce fracture risk in postmenopausal women, especially those with inadequate calcium intake; however, for other groups the benefits aren't clear.

There has been some controversy on the cardiovascular risks of calcium supplementation.

3. Pharmacological measures. These medications should be prescribed in:
   - those with minimal trauma fracture
   - those 70 years or more with a T-score of 3.0 or less
   - those on 7.5 mg/day or more prednisolone (or equivalent dose of an alternate corticosteroid) for at least 3 months and with a T-score of −1.5 or less

Q: What medications can be used (Honig *et al.*, 2013; Bell *et al.*, 2012; Sweet *et al.*, 2009)?

1. **Bisphosphonates** inhibit bone resorption by inhibiting osteoclast activity. They can be administered orally or intravenously. Alendronate, zoledronic acid and risedronate are PBS listed for the first-line therapy in men and women for both primary and secondary prevention of hip, nonvertebral and vertebral fractures. The main problem with oral bisphosphonates is that they can cause oesophagitis. Therefore, an individual has to:
   - take it in the morning with a glass of water
   - take it 30 minutes before other food or drink is consumed
   - remain seated upright for 30 minutes after taking it.

   Alendronate can be taken as a weekly dose (70 mg) or a daily dose (10 mg). Both regimens are equally efficacious.

   IV bisphosphonates include zoledronic acid, which only has to be given once a year! A serious and highly publicised side effect of bisphosphonates is radionecrosis of the jaw, although this is very rare and tends to affect cancer patients receiving frequent IV bisphosphonates.

2. **Raloxifene** (selective oestrogen receptor modulator). This is PBS listed for use in postmenopausal women with a minimal trauma fracture.

3. **Strontium**. This is an antiresorptive medication that is PBS listed for primary and secondary prevention of vertebral fractures in postmenopausal women.

4. **Desonumab**. This monoclonal antibody inhibits receptor activator of nuclear factor kappa B ligand (RANKL). It is administered every 6 months subcutaneously and reduces bone resorption and increases bone density.

5. **Calcitonin nasal spray or injection**. This decreases the incidence of vertebral compression fractures only. However, the US FDA felt that its risks outweighed its benefits in treating osteoporosis.

213

6. **Teriparatide.** This recombinant human parathyroid hormone is injected subcutaneously and reduces fracture rates in osteoporosis. It is PBS listed for patients who are at very high risk of fractures and in whom other medications have failed or not been tolerated.

The rheumatologist did, in fact, commence Mrs Panetta on weekly alendronate.

Achievements

You now:

- know the clinical features of giant-cell arteritis (GCA)
- understand the urgency of making a diagnosis of GCA to avoid blindness
- can calculate the ESR for people of different ages
- realise that all patients with suspected GCA need a temporal artery biopsy
- know how to treat GCA
- are aware of the side effects of corticosteroids
- know the criteria for diagnosing osteoporosis
- appreciate the morbidity and mortality associated with osteoporosis
- know the risk factors and secondary causes of osteoporosis
- understand the role of a Z score in osteoporosis
- can investigate patients for secondary osteoporosis
- realise that low doses of corticosteroids of short duration can lead to osteoporosis
- know the role of pharmacotherapy in osteoporosis.

References

Bell, J.S., Blacker, N., Edwards, S., *et al.* (2012), 'Osteoporosis: Pharmacological prevention and management in older people', *Australian Family Physician*, vol. 41, no. 3, pp. 110–118.

Kawasaki, A. and Purvin, V. (2009), 'Giant cell arteritis: An updated review', *Acta Ophthalmologica*, vol. 87, no. 1, pp. 13–32.

Miller, A., Green, M. and Robinson, D. (1983), 'Simple rule for calculating normal erythrocyte sedimentation rate', *British Medical Journal Clinical Research*, Ed 286(6361), 266.

Mourad, O., Palda, V. and Detsky, A.S. (2003), 'A comprehensive evidence-based approach to fever of unknown origin', *Archives of Internal Medicine*, vol. 163, no. 5, pp. 545–551.

Salvarani, C. *et al.* (2002), 'Polymyalgia rheumatica and giant-cell arteritis', *New England Journal of Medicine*, vol. 347, no. 4, pp. 261–271.

Sambrook, P.N. *et al.* (2001), 'Corticosteroid induced osteoporosis: Guidelines for treatment', *Australian Family Physician*, vol. 30, no. 8, pp. 793–796.

Seale, J.P. and Compton, M.R. (1986), 'Side-effects of corticosteroid agents', *Medical Journal of Australia*, vol. 144, no. 3, pp. 139–142.

Srivastava, M. and Deal, C. (2002), 'Osteoporosis in elderly: Prevention and treatment', *Clinics in Geriatric Medicine*, vol. 18, no. 3, pp. 529–555.

Sweet, M.G., Sweet, J.M., Jeremiah, M.P. and Galazka, S.S. (2009), 'Diagnosis and treatment of osteoporosis', *American Family Physician*, vol. 79, no. 3, pp. 193–200.

Tuck, S.P. and Francis, R.M. (2002), 'Osteoporosis', *Postgraduate Medical Journal*, vol. 78, no. 923, pp. 526–532.

Weyand, C.M. and Goronzy, J.J. (2014), 'Giant-cell arteritis and polymyalgia rheumatica', *New England Journal of Medicine*, vol. 371, no. 1, pp. 50–57.

Writing Group for the Women's Health Initiative Investigators (2002), 'Risks and benefits of estrogen plus progestin in healthy postmenopausal women: Principal results from the Women's Health Initiative randomised controlled trial', *Journal of the American Medical Association*, vol. 288, no. 3, pp. 321–333.

Chapter 20
Emmanuel suffers a needlestick injury

Scenario

You are paged by Emmanuel, the ward blood collector. He informs you that he has received a needlestick injury while taking venous blood from a patient.

Q: What is your approach?

A: You must assess the following 4 factors:

1. risk of transmission of bloodborne viruses
2. risk of the source having bloodborne viruses
3. immunisation status of the health care worker
4. timing of the injury, as prophylaxis for hepatitis B and human immunodeficiency virus (HIV) is beneficial only within a certain time.

To ascertain the risk of the injury, simply take a history of what happened.

Q: What factors increase the risks associated with a needlestick injury?

A: Increased risks relate to:

- what the needle was used for (i.e. an injury from a needle used for an IV injection would have a higher risk than one from a needle that had been used for a subcutaneous injection)
- whether the needle was solid or hollow-bore (i.e. the risk from a suturing needle is lower than that from a hollow-bore needle used for venepuncture or administration of an injection)
- whether any blood was visible in the syringe or at the top of the needle at the time of the injury
- how deep the injury is (i.e. the deeper the injury, the higher the risk)
- how much blood was involved (i.e. the larger the volume of blood, the higher the risk)
- when the injury occurred (i.e. the risk is higher if the blood was injected at the time of injury).

Q: What factors increase the risk of transmission of bloodborne viruses?

A: The risk of transmission is higher if the source tests positive for hepatitis B, hepatitis C or HIV. If the person is positive for hepatitis B or hepatitis C, the presence of a positive viral DNA and a positive viral RNA, respectively, increases the risk. The higher the viral load in the blood of someone who is HIV positive, the higher the risk.

Q: Emmanuel tells you that he had just taken a venous blood sample from the source. The needle slipped and pricked his left index finger, probably penetrating only a few millimetres. Nevertheless, on removing his glove, he found that his finger was bleeding freely. He washed his finger under running water and then called you. What do you think of the injury?

A: You should regard the injury as fairly high risk because a hollow-bore needle was being used to take IV blood. Additionally, there was blood in the syringe and needle at the time of the injury.

Q: What is your next step?

A: You quite correctly ask Emmanuel when the incident occurred. He tells you that it occurred about 15 minutes ago.

Q: Now what do you ask?

A: You now need to ascertain the risk of the source. This involves looking at the results of previous and current blood tests on the hospital computer system to see if hepatitis B, hepatitis C and HIV serology have been performed.

Keep in mind, however, that even if the source was negative in the past, this may no longer be the case. Any of these bloodborne viruses could have been acquired recently and still be in a 'window period'. During this period, the body is infected but hasn't had time to mount an antibody response, rendering serological testing ineffective. Consequently, you need to read the source's medical notes to look for risk factors for bloodborne viruses and then take a history from the source regarding the same.

The best way to approach the source is to introduce yourself and explain that a needlestick injury has occurred. Explain that as part of hospital protocol you need to ask some personal questions and request some blood tests. You should also reassure the person that this discussion is confidential and will not be discussed with friends or family. Tell the source that hepatitis B, hepatitis C and HIV can be acquired by:

- injecting drug use
- blood transfusions[1]

---

[1] In Australia, blood has been screened for hepatitis B since 1972, HIV since 1985 (in 1984, just before the introduction of HIV testing kits, hepatitis B cAb was used as a test for HIV) and hepatitis C since 1990. However, a blood transfusion received overseas, even recently, may have put the individual at risk of transmission of bloodborne viruses.

- unprotected sexual intercourse with a partner at risk for hepatitis B, hepatitis C or HIV (mention in particular sex workers, sexual encounters overseas, sexual encounters with foreign nationals, men who have sex with men)
- tattooing or body piercing
- living in an endemic country (e.g. hepatitis B is endemic in some regions of Asia).

   Then ask the source if any of these criteria would apply. (Assessing risk factors this way is often less offensive than directly asking, 'Do you inject drugs?' or 'Do you sleep with sex workers?')

Q: The source is a 62-year-old woman who has been married for 42 years. She has 3 adult children and 6 grandchildren. She moved to Australia from mainland China 30 years ago. She has been admitted for investigation of chest pain. She tells you that she does not meet any of the criteria you mention for bloodborne viruses, apart from living in China before. She does recall being jaundiced as a young girl in China. She has never had blood tests for hepatitis. How do you assess her as a source of transmission of bloodborne viruses?

A: While it is possible that an episode of jaundice in childhood in mainland China could represent hepatitis B, she is otherwise a low-risk source.

Q: The final factor you need to assess before deciding how to manage the needlestick injury is to work out the vaccination status of the health care worker. Are there vaccines for hepatitis B, hepatitis C and HIV?

A: Hepatitis B is the only one of the 3 for which there is a vaccine. All health care workers should generally have been immunised against hepatitis B. This involves 3 vaccination shots administered over several months.

   A sign of immunity is the production of hepatitis B surface antibodies (Hep B sAb) in response to the vaccine. Immunity is considered lifelong. Therefore, if previous postvaccination Hep B sAb levels were above 10 mIU/mL, a person can be considered immune.

Q: Although Emmanuel is absolutely sure that he had his full hepatitis B vaccination about 5 years ago through the hospital employee health clinic, he is not sure if his antibody levels were tested. Now that you have elicited all the appropriate information, what is your assessment of the needlestick injury?

A: You conclude that:
- the mechanism of injury was high risk
- the source history raises concerns about childhood hepatitis B

- the health care worker has an unknown hepatitis B surface antibody status
- the injury is now only 45 minutes old.

Q: Why is the timing of the injury important?

A: Hepatitis B immunoglobulin and HIV post-exposure prophylaxis (PEP) should be administered within 72 hours of the injury (ideally as soon as possible) to provide any benefit. (Some physicians, however, may commence HIV PEP outside this period if the exposure was very high risk.)

Q: Emmanuel now asks you what the risk of transmission of bloodborne viruses from a needlestick injury is. What do you tell him?

A: Think of the '3s' to help you remember the risk of transmission of hepatitis B and HIV:

- 0.3% risk of transmission of HIV from a positive source
- 3% risk of transmission of hepatitis B from hepatitis surface antigen (sAg) positive/e antigen (eAg) negative source
- 30% risk of transmission of hepatitis B from hepatitis B sAg positive/eAg positive and/or hepatitis B virus (HBV) DNA positive source.

The risk of transmission of hepatitis C is:

- 2% from a hepatitis C antibody positive/hepatitis C virus (HCV) RNA negative source
- 10% from a hepatitis C antibody positive/HCV RNA positive source.

Q: What do you do now?

A: You should not only check Emmanuel's hepatitis B sAb levels, but also his baseline HIV and hepatitis C levels in case subsequent blood tests are positive. It can then be ascertained if he was positive before the injury or seroconverted only after it. In a major teaching hospital you should have these results within a few hours of collecting the specimen.

You should also check the source's hepatitis B sAg and core antibody (cAb) levels. The hepatitis B sAg is a marker of active viral infection with hepatitis B. The hepatitis B cAb is a marker of previous infection with hepatitis B and not immunisation. People who are immunised produce only surface antibodies (sAb). Therefore, a person who is hepatitis B sAg negative but hepatitis B cAb positive has had previous infection, but is not likely to be currently infected.

Q: Would you test for hepatitis C and HIV on the source?

A: Theoretically, given the source's low-risk history for HIV and hepatitis C, it would be reasonable not to test the source for these viruses.

Nevertheless, in reality health care workers are usually so anxious, despite reassurance, that you would test the source to allay their fears.

Q: How do you test for HIV?

A: Many labs in Australia test for HIV via a combined antigen-antibody test. One problem of the test kits that only detected antibodies was that false negative results can occur during the window period. The window period is taken to be within 3 months of infection, although a positive ELISA is observed within 3–6 weeks in most cases. The advent of the combined antigen-antibody tests is thought to reduce false negatives in the window period by detecting p24 antigen; however, it still isn't considered 100% sensitive.

Although false positives can also occur with testing, they are rare. In fact, the specificity of the test is more than 99.8%.

The causes of false positive ELISA results include:
- human leukocyte antigen (HLA) class II antigens
- recent influenza vaccination
- acute viral infections
- liver disease
- autoantibodies.

Q: Is a positive HIV antigen-antibody test sufficient to make a diagnosis of HIV?

A: As discussed earlier, an ELISA for HIV is merely a screening test. A positive ELISA test must be followed by a Western Blot test. A positive Western Blot will confirm a diagnosis of HIV.

Q: You should get consent from and give pretest counselling to a person being tested for bloodborne viruses such as hepatitis B, hepatitis C and HIV. What would you tell the source?

A: Pretest counselling is poorly understood by most medical practitioners. There is a lot more to it than simply asking the patient's permission to perform the test.

According to NSW Health (1992), pretest counselling for HIV should include the following:

1. **Confidentiality**. You need to explain who will and who will not have access to the test results.
2. **Informed consent**. You need to explain:
   a. the mode of transmission of HIV
   b. the meaning of the window period
   c. the significance of a positive, negative or indeterminate result

    d. the prognostic and therapeutic implications of a positive result

    e. the methods of reducing transmission of HIV.

3. **Assessing risk factors.** This is discussed above.

4. **Assessing the patient's mental and emotional state.** A diagnosis of HIV or waiting for the result of an HIV test can be extraordinarily stressful. It is important to understand how the patient is likely to cope with these events. For example, if the patient is extremely stressed and you feel a diagnosis of HIV will result in suicide, you may have to defer testing until you feel the person is more able to cope, or ensure that a good support system is available.

Ways of assessing a patient's emotional state include:

    a. checking how the person has coped with stressful situations in the past

    b. finding out if the person is currently under stress

    c. asking the person to tell you how they would react to a negative or positive result

    d. exploring what support is currently available to the person

    e. finding out whether the patient might want to share the result with anyone.

Q: Both Emmanuel and the source consent to HIV testing, as well as serology for hepatitis B and hepatitis C. The source's blood tests reveal the following:

Hep B cAb: positive

Hep B sAg: negative

Hep C antibody: negative

HIV antibody: negative

How would you interpret this?

A: The source has had, but is no longer infected with, hepatitis B. This may well have been the cause of her childhood illness in China.

Q: Does this mean the source definitely is not infected with hepatitis C or HIV?

A: Although theoretically she could still be in the window period, in this case the source is at extremely low risk for having these bloodborne viruses. It would be reasonable to assume that her negative hepatitis C and HIV serology is a true reflection of her current infection status.

Q: Emmanuel's serology is as follows:

Hep B sAb: 22 mIU/mL

Hep B sAg: negative
Hep C antibody: negative
How would you interpret this?

A: Adequate immunity against hepatitis B is reflected by post-vaccination hepatitis B sAb levels greater than 10 IU/mL. Therefore, Emmanuel would be considered immune to hepatitis B.

Q: If a person who has not been vaccinated against hepatitis B or who has suboptimal post-vaccination sAb levels receives a high-risk needlestick injury from a high-risk source, how would you prevent transmission of hepatitis B?

A: The person would require hepatitis B immunoglobulin intramuscularly within 72 hours of the injury. You would also start the hepatitis B vaccination course as soon as possible, but ideally within 24 hours of the exposure (Antibiotic Expert Group, 2014). However, only the immunoglobulin would provide immediate protection. The vaccine would provide protection in the longer term.

Q: The lab calls you urgently with Emmanuel's HIV result: it is positive. You inform Emmanuel and he is understandably worried. 'But it doesn't make sense. I was being honest when I told you that I have no risk factors for HIV. I lead the most boring life! I can't believe this!' You explain to him that he is still likely to be negative when the confirmatory Western Blot result returns. But Emmanuel is not convinced. 'After all, aren't the sensitivity and specificity of this test around 99%? It's an accurate test.'

You tell him that the key to all this is the positive predictive value (PPV), and not just the sensitivity and specificity. What is the PPV?

A: First, remember that the sensitivity of a test is the percentage of those WITH the disease who test positive. The specificity of a test is the percentage of those WITHOUT the disease who test negative. On the other hand, the PPV is the likelihood that a person with a positive test actually has the disease. Unlike sensitivity and specificity, the PPV is affected by the prevalence of a disease in the population. Mathematically, it is represented by: True positives/(True positives + False positives).

For example, make the following assumptions:

1. The sensitivity and specificity of the HIV screening test is 99%.
2. The prevalence of HIV in the Australian population is about 1 in 1000 (Emmanuel's risk).

Therefore, in a population of 100 000, there would be 100 people with HIV and the following could be calculated:

	Test +	Test −	Total
Disease +	99	1	100
Disease −	999	98 901	99 900
	1 098	98 902	100 000

The PPV = 99/(99 + 999) = 9%. Therefore, the likelihood that Emmanuel's positive test truly represents HIV is only 9%. You explain this to Emmanuel, who is reassured.

If Emmanuel came from a high-risk population where the prevalence of HIV was 1 in 10, then the PPV would be different in a population of 100 000 as there would be 10 000 people living with HIV:

	Test +	Test −	Total
Disease +	9 900	100	10 000
Disease −	900	89 100	90 000
	10 800	89 200	100 000

The PPV would then = 9900/(9900 + 900) = 92%.

Q: If you had been concerned about HIV transmission from this exposure, what could you have offered Emmanuel?

A: To prevent transmission of HIV from a high-risk injury from a high-risk source, commence HIV post-exposure prophylaxis (PEP) as soon as possible, but ideally within 72 hours of the injury (Antibiotic Expert Group, 2014). This involves the use of 2 antiretroviral medications (usually 2 nucleoside analogues) for 1 month: for example, emtricitabine/tenofovir (200/300 mg) 1 daily or lamivudine/zidovudine (150/300 mg) 1 bd.

If the exposure to HIV is considered high-risk, then a third antiretroviral can be added, for example, lopinavir/ritonvavir (400/100 mg) bd or raltegravir 400 mg bd.

If the source is known to have HIV and their viral resistance profile is available, then that will also guide the choice of antiretroviral PEP.

Q: The Western Blot is performed and, as you predicted, Emmanuel is negative for HIV. Returning to the original needlestick injury, does Emmanuel have to be followed up?

A: If the source is seronegative for HBsAg, HCV and HIV, and unlikely to be in a window period, then further follow-up of the healthcare worker isn't necessary. But if the source tests positive or has a history suggesting that they might be in a window period, then testing could be done in the following way (Department of Health, Victoria, 2007):

3 months after the injury:
  a. hepatitis B sAg
  b. hepatitis C Ab*
  c. HIV ELISA

6 months after the injury:
  a. hepatitis B sAg
  b. hepatitis C Ab
  c. HIV ELISA (only if PEP was used, as this may prolong time to seroconversion)

During this period of testing, the healthcare worker should be advised to minimise chances of transmitting a bloodborne virus (e.g. by not donating blood, not sharing razors, practising safe sex).

Given the low risk of the source and Emmanuel's immunity to hepatitis B infection, he is not required to have further follow-up.

Achievements

You now:
- know the 4 factors to assess in any occupational exposure
- understand the factors that make a needlestick injury itself high risk
- know how to explore risk factors for bloodborne viruses in the source
- know when blood was screened for bloodborne viruses in Australia
- realise that even recent blood transfusions overseas may have used unscreened blood
- know that there is a vaccine for hepatitis B, but not for hepatitis C or HIV
- appreciate the timing of the injury and its relationship to commencing PEP for hepatitis B or HIV
- can explain the risk of transmission of hepatitis B, hepatitis C and HIV with needlestick injuries
- can differentiate between past and current hepatitis B infection and immunisation using serology
- know that an HIV diagnosis requires a screening ELISA and confirmatory Western Blot test
- know the definitions of sensitivity and specificity

---

*There may be a role for HCV polymerase chain reaction assays in certain circumstances too (Antibiotic Expert Group, 2014).

- know how the prevalence of a disease in a population affects the PPV of a test
- know the causes of a false positive and negative HIV ELISA
- know how to perform pretest counselling for HIV
- know which individuals should receive hepatitis B immunoglobulin or a booster
- know when these individuals should have follow-up testing.

References

Antibiotic Expert Group (2014), *Therapeutic Guidelines: Antibiotic*, Version 15, Therapeutic Guidelines Ltd, Melbourne.

Department of Health, Victoria (2007), 'Appendix 4: Procedure for managing an exposure to blood/body fluids/substances', at <http://ideas.health.vic.gov.au/bluebook/appendix4.asp>, accessed 21 November 2014.

NSW Health (1992), 'Guidelines for counselling associated with HIV antibody testing', Circular No. 92/20, Sydney.

NSW Health (2005), 'HIV, hepatitis B and hepatitis C—management of health care workers potentially exposed', PD2005_311, Sydney.

Oelrichs, R. (2003), 'Diagnostics', in J. Hoy and S. Lewin (eds), *HIV Management in Australasia: A Guide for Clinical Care*, Australasian Society for HIV Medicine Inc., Sydney, pp. 51–71.

Chapter 21
McGyver has postoperative fever

Scenario

You are working another overtime shift, and have just been paged to see a patient with a fever on the surgical ward. Mr Wilson ('just call me McGyver') is a 52-year-old man who underwent an anterior resection for Duke's A colorectal cancer 7 days ago. He takes omeprazole for oesophagitis, but otherwise has been well.

Although his postoperative course had been uneventful to this point, this evening McGyver felt very cold and started shivering before breaking out in a sweat. The nurse checked his temperature, which was 39.1 °C. She then paged you to review the patient.

Q: What are the likely sources of fever in a postoperative patient such as McGyver?

A: Infective causes would include:
- chest infection
- UTI
- surgical site infection
- IV line infection
- endocarditis
- meningitis (uncommon outside neurosurgical patients).

Non-infective causes include:
- atelectasis
- pulmonary embolism (PE)[1]
- drug fever
- deep venous thrombosis (DVT)[2]

---

[1]Stein *et al.* (2000) found that fever could occur in PE in the absence of pulmonary haemorrhage or infarction. Although the fever is usually low-grade, high fevers can occur.

[2]In a review of fever of unknown origin, Mourad *et al.* (2003) found that 3% of cases of pyrexia of unknown origin were due to DVT.

Q: You take a history from McGyver. He has no focal symptoms of infection apart from some pain around his IV cannula site. It had not become painful until yesterday and had been fine for the previous 3 days. You proceed to examine McGyver. He looks tired, and has a fever of 39 °C and a tachycardia of 100 beats/minute. He has no peripheral stigmata of endocarditis and no murmurs. His abdominal wound looks clean and his abdomen is not tender. The respiratory examination is unremarkable. His oxygen saturation is 98% on room air. Nevertheless, there is erythema and tenderness around the cannula entry site on his right forearm. With gentle pressure, a thick yellow exudate discharges from the site. Why do you think McGyver has a fever?

A: McGyver has a peripheral venous catheter infection. This is almost certainly responsible for his fever.

Q: From the history he has given, what factor do you think has contributed to McGyver's cannula infection?

A: McGyver has indicated that his peripheral cannula has been in place for 5 days.

The 2002 guidelines from the Centers for Disease Control and Prevention (CDC, Atlanta) recommend that IV peripheral catheters be replaced every 72–96 hours. After this time, there is an increased incidence of phlebitis and bacterial colonisation, and so an increased risk of infection. In Australia, most hospitals recommend changing peripheral intravascular catheters every 48–72 hours, and sometimes even more frequently (< 24 hours) for those inserted in ambulances and in emergency situations.

As an intern or resident, you must ensure that your patients' cannulae are replaced as often as recommended. Infections due to cannulae not being replaced within 72 hours are not acceptable! Many hospitals use labels on which the date a cannula was inserted is written. One part of the label is placed in the patient's notes and the other at the cannula site.

Q: What investigations should you perform?

A: Now that you have established that McGyver has a peripheral cannula infection, you should swab the yellow discharge from the cannula site and send it for culture.

1. Take 2 sets of blood cultures at different times from different sites.
2. Undertake a full blood count, electrolytes and liver function tests.

Q: Does the patient have to be febrile while you take the blood culture?

A: No. There is no problem in taking the blood culture while McGyver is afebrile.

Q: What organisms are most commonly associated with peripheral line infections?

A: Skin commensals, not surprisingly, are the usual pathogens. Other organisms associated with these infections are:

- coagulase-negative staphylococci (35%)
- *Staphylococcus aureus* (25%)
- enteric gram-negative bacilli (15%)
- yeasts (10%)
- streptococci and enterococci (10%)
- *Pseudomonas* spp. (5%)
- other (5%).

Q: Are blood cultures really necessary for an intravascular catheter infection?

A: Definitely! The most common cause of bloodstream infections in Australia is sepsis arising from intravascular catheter infections.

The rate of bloodstream infections attributable to peripheral venous catheters is 0.36 per 1000 catheters. Given the absolute number of patients who receive peripheral venous catheters in Australia, however, this is a significant number.

The rate of bloodstream infections for percutaneous central venous catheters is 23 per 1000. In an Australian study, Blyth *et al.* (2002) discovered that 51% of hospital-acquired cases of *S. aureus* bacteraemia were due to infected IV lines.

Q: If McGyver had an infected central venous catheter (CVC) rather than a peripheral cannula, what other investigation might you perform?

A: In addition to peripheral blood cultures, blood cultures should be taken directly and simultaneously from the CVC. The idea here is that because the source of sepsis (the CVC) will have a higher density of organisms than the peripheral venous sample, it may become positive more quickly (often 2 hours earlier using the 'Bactec' blood culture system).

Q: If the source of fever is not clear after clinically assessing McGyver, what other investigations would you perform?

A:

1. chest X-ray
2. midstream urine
3. a work-up for PE and DVT if the preliminary investigations for infection are negative.

Q: What empirical antibiotic therapy would you commence?

A: If he has no antibiotic allergies, commence an antibiotic that targets *S. aureus*. If you work in a hospital where methicillin-resistant *S. aureus* (MRSA) is prevalent, you should commence IV vancomycin (unfortunately this applies to most major teaching hospitals in Australia). However, if McGyver's infection is due to a methicillin-sensitive *S. aureus* (MSSA) strain, then you should also add IV flucloxacillin (assuming no allergies) to the IV vancomycin. The reason for this is that, although MSSA is sensitive to vancomycin, vancomycin is nowhere near as effective as flucloxacillin (Corey, 2009). Patients who receive vancomycin as initial empirical therapy for MSSA bacteraemia are more likely to have delayed clearance of bacteria (Khatib *et al.*, 2006). In addition, given the lower risk of a Gram-negative infection, it would be reasonable to use an antibiotic combination with Gram-negative cover too.

Q: You remove the IV cannula and send the appropriate cultures. Given the large prevalence of MRSA in your hospital, you commence both IV vancomycin and IV piperacillin-tazobactam 4.5 g q8h. What dose of vancomycin should you prescribe?

A: In patients where the antibiotics don't have to be adjusted for impaired renal function, it would be reasonable to prescribe (Antibiotic Expert Group, 2014):

- IV vancomycin loading dose of 25–30 mg/kg followed 12 hours later by regular dosing of 15–20 mg/kg q12h.
- The vancomycin trough level should be checked before the fourth dose.

Q: Within 24 hours, the blood and yellow discharge all grow clusters of Gram-positive cocci. Within 48 hours, they are identified as MSSA. You cease IV vancomycin and piperacillin-tazobactam, instead switching to IV flucloxacillin 2 g q6h. What investigation should every patient with *S. aureus* bacteraemia undergo?

A: A transthoracic echocardiogram (TTE) or a transoesophageal echocardiogram (TOE) should be performed after a few days of IV therapy to exclude infective endocarditis (IE).

Unfortunately, it is quite common for *S. aureus* bacteraemia to be complicated by IE and other metastatic infections. One large series found that a third of all patients with *S. aureus* bacteraemia developed metastatic infection while 12% developed endocarditis (Fowler *et al.*, 2003).

Q: Which investigation is better in evaluating the presence of IE in *S. aureus* bacteraemia: TTE or TOE?

A: A TOE is the investigation of choice. Overall, in IE, TOE is more sensitive than TTE (75–95% versus 60–70%) and has similar specificity (up to 98%). However, in some hospitals you may have to use TTE due to restricted access to TOE.

Q: How long would you treat McGyver for?

A: Consult the infectious diseases or microbiology team for guidance on this issue. There are consensus recommendations for the treatment of *S. aureus* bacteraemia (Fowler *et al.*, 1998) based on the risk of metastatic infection. However, you do not have to memorise these. What you need to remember is that the minimum duration of antibiotic therapy for a simple or uncomplicated bacteraemia is often 2 weeks and certainly no less than 1 week. Bacteraemia complicated by metastatic infection will require therapy for a much longer period.

The whole antibiotic course should be IV rather than oral. This has both an economic and psychological impact on the hospital and patient.

Q: A pure growth of MSSA is isolated from McGyver's midstream urine specimen. Does this mean that McGyver has an MSSA UTI?

A: Lee *et al.* (1978) demonstrated a relationship between *S. aureus* bacteraemia and bacteriuria. They concluded that, in most cases, the bacteriuria was secondary to bacteraemia. Although *S. aureus* UTIs certainly occur, they are uncommon.

And note ...

The important message is that *S. aureus* bacteriuria is usually secondary to bacteraemia. Therefore, you must take blood cultures in all patients with *S. aureus* in the urine.

Q: You feel that McGyver's bacteriuria is secondary to his line-related bacteraemia. He continues on IV flucloxacillin, but still spikes fevers above 38 °C. You now can hear a soft pansystolic murmur, which you feel wasn't there when you first assessed him. A repeat blood culture on day 4 again isolates MSSA. On day 6 of treatment, a TTE demonstrates mild mitral regurgitation. A TOE is therefore performed. It demonstrates a mitral valve vegetation with moderately severe mitral regurgitation. Does McGyver have IE?

A: Yes. The combination of ongoing MSSA bacteraemia despite adequate IV flucloxacillin therapy and a TOE appearance consistent with a mitral valve vegetation makes IE a highly likely diagnosis.

Nevertheless, it is worth being aware of the Modified Duke Criteria (described by Li *et al.*, 2000). These are a number of major and minor criteria that can be used to support a diagnosis of IE.

McGyver's bacteraemia and TOE findings would provide the 2 major criteria required to make a diagnosis of IE. The criteria can be especially useful when a diagnosis is not obvious.

Q: Is *S. aureus* a common cause of IE?

A: Definitely. *S. aureus* is now the leading cause of IE (Murdoch *et al.*, 2009).

Q: What major complications of IE could McGyver face?

A:

1. **Cardiac complications**, including:
   a. cardiac failure, usually secondary to valvular disease
   b. MI, usually secondary to septic emboli
   c. arrhythmias, including heart block, usually secondary to invasion of the septum
   d. pericarditis and tamponade.
2. **Neurologic complications**, including:
   a. stroke, usually secondary to septic emboli and ruptured mycotic aneurysms
   b. intracranial haemorrhage, usually secondary to ruptured mycotic aneurysms.
3. **Systemic emboli and splenic abscess**, which are found most commonly on the kidneys, spleen, liver and iliac or mesenteric arteries.
4. **Prolonged fever**.

Q: McGyver becomes upset as you explain the complications of IE to him. Given that many of these complications are related to septic emboli arising from the valvular vegetation, shouldn't you anticoagulate him?

A: Although anticoagulation of a native valve sounds like a sensible suggestion, it has not been shown to prevent embolic phenomena and may even increase the risk of intracerebral bleeding.

On the other hand, anticoagulation for prosthetic valve endocarditis (PVE) of mechanical valves is usually recommended. In this setting, good anticoagulation will decrease the risk of stroke without increasing the frequency of haemorrhagic complications. The only exception is in those people with mechanical valve PVE due to *S. aureus* who have experienced a recent embolus to the central nervous system, where anticoagulation should be avoided in the first 2 weeks of therapy (Baddour *et al.*, 2005). However, anticoagulation for PVE of bioprosthetic valves is not recommended.

Q: McGyver now wants to know how long he will need to take antibiotics. What do you tell him?

A: He will need 4–6 weeks of IV flucloxacillin in total at an increased dose of 2g q4h (may need renal adjustment).

Q: 'If I have 6 weeks of antibiotics, I will definitely be cured, right?'

A: Unfortunately, you cannot guarantee that; *S. aureus* IE has a staggering mortality rate of around 25% (Fowler *et al.*, 2005). The overall mortality rate for IE from all causes is around 20% (Murdoch *et al.*, 2009).

Q: 'So, we're about 5½ weeks into treatment, aren't we?'

A: No, the 6 weeks of therapy begins from when McGyver first has negative blood cultures (Baddour *et al.*, 2005). McGyver's blood cultures were still positive on day 4 of therapy. In other words, blood cultures must be taken every day or so until they become negative. This is because, unfortunately, bacteraemia can persist even while on appropriate antibiotic therapy. This usually means that there is an abscess or endovascular source that may require surgery and possibly a change in antibiotic therapy.

Q: 'Can surgery fix me, Doctor?'

A: There certainly is a role for surgery in IE. Common procedures include valve replacement and vegetectomy (removal of the vegetation without replacing the valve).

Common indications for surgery include:
- congestive cardiac failure
- perivalvular invasive disease
- uncontrolled infection despite appropriate antibiotic treatment
- prosthetic valve infection
- ongoing embolic phenomena.

However, you hope that antibiotic therapy alone will be sufficient to cure McGyver.

Q: Thankfully, McGyver does recover. However, due to worsening mitral regurgitation and heart failure, he required a mitral valve replacement with a mechanical valve. He will require lifelong warfarin. 'Doc, surely this mechanical valve can't get infected?' What is your response?

A: Unfortunately, PVE is responsible for some 10–15% of all cases of endocarditis. However, the lifelong rate of infection is low, at 0.4% per year (but slightly higher in the first 6–12 months after the valve replacement surgery).

Q: Should patients with prosthetic valves have prophylactic antibiotics before any invasive procedure?

A: It is recommended that patients with prosthetic valves should have prophylactic antibiotics for certain procedures. This is to prevent bacteraemia and endocarditis.

And note ...

IE is a difficult disease to manage. It is much easier to change peripheral venous catheters every 48–72 hours and avoid *S. aureus* bacteraemia in the first place!

Q: What empirical antibiotic therapy would you commence in native valve IE before blood culture results are available?

A: IV flucloxacillin and penicillin and gentamicin. If the patient has penicillin hypersensitivity, use: IV vancomycin and gentamicin +/− IV cephalothin or cephazolin (avoid the first-generation cephalosporins if there's a history of type 1 hypersensitivity to penicillins).

Achievements

You now:

- know the infective and non-infective sources of fever in postoperative patients
- are aware that PE can cause fevers
- understand the importance of replacing peripheral IV catheters regularly
- know how to investigate a patient with an IV catheter infection
- know the most common bacterial causes for IV catheter infections
- realise that *S. aureus* bacteriuria is often secondary to bacteraemia rather than being a primary UTI
- can chart appropriate empirical therapy for IV catheter infections
- realise that TOE or TTE must be performed to exclude IE in *S. aureus* bacteraemia
- appreciate that *S. aureus* bacteraemia requires a minimum of 1 week of IV antibiotic therapy
- are aware of the existence of the Modified Duke Criteria for diagnosis of IE
- realise that *S. aureus* is the most common cause of IE in most parts of the world
- know the complications of IE

- know the role of anticoagulation in native and prosthetic valve endocarditis (PVE)
- know that a minimum of 4–6 weeks of antibiotic therapy is required for left-sided *S. aureus* IE
- know that the duration of antibiotic therapy for IE begins from when blood cultures first become negative
- understand the role of surgery in IE
- are aware of which procedures require prophylaxis against PVE
- know an appropriate empirical antibiotic regimen for IE while waiting for culture results.

References

Antibiotic Expert Group (2014), *Therapeutic Guidelines: Antibiotic*, Version 15, Therapeutic Guidelines Ltd, Melbourne.

Baddour, L. M., Wilson, W.R., Bayer, A.S., *et al.* (2005), 'Infective endocarditis: diagnosis, antimicrobial therapy, and management of complications: A statement for healthcare professionals from the Committee on Rheumatic Fever, Endocarditis, and Kawasaki Disease, Council on Cardiovascular Disease in the Young, and the Councils on Clinical Cardiology, Stroke, and Cardiovascular Surgery and Anesthesia, American Heart Association: endorsed by the Infectious Diseases Society of America.' *Circulation*, vol. 111, no. 23, pp. e393–434.

Blyth, C.C. *et al.* (2002), 'Evaluation of clinical guidelines for the management of Staphylococcus aureus bacteraemia', *Internal Medicine Journal*, vol. 32, nos 5–6, pp. 224–232.

Corey, G.R. (2009), 'Staphylococcus aureus bloodstream infections: Definitions and treatment', *Clinical Infectious Diseases*, vol. 48, suppl. 4, S254–259.

Fowler, V.G. Jr *et al.* (1998), 'Outcome of Staphylococcus aureus bacteremia according to compliance with recommendations of infectious diseases specialists: Experience with 244 patients', *Clinical Infectious Diseases*, vol. 27, no. 3, pp. 478–486.

Fowler, V.G. Jr, Miro, J.M., Hoen, B. *et al.* (2005), 'Staphylococcus aureus endocarditis: A consequence of medical progress', *Journal of the American Medical Association*, vol. 293, no. 24, pp. 3012–3021.

Fowler, V.G. Jr, Olsen, M.K., Corey, G.R. *et al.* (2003), 'Clinical identifiers of complicated Staphylococcus aureus bacteraemia', *Archives of Internal Medicine*, vol. 163, no. 17, pp. 2066–2072.

Horvarth, R. and Collignon, P. (2003), 'Controlling intravascular catheter infections', *Australian Prescriber*, vol. 26, no. 2, pp. 41–43.

Karchmer, A.W. (2000), 'Infections of prosthetic valves and intravascular devices', in G.L. Mandell, J.E. Bennett and R. Dolin (eds), *Principles and Practice of Infectious Diseases*, Churchill Livingstone, Philadelphia, pp. 903–917.

Khatib, R., Saeed, S., Sharma, M., Riederer, K., Fakih, M.G. and Johnson, L.B. (2006), 'Impact of initial antibiotic choice and delayed treatment on the outcome of Staphylococcus aureus bacteremia', *European Journal of Clinical Microbiology & Infectious Diseases*, vol. 25, no. 3, pp. 181–185.

Lee, B.K., Crossley, K. and Gerding, D.N. (1978), 'The association between Staphylococcus aureus bacteremia and bacteriuria', *American Journal of Medicine*, vol. 65, no. 2, pp. 303–306.

Li, J.S., Sexton, D.J. and Mick, N. *et al.* (2000), 'Proposed modifications to the Duke criteria for the diagnosis of infective endocarditis', *Clinical Infectious Diseases*, vol. 30, no. 4, pp. 633–638.

MMWR (2002), 'Guidelines for the prevention of intravascular catheter-related infections', at <www.cdc.gov/mmwr/preview/ mmwrhtml/rr5110a1.htm>.

Mourad, O., Palda, V. and Detsky, A.S. (2003), 'A comprehensive evidence-based approach to fever of unknown origin', *Archives of Internal Medicine*, vol. 163, no. 5, pp. 545–551.

Murdoch, D.R., Corey, G.R., Hoen B. *et al.* (2009), 'Clinical presentation, etiology, and outcome of infective endocarditis in the 21st century: The International Collaboration on Endocarditis-Prospective Cohort Study', *Archives of Internal Medicine*, vol. 169, no. 5, pp. 463–473.

Mylonakis, E. and Calderwood, S.B. (2001), 'Infective endocarditis in adults', *New England Journal of Medicine*, vol. 345, no. 18, pp. 1318–1330.

Stein, P.D. *et al.* (2000), 'Fever in acute pulmonary embolism', *Chest*, vol. 117, no. 1, pp. 39–42.

Tornos, P. *et al.* (1999), 'Infective endocarditis due to Staphylococcus aureus: Deleterious effect of anticoagulant therapy', *Archives of Internal Medicine*, vol. 159, no. 5, pp. 473–475.

Chapter 22
Bobby presents with HIV and fever

Scenario

You are in the Emergency Department reading the newspaper. Having successfully managed an elderly woman with NSTEMI and a man with pneumonia, you are feeling calm and in control. Then the emergency registrar taps you on the shoulder. 'There's a young man with fevers in Room 2. Could you please see him?'

You confidently walk into Room 2 thinking of all the likely causes of fevers in a young man.... could it be endocarditis in an injecting drug user, pneumococcal pneumonia or perhaps meningitis? Whatever it is, you know you can handle it.

As you walk into the room, an unwell-looking young man says, 'Hi Doctor. I have had untreated HIV for 10 years. Now I'm losing weight and I have horrible chills. Please help me'. You feel your confidence slipping very quickly.

The patient's name is Bobby. He hands you a letter from a GP in the area.

Dear Doctor,

Re: Bobby X

He is a 35-year-old man who came to my practice last week. He told me that he was diagnosed with HIV 12 years ago. However, he never sought treatment because he was in denial. Now he presents with fevers and deterioration in the past 2 months.

I repeated the HIV ELISA and Western Blot; both were positive. I checked the CD4 count (20) and viral load (>100 000).

I don't see enough HIV patients to feel confident managing Bobby.

Could you please sort him out?

Many thanks,

Dr Wang

Q: Could it really be 12 years between the time of diagnosis and Bobby's present illness?

A: Surprisingly, it could be. It is a common myth that HIV will kill within 1 year. Actually, in most cases untreated HIV will progress to acquired immune deficiency syndrome (AIDS) over 8–12 years. However, there is considerable variation between individuals.

Q: What do you think of a CD4 count of 20?

A: In HIV, depletion of CD4 cells by the virus makes individuals susceptible to opportunistic infections and malignancies. A normal CD4 count in adults is over 500 cells/μL.

Patients with HIV are usually at risk from opportunistic infections when the CD4 count is under 200 cells/μL. In fact, when the CD4 count is under 50/μL, almost any opportunistic process can occur.

With a CD4 count of 20/μL, Bobby is in big trouble.

Q: What is 'Ockham's razor'?

A: William of Ockham was an English philosopher. One of his famous teachings was that if you can explain a situation with a single explanation rather than many, you should do so. This was referred to as his 'razor', apparently because he wielded it sharply!

In medicine, we constantly apply Ockham's razor: it is better to assign a constellation of symptoms and signs to a single diagnosis rather than multiple diagnoses. For example, we would diagnose a patient with central crushing chest pain, shortness of breath and sweating with acute coronary syndrome rather than attributing the chest pain to pericarditis, the shortness of breath to lung fibrosis and the sweating to diabetic autonomic neuropathy.

However, in severely immunocompromised individuals such as those with HIV, Ockham's razor should be tossed into the philosopher's sharps container. Patients like Bobby, with his 20 CD4 cells, can have more than 1 infection and malignancy simultaneously. If you tried to tie all the clinical features down to a single diagnosis in a case like Bobby's, you could miss the presence of another serious disease.

Q: You take a history from Bobby. What do you ask him or any patient with a diagnosis of HIV?

A:

1. When was he diagnosed?
2. What was the mode of transmission (sex, injecting drug use, blood transfusion, needlestick injury or other occupational exposure)?
3. Did he experience a seroconversion illness?[1]

---

[1] This mononucleosis-like syndrome occurs 10–42 days after infection. Typical symptoms include fever, sore throat, headache, rash, lymphadenopathy, arthralgia, diarrhoea and myalgia. However, a wide variety of symptoms have been described.

4. Has he ever been on antiretroviral medications (ARVs) for HIV? If so, which ones and why did he cease them?
5. Has he ever taken medications for prophylaxis of opportunistic infections?
6. What is his current CD4 count and viral load, and what is the lowest the CD4 count and the highest the viral load have been?
7. Has he ever had an opportunistic infection or malignancy?
8. Who is aware of his diagnosis of HIV?[2]
9. Of course, you would also take a complete history in addition to asking the above questions.

Scenario

Bobby tells you that he got HIV after unsafe sex with a number of male partners 12 years ago. He sought medical treatment when he had a febrile illness about 3 weeks after one of these encounters (probably a seroconversion reaction). He was diagnosed with HIV shortly thereafter. However, he didn't want to deal with the disease, so he stayed away from doctors. He has practised safe sex since his diagnosis so he would not put anyone else at risk. Only his partner of 5 years (who is HIV negative) knows of his diagnosis.

He certainly hasn't been on ARVs or prophylactic therapy. In fact, he has been so well that his deterioration has come as a surprise to him. About 5 weeks ago he developed a mild, dry cough and in the past week he has become slightly short of breath on exertion. Additionally, he has experienced sweats and chills in the past 2 weeks. These have been associated with anorexia and lethargy. He has not taken antibiotics.

You examine Bobby and discover the following findings: respiratory rate of 22/minute, heart rate 110/minute, blood pressure 110/60, oxygen saturation on room air of 93%. His temperature is 38 °C. He has a few bibasal crackles, but no other respiratory or cardiac findings. His abdominal and neurological examinations are unremarkable. There is no lymphadenopathy. He has a white lesion on the side of his tongue.

Q: How do you interpret your findings so far?
A: Bobby is febrile, tachycardic and tachypnoeic with bibasal crackles. He most likely has an underlying chest infection.

---

[2]This is very important, as some individuals do not tell anyone their diagnosis, whereas others are happy for all their friends and family to know. Breaching confidentiality accidentally when it comes to HIV can be an extremely distressing situation.

Q: The tongue lesion is likely to be oral hairy leukoplakia (OHL). What organism is responsible for OHL?

A: The Epstein–Barr virus causes OHL.

Q: Is OHL dangerous?

A: Although it is not dangerous in itself, HIV patients with OHL are more likely to progress to AIDS than those who do not have OHL.

Q: What investigations are you going to order to find the cause of Bobby's illness?

A:

1. Full blood count, electrolytes, urea, creatinine and liver function tests
2. CD4 count and HIV viral load (if you feel the hospital laboratory is more reliable than the commercial lab Dr Wang used)
3. blood cultures
4. arterial blood gas
5. cryptococcal antigen
6. Mycobacterium avium complex (MAC) blood cultures[3]
7. chest X-ray
8. sputum culture.

Q: The chest X-ray demonstrates diffuse bilateral alveolar airspace consolidation. The full blood count is unremarkable apart from a lymphopaenia (which most likely reflects HIV-mediated depletion of CD4 cells). The electrolytes and liver function are normal.

The arterial blood gas is as follows: pH: 7.38 PaO_2: 68 mm Hg $PaCO_2$: 40 mm Hg. What is the most likely cause of Bobby's chest infection?

A: Once again, given Bobby's level of immunosuppression, there are a number of possible causes of his chest infection. Nevertheless, the subacute presentation with fevers, the dry cough and minimal chest signs despite marked hypoxia and the chest X-ray changes would all be consistent with Pneumocystis pneumonia (PCP) (due to Pneumocystis jiroveci). You therefore place Bobby on supplemental oxygen.

PCP tends not to be an acute illness. People often insidiously decline over several weeks. The chest X-ray appearance of PCP is variable and can include:

• Perihilar interstitial infiltrates.
• Diffuse alveolar shadowing (which Bobby has). It looks like pulmonary oedema because it is in fact non-cardiogenic pulmonary

---

[3]Both *Cryptococcus* (a yeast) and MAC typically affect HIV patients with a CD4 count under 50/µL.

oedema! (In the past, patients with PCP were mistakenly treated for pulmonary oedema on the basis of the chest X-ray.)

- Pneumothoraces.
- Normal chest X-ray (10% of cases).[4]

Q: Is PCP the most common cause of lower respiratory infections in HIV patients?

A: In fact, pneumococcal (Streptococcus pneumoniae) pneumonia is far more common than PCP in HIV-positive patients. HIV-positive patients have rates of pneumococcal pneumonia that are 5–17 times higher than the general population. The risk of pneumococcal infection increases with CD4 counts < 500/uL but are highest at < 200/uL.

Q: What do you need to find the definitive cause of Bobby's lung pathology?

A: Bobby needs to provide a sputum sample. This is because many patients with PCP (if that is what Bobby has) will not have a productive cough.

An induced sputum specimen is acquired by administering nebulised hypertonic saline to the patient. This stimulates coughing and production of sputum from the lower respiratory tract. Because tuberculosis (TB) is another possible cause of Bobby's lung disease and is highly infectious, the acquisition of induced sputum should be performed using appropriate respiratory precautions.

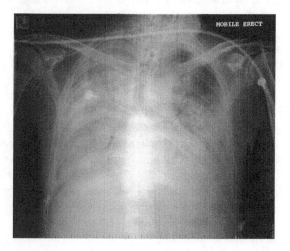

Figure 22.1 Chest X-ray of a man with PCP with diffuse alveolar airspace consolidation

---

[4]A high-resolution CT may identify PCP in patients with a consistent clinical picture who have a normal chest X-ray.

PCP in sputum can be identified through immunofluorescence with monoclonal antibodies and less sensitive staining methods (e.g. silver stains). Polymerase chain reaction (PCR) assays are also used although they might have to be sent away to reference laboratories.

Q: The HIV physiotherapist is able to get Bobby to provide an induced sputum. You order immunofluorescence and staining and PCR for PCP. What other tests will you order on the sputum?

A:

1. Mycobacterial staining and culture (cultures can take up to 8 weeks to become positive)
2. microscopy, culture and sensitivity
3. influenza and parainfluenza testing (hospitals often have a PCR panel of common respiratory viral pathogens that includes influenza)
4. legionella immunofluorescence and cultures

Q: While waiting for the results of the sputum examination, you give Bobby oxygen supplementation. You also realise that you forgot to order a number of screening tests for him. What are they? (The clue here is to think about how Bobby contracted HIV.)

A: Bobby should be screened for other sexually transmitted infections (STIs). He acquired HIV through unprotected sex so it is possible that he contracted other STIs as well.

Syphilis, in particular, bears a close relationship to HIV. The genital ulcer disease of primary syphilis increases the risk of transmission of HIV. Also, the prevalence of 1 disease often mirrors trends in the other (e.g. increasing syphilis numbers in a community often indicate increasing HIV numbers).

You should order the following tests:

1. serology for syphilis, hepatitis A, hepatitis B and hepatitis C
2. urinary PCR for *Neisseria gonorrhoea* and *Chlamydia trachomatis*
3. rectal swab for *N. gonorrhoea*.
4. Other important tests for HIV in general include (Aberg *et al.*, 2014): CMV serology, varicella serology, HIV resistance assay, toxoplasmosis serology, HLA B*5701 assay (assesses the risk of hypersensitivity to an ARV called abacavir), screening for latent TB, EUC and urinalysis (for HIV nephropathy), LFTs, fasting glucose (or HbA1C) and lipids (due to an increased risk of cardiovascular disease).

Q: The immunofluorescence for PCP on the sputum returns positive. What are you going to treat Bobby with?

A: The first-line therapy is cotrimoxazole. (You do not need to know this, but patients with PCP and a PaO_2 under 70 mm Hg should receive corticosteroids, as this improves prognosis. With a PaO_2 of 68 mm Hg, Bobby meets this criterion.)

Q: Bobby is relieved to have a diagnosis and further relieved to hear that treatment is available. He commences cotrimoxazole and prednisone therapy. Although his respiratory symptoms significantly improve over the next 5 days, his high fevers persist. Why isn't the PCP responding?

A: Remember that Ockham's razor does not apply to advanced HIV. More than 1 disease process can be present simultaneously.

Sure enough, the MAC blood cultures become positive. In addition to PCP, Bobby has disseminated MAC infection. Once again, you do not need to know this, but a reasonable treatment regimen for MAC would be clarithromycin and ethambutol plus or minus rifabutin.

Q: Bobby's CD4 count returns on the computer display as $0.02 \times 10^9/L$. What is his CD4 count in more common terms?

A: This can be a bit confusing, as most labs do not display CD4 counts in the familiar '20' or '250' format. However, Bobby's CD4 count is 20. If the figure had been $0.2 \times 10^9/L$, then his CD4 count would have been 200.

Q: Now that his PCP and MAC infections are being successfully addressed, Bobby wants to talk with you. The first question he asks is, 'Do I have AIDS?'

A: AIDS reflects advanced HIV disease. Individuals are given a diagnosis of AIDS if they suffer from an 'AIDS-defining illness'. These illnesses consist of a combination of malignancies, infections and neurologic disorders.

As both PCP and disseminated MAC infections are AIDS-defining conditions, Bobby does have AIDS.

Q: Bobby is very upset. You start reassuring him by telling him about ART. By the way, what is ART?

A: ART refers to 'active antiretroviral therapy'. This is a combination of 3 ARVs that has profoundly changed the prognosis of HIV patients.

In the early days of HIV, when no ARVs or only monotherapy was available, HIV was a disease that people died from. Since the advent of combination therapy and so many different types of ARVs, HIV is a disease that people can live with. Certainly, there are still patients who die from HIV due to the development of resistant strains of the virus or an inability to tolerate the side effects of ARVs, but the overall outlook is much better.

Q: Bobby wants to know what drugs are available for HIV?

A: ARV therapy is a very complex field full of drugs with complicated names and interactions. Do not try to learn about them in detail—you will be overwhelmed. In fact, you will find that very few doctors outside the HIV spectrum have a good knowledge of these agents.

Nevertheless, you should know the 6 broad categories of ARVs:
1. nucleoside reverse transcriptase inhibitors (NRTIs or 'nukes')
2. non-nucleoside reverse transcriptase inhibitors (NNRTIs or 'non-nukes')
3. protease inhibitors (PIs)
4. entry inhibitors
5. fusion inhibitors
6. integrase inhibitors.

All these drugs have a long list of side effects and interactions.

Q: Bobby asks you how you will know if the ARVs are working. What do you tell him?

A: The best way to monitor Bobby's response to therapy is by serial measurement of the CD4 count and HIV viral load. This is usually done regularly in the outpatient setting. The initial goal of ART is to achieve a 1 log reduction in viral load after 4 weeks of ART and have an undetectable viral load after 24 weeks of therapy (Vujovic and Pierce, 2009).

Q: When can he begin treatment?

A: There are different opinions on this topic. In general, however, commence ART in the following circumstances (Antibiotic Expert Group, 2014):
- CD4 count < 500 cells/uL
- the person is at risk of transmitting HIV to others
- pregnancy and HIV
- co-infection with hepatitis B infection that needs treatment
- the presence of an HIV-associated complication irrespective of the CD4 count (e.g. thrombocytopaenia, nephropathy, neurological disease, opportunistic infection).

Q: 'Doctor, I don't want to get this PCP or MAC stuff again. It was awful! What can I do to stop it?'

A: Bobby is asking you about secondary prophylaxis. Secondary prophylaxis refers to preventing repeat infection in patients who have already suffered from the disease. Primary prophylaxis refers to preventing the disease in patients who have never had it.

The table below gives an indication of appropriate primary and secondary prophylaxis for common opportunistic infections. Once his treatment for PCP and MAC has been completed, Bobby will need cotrimoxazole and azithromycin prophylaxis until he meets the cessation criteria set out in the following table.

Infection	Primary prophylaxis	Secondary prophylaxis	Cease prophylaxis	Main agent
Pneumocystis	CD4 < 200	CD4 < 200	CD4 > 200 and > 14% of the total lymphocyte count for over 3 months	Cotrimoxazole
Cryptococcus	No	CD4 < 200	CD4 > 200 for over 6 months	Fluconazole
Toxoplasma	CD4 < 200	CD4 < 200	CD4 > 200 for over 3 months (primary prophylaxis only)	Cotrimoxazole
MAC	CD4 < 50	CD4 < 100	CD4 > 100 for over 3 months (primary prophylaxis) and after 12 months of Rx in those on maintenance Rx	Azithromycin

Source: Adapted from Clezy (2009a, b) and Post (2009a, b).

Scenario

After a week Bobby is almost back to normal. The infectious diseases specialist commences him on ART, in addition to specific MAC and PCP therapy.

Six weeks later, however, Bobby is back in the Emergency Department. He presents with fevers. Examination reveals axillary lymphadenopathy. He assures you that he has been compliant with his therapy, which currently includes azithromycin, cotrimoxazole and 3 ARVs.

Q: What could be the cause of fever and lymphadenopathy at this stage of Bobby's treatment?

A: This is a difficult problem for you to solve! The possibilities are:
- immune restoration disease
- opportunistic infection
- malignancy (in particular lymphoma).

Q: What is immune restoration disease (IRD)?

A: Again, this is an issue you should be aware of without going into too much detail. ART restores the immune response that has been lost to the HIV disease process. This often leads to resolution of current infections and ends the need for prophylaxis. However, the revitalised immune system can harm the individual by causing excessive inflammatory responses. These damaging inflammatory responses are the basis for IRD.

IRD has been described during the treatment of MAC in HIV patients on ART. It can present with fever and lymphadenitis. Therefore, this could be the cause of Bobby's deterioration.

Q: Is lymphoma more common in HIV?

A: Definitely. Non-Hodgkin's lymphoma (NHL) is a staggering 134 times more common in HIV patients than in non-HIV patients. It is usually seen when CD4 is under $150/\mu L$. Hodgkin's lymphoma (HL) is 13 times more likely to occur in HIV patients than in the general population. Other malignancies commonly associated with HIV include Kaposi's sarcoma anal cancer, cervical cancer and possibly lung cancer.

Q: You have a number of possible diagnoses for Bobby's fever and lymphadenopathy. What is the best investigation for finding a cause?

A: A lymph node biopsy, which can be done percutaneously under radiologic guidance, or a complete excisional node biopsy, which can be performed under general anaesthetic.

Q: A percutaneous lymph node biopsy of one of the enlarged axillary nodes is performed under ultrasound guidance. You request histology, immunophenotyping, staining for acid-fast bacilli, fungal and mycobacterial cultures, standard microscopy and culture. Unfortunately, the biopsy result demonstrates a B-cell form of NHL. What do you do next?

A: As with any newly diagnosed malignancy, the lymphoma must be staged.

Q: How do you stage lymphoma?

A: Although it was originally developed for HL, the Ann Arbor system is used for both NHL and HL (adapted from Armitage and Longo, 2002).
- **Stage I:** Involvement of single lymphoid structure or single lymph node region.
- **Stage II:** Involvement of 2 or more lymph node regions on the same side of the diaphragm.

- **Stage III**: Involvement of lymphoid structures or lymph node regions on both sides of the diaphragm.
- **Stage IV**: Involvement of extranodal site(s) beyond localised, solitary involvement of extralymphatic tissue (excluding liver and bone marrow); any involvement of liver or bone marrow; more than 1 extranodal deposit at any location.

Q: What are B symptoms?

A: B symptoms consist of fevers, night sweats and weight loss of more than 10% of the body weight. B symptoms can be applied to staging and they tend to have an adverse effect on prognosis.

Q: What investigations would you use to stage lymphoma?

A:

1. CT chest/abdomen/pelvis
2. PET scan
3. CT or MRI brain
4. lumbar puncture[5]
5. bone marrow biopsy.

Q: The CT, PET scan and bone marrow biopsy demonstrate widespread involvement of the lymphoma, which is finally classified as a diffuse large B-cell lymphoma. Bobby has stage IV of the disease, which is finally classified as a diffuse large B-cell lymphoma (DLBCL). What treatment is available?

A: Due to the success of ART in HIV, the treatment for NHL in HIV is now becoming comparable to therapy of immunocompetent people with regard to toxicity and outcomes (Kaplan, 2012). The options for therapy include (Krishnan, 2009; Ribera *et al.*, 2008):

1. Combination chemotherapy (the regimen you will probably hear about most often is cyclophosphamide, doxorubicin, vincristine and prednisone (CHOP), especially in non-HIV NHL).
   Also, these days, the chemotherapy is often combined with rituximab (an anti-CD20 monoclonal antibody)—so-called 'immunochemotherapy'.
2. Peripheral stem cell transplantation.
3. Radiotherapy for very bulky disease.

---

[5]Almost 30% of NHL in HIV patients are primary central nervous system lymphomas and there is a high incidence of central nervous system involvement with stage IV of the disease. A CT or MRI brain scan and a lumbar puncture are therefore warranted.

Bobby is referred to an oncologist for etoposide, prednisone, vincristine, cyclophosphamide and doxorubicin (dose-adjusted EPOCH) combination chemotherapy + rituximab. You wish him well.

Achievements

You now:
- know that the progression from HIV to AIDS is gradual, over 8–12 years
- know what a normal CD4 count is
- realise that Ockham's razor does not apply to advanced HIV
- can take a thorough history in a patient with HIV
- understand what OHL is and its significance
- know how to recognise, diagnose and treat PCP
- understand the importance of screening for other STIs in a newly diagnosed HIV patient
- know what ART is
- can recognise the various groups of ARVs
- know the indications for commencing ARV therapy
- know indications for primary and secondary prophylaxis for common opportunistic infections in HIV
- understand what immune restoration disease is
- realise how much more common lymphoma is in HIV
- know how to diagnose, stage and treat lymphoma.

References

Aberg, J.A., Gallant, J.E., Ghanem, K.G., Emmanuel, P., Zingman, B.S. and Horberg, M.A. (2014), 'Primary care guidelines for the management of persons infected with HIV: 2013 update by the HIV Medicine Association of the Infectious Diseases Society of America', *Clinical Infectious Diseases*, vol. 58, no. 1, pp. e1–34.

Antibiotic Expert Group (2014), *Therapeutic Guidelines: Antibiotic*, Version 15, Therapeutic Guidelines Ltd, Melbourne.

Armitage, J.O. and Longo, D.L. (2002), 'Malignancies of lymphoid cells', in E. Braunwald, A.S. Fauci, D.L. Kasper, S.L. Hauser, D.L. Longo and J.L. Jameson (eds), *Harrison's Principles of Internal Medicine*, McGraw-Hill, New York, pp. 715–727.

Chipman, M. and Workman, C. (2009a), 'Oncological conditions', in J. Hoy and S. Lewin (eds), *HIV Management in Australasia: A Guide for Clinical Care*, Australasian Society for HIV Medicine Inc., Sydney, pp. 207–216.

Clezy, K. (2009a), 'Cryptococcosis', in J. Hoy and S. Lewin (eds), *HIV Management in Australasia: A Guide for Clinical Care*, Australasian Society for HIV Medicine Inc., Sydney, pp. 156–158.

Clezy, K. (2009b), 'Toxoplasmosis', in J. Hoy and S. Lewin (eds), *HIV Management in Australasia: A Guide for Clinical Care*, Australasian Society for HIV Medicine Inc., Sydney, pp. 154–155.

Gazzard, B.G. and BHIVA Treatment Guidelines Writing Group (2008), 'British HIV Association Guidelines for the treatment of HIV-1-infected adults with antiretroviral therapy 2008', *HIV Medicine*, vol. 9, no. 8, pp. 563–608.

Kaplan, L.D. (2012), 'HIV-associated lymphoma', Best Practice & Research, *Clinical Haematology*, vol. 25, no. 1, pp. 101–117.

Kelly, M. (2009), 'Immune restoration disease', in J. Hoy and S. Lewin (eds), *HIV Management in Australasia: A Guide for Clinical Care*, Australasian Society for HIV Medicine Inc., Sydney, pp. 287–294.

Krishnan, A. (2009), 'Stem cell transplantation in HIV-infected patients', *Current Opinion in HIV and AIDS*, vol. 4, no. 1, pp. 11–15.

Pett, S. and Pierce, A. (2009), 'Antiretroviral therapy', in J. Hoy and S. Lewin (eds), *HIV Management in Australasia: A Guide for Clinical Care*, Australasian Society for HIV Medicine Inc., Sydney, pp. 59–72.

Post, J.J. (2009a), 'Mycobacterium avium complex', in J. Hoy and S. Lewin (eds), *HIV Management in Australasia: A Guide for Clinical Care*, Australasian Society for HIV Medicine Inc., Sydney, pp. 145–148.

Post, J.J. (2009b), 'Pneumocystis carinii', in J. Hoy and S. Lewin (eds), *HIV Management in Australasia: A Guide for Clinical Care*, Australasian Society for HIV Medicine Inc., Sydney, pp. 133–137.

Ribera, J.M., Oriol, A., Morgades, M. *et al.* (2008), 'Safety and efficacy of cyclophosphamide, adriamycin, vincristine, prednisone and rituximab in patients with human immunodeficiency virus-associated diffuse large B-cell lymphoma: Results of a phase II trial', *British Journal of Haematology*, vol. 140, no. 4, pp. 411–419.

Sonnenberg, A. (2001), 'When William of Ockham meets Thomas Bayes: Finding a few diagnoses among a great many symptoms', *Alimentary Pharmacology & Therapeutics*, vol. 15, no. 9, pp. 1403–1407.

Vujovic, O. (2009), 'Initiation of antiretroviral therapy in the naïve patient', in J. Hoy and S. Lewin (eds), *HIV Management in Australasia: A Guide for Clinical Care*, Australasian Society for HIV Medicine Inc., Sydney, pp. 77–92.

Vujovic, O. and Pierce, A. (2009), 'Managing the patient on antiretroviral therapy', in J. Hoy and S. Lewin (eds), *HIV Management in Australasia: A Guide for Clinical Care*, Australasian Society for HIV Medicine Inc., Sydney, pp. 93–102.

Woolley, I. and Workman, C. (2009b), 'Respiratory infections', in J. Hoy and S. Lewin (eds), *HIV Management in Australasia: A Guide for Clinical Care*, Australasian Society for HIV Medicine Inc., Sydney, pp. 176–179.

Chapter 23
Sachin presents with fever and headache

Scenario

A young man is sent in by his local doctor with headache and fever.

Dear Doctor,

Sachin Dravid is a 24-year-old bank clerk. He has been unwell for the past 48 hours with fevers and a headache. I am concerned about meningitis. I was going to prescribe antibiotics but thought it better to send him to you first.

Please assess.

Regards,

Dr Rex Riviera MD

Sachin looks unwell and is wearing sunglasses. He tells you that he has never seen a doctor in his life, apart from when he had 1 or 2 minor cricketing injuries. Two days ago, he woke up feeling quite tired. He had no appetite. As the day progressed, he started to experience chills and sweats. Last night, he developed a severe bifrontal headache. Today he found that he cannot tolerate bright light (hence the sunglasses) and that his headache has worsened in severity. He denies any upper respiratory tract symptoms.

Sachin has lived in Perth all his life and has never been outside Western Australia. He denies known contact with anyone with TB.

A physical examination reveals a tachycardia, high fever and neck stiffness. There is no rash and there are no focal neurological signs. Sachin is completely oriented. The ears and throat are normal and the sinuses nontender. The remainder of the examination is normal.

Q: What is your provisional diagnosis?
A: The fevers, headache, photophobia and neck stiffness are all consistent with acute meningitis.

Q: How will you investigate Sachin?

A: The most critical test is a lumbar puncture (LP) to examine the cerebrospinal fluid (CSF). Other investigations include:

- blood cultures (2 sets taken at different times from different sites)—although a LP is the gold standard investigation for meningitis, blood cultures can be very valuable and should be taken within 30 minutes of first seeing the patient (Antibiotic Expert Group, 2014)
- full blood count
- electrolytes, urea, creatinine
- blood sugar
- liver function tests
- coagulation studies[1]
- meningococcal polymerase chain reaction on blood
- chest X-ray (pneumococcal meningitis may be associated with pneumonia; sometimes, atypical pneumonia may present with symptoms of meningitis and a normal LP).

Q: Why would you order a blood sugar level in suspected acute meningitis?

A: An indicator of bacterial meningitis is a low CSF/serum glucose ratio. Therefore, serum and CSF glucose levels must be ordered.

Q: Martin, one of the medical students, asks you if Sachin needs a CT brain scan before an LP. What do you tell him?

A: Martin has raised a relevant issue. Herniation (or 'coning') is one of the risks of an LP in the presence of raised intracranial pressure.

CT brain scans are used to identify patients with raised intracranial pressure. However, the scans have limitations, as a normal result does not exclude raised intracranial pressure.

In practical terms, an alert patient without focal neurological signs or papilloedema should not require a CT brain scan before an LP.

A study by Hasbun et al. (2001) found that patients with suspected meningitis were unlikely to have an abnormal CT brain scan if the following baseline characteristics were absent:

- age at least 60 years
- immunocompromised state
- history of a central nervous system disease
- seizure within 1 week of presentation
- abnormal level of consciousness
- inability to follow 2 consecutive commands correctly

---

[1]A full blood count, electrolytes, urea, creatinine, liver function tests and coagulation studies are useful baseline markers, but will not assist you with diagnosis.

- gaze palsy
- abnormal visual fields
- facial palsy
- arm drift
- leg drift
- abnormal language.

If a patient has any of these features, they should undergo a CT brain scan. If the CT brain scan does not show any gross evidence of raised intracranial pressure, then it is safe to proceed to a LP (Tunkel *et al.*, 2004). (But still, speak to a more senior doctor first.)

Q: Sachin is oriented and has no papilloedema or focal neurological signs. You feel that he is unlikely to be at risk of herniation. Why do you want to do an LP?

A: In this situation, an LP will:

- confirm whether or not Sachin has meningitis
- distinguish between viral and bacterial meningitis
- allow you to find the causative agent and focus antibiotic therapy on the organism. Otherwise, you will have to use broad-spectrum antibiotic therapy, which is more extensive and carries risks of adverse drug reactions and resistance.

However, if a patient looks extremely unwell (haemodynamically or neurologically unstable) you may have to commence antimicrobial therapy before the CT brain scan or LP. This will reduce the chances of identifying the causative organism, but this is still a better outcome than death! Remember that there are always more senior staff available with whom you can discuss this issue.

Q: How will you use the LP to distinguish between viral and bacterial meningitis?

A:

	Normal range	Bacterial	Viral
CSF pressure	<30 mm H_2O	Raised	Normal
Colour	Clear	Sometimes turbid	Clear
Cell count	<5 × 10^6/L	Increased	Increased
	Normal range	Bacterial	Viral
Differential	L (60–70%), M (30–50%), no N	N predominance	L predominance
Protein	0.15–0.45 g/L	Increased a lot	Normal or slight increase

	Normal range	Bacterial	Viral
CSF/serum glucose ratio	>60%	Reduced	Normal or slight increase
Gram stain		Sometimes positive	Negative

L = lymphocytes, M = monocytes, N = neutrophils.
Source: Adapted from Beaman and Wesselingh (2002).

However, you should be aware that:

- 3% of cases of bacterial meningitis have a normal CSF on presentation
- viral meningitis may have a neutrophil predominance in CSF before the lymphocytic pleocytosis
- *Listeria monocytogenes* (a bacterium) may be associated with a lymphocytic predominance in CSF.

Q: What other tests (not included in the preceding table) would you order on the CSF?

A:

1. **Culture and sensitivities.**
2. **Meningococcal polymerase chain reaction (PCR)** (if available, can be very useful if antibiotics were given prior to the LP).
3. *Streptococcus pneumoniae* antigen.
4. **PCR for common viral causes of meningitis (enterovirus, herpes simplex virus and varicella zoster virus).**

Most LP kits will come with 3 small bottles for CSF specimens. Please use all 3 bottles.

And note ...

Patients with a travel or contact history that might put them at risk of exposure to tuberculosis should undergo Ziehl–Neelsen staining, TB PCR and mycobacterial cultures of CSF.

Q: What are the most common causes of viral meningitis?

A: Enteroviruses (85–95%) are by far the most common cause. Other herpes viruses (e.g. herpes simplex virus 1 and 2, varicella zoster virus, cytomegalovirus, Epstein–Barr virus, human herpes virus 6–8) and HIV are less common causes.

Q: What are the most common causes of bacterial meningitis?

A: The triad of encapsulated bacteria (*Streptococcus pneumoniae, Neisseria meningitidis* and *Haemophilus influenzae* type b[2]) account for 80% of cases.

In neonates, *Escherichia coli* and group B streptococci are important causes.

The CSF is turbid and the opening pressure is 32 mm H_2O. You send the CSF off to the lab.

And note ...

Most pathology laboratories in Australia will process CSF as a matter of urgency. Nevertheless, you should always call and warn the lab of the impending arrival of CSF so it can be processed quickly. Give your name and ask to be called in the Emergency Department with the result. The results of the protein, glucose, cell count and differential and Gram stain should be available within 60 minutes.

Q: The medical registrar tells you to commence empirical antibiotic therapy. What therapy are you going to initiate?

A: Sachin has no antibiotic allergies. Therefore, you will commence a third-generation cephalosporin (Antibiotic Expert Group, 2014):

- ceftriaxone (4 g daily or 2 g q12h) OR
- cefotaxime 2 g q6h.

(A third-generation cephalosporin in Australia will cover *N. meningitidis, H. influenzae* and most strains of *S. pneumoniae*.)

Q: You ask the registrar whether the ceftriaxone will cover *Listeria monocytogenes*. What does he say?

A: *Listeria* is resistant to cephalosporins. If you want to cover the organism, then use benzylpenicillin 2.4 g q4h IV; however, you don't have to cover *Listeria* unless the patient (Antibiotic Expert Group, 2014):

- is immunocompromised
- is aged over 50 years
- uses alcohol heavily
- is pregnant
- is debilitated.

In Sachin, it would be reasonable not to cover *Listeria* as he is an otherwise healthy young man.

---

[2]*Haemophilus influenzae* type b meningitis has become extremely uncommon due to the introduction of a vaccination program.

Q: The registrar gets called away to a MET. As he rushes off, he shouts back to you, 'Don't forget the roids!' What is he talking about?

A: He is referring to corticosteroids, specifically dexamethasone, which should be given BEFORE or WITH the first dose of IV antibiotic. The rationale behind this is that it is thought that the inflammatory response to the meningitis, especially to bacterial products released from dead organisms, is itself highly detrimental to the patient, hence the recommendation to use an agent that dampens the inflammatory response. The standard dose is dexamethasone 10mg q6h IV for 4 days. If the cause of the meningitis ends up being listeria, then there is no role for corticosteroids and they can be ceased (Antibiotic Expert Group, 2014).

Q: The lab calls you. The CSF shows the following:
- protein: 1.2 g/L
- CSF glucose 2.0 mM/serum glucose 6.0 mM = ratio of 0.3
- cell count: 200 red blood cells, 300 white cells $\times$ 10^6/L (90% neutrophils)
- Gram stain: Gram-positive diplococci

What do you conclude?

A: Sachin has turbid CSF with raised CSF pressure, elevated CSF protein and neutrophils and reduced CSF/serum glucose ratio. These results are consistent with acute bacterial meningitis. The presence of Gram-positive diplococci mean that the likely cause is pneumococcus (*S. pneumoniae*); until sensitivities are available, you add IV vancomycin to the ceftriaxone and dexamethasone (give a loading dose of vancomycin of 25–30 mg/kg and 12 hours later, commence 15–20 mg/kg q12h).

Q: Why do you add vancomycin?

A: If pneumococcal meningitis is confirmed or strongly suspected (e.g. presence of sinusitis, otitis media, Gram-positive diplococci in CSF), then vancomycin should be added until sensitivities are available due to the presence of beta-lactam resistance (Antibiotic Expert Group, 2014), although this is much less of an issue in Australia compared to some other parts of the world.

Q: Martin says, 'But there are red cells in the CSF because it is a traumatic tap. Therefore, the white cells in the CSF just reflect contamination with blood. He doesn't have meningitis'. How do you respond to this?

A: Martin is referring to a 'traumatic tap'. If a blood vessel is damaged while performing the LP, blood can contaminate the CSF. Hence both red and white blood cells will appear in the CSF although, in truth, they are from blood.

Nevertheless, there is a way of determining whether the white cells are mainly from the CSF or the blood. It involves simple mathematics. Examine Sachin's full blood count. Look at the white cell count and the red cell count (not the haemoglobin):

White cell count: $12 \times 10^9/L$ (normal range: $3.5-11 \times 10^9/L$)

Red cell count: $6 \times 10^{12}/L$ (normal range: $4.5-6.5 \times 10^{12}/L$)

The ratio of white cells : red cells $= 12/6 \times 10^3 = 1/500$

In other words, in the peripheral blood there is 1 white cell for every 500 red cells.

Now look at the CSF white cell : red cell ratio for Sachin.

White cell : red cell ratio in CSF for Sachin $= 300 : 200 = 3 : 2$

In other words, in the CSF, there are 3 white cells for every 2 red cells.

This ratio is much higher than Sachin's white cell to red cell ratio in the peripheral blood (3 : 2 versus 1 : 500). Therefore, you can conclude that the white cells in the LP are from the CSF and not just blood. You can still say that this result supports your diagnosis of meningitis.

It is worth knowing this because during your career you will encounter many traumatic taps with mixtures of red and white cells. (Of course, there are occasions when red blood cells from a LP actually do arise from the CSF; e.g. subarachnoid haemorrhage.)

Martin is awestruck by your 'intern brain'.

Q: Sachin starts to improve within 24 hours of therapy. At this stage, the CSF cultures grow *S. pneumoniae*. You are therefore satisfied with your empirical therapy. Martin asks whether the public health unit (PHU) needs to be notified about pneumococcal meningitis.

A: Yes. Invasive pneumococcal disease, meningococcal and *Listeria* infections (including meningitis) are notifiable diseases in Australia. The hospital switchboard will be able to connect you to the on-call staff at the PHU. (See Chapter 24 for more information about notifying meningococcal disease to the public health unit.)

Q: What is the likely source of Sachin's pneumococcal infection?

A: One study examined the source of pneumococcal meningitis cases (Ostergaard *et al.*, 2005). They found that 42% of cases had no obvious focus. In the remainder they found 30% with an otogenic focus, 18% with a pulmonary focus, 8% with sinusitis and 2% miscellaneous foci. Therefore, examine Sachin's middle ear, sinuses and lungs for a focus of pneumococcal disease outside the meninges as this may require surgical intervention or a longer duration of antibiotics.

Q: Can you narrow your antibiotic therapy?

A: Yes. Unfortunately, penicillin-resistant *S. pneumoniae* has become a problem in Australia. You therefore need to wait until the lab has tested the minimum inhibitory concentration (MIC) for the organism. If the MIC is under 0.125 mg/L, benzylpenicillin monotherapy is indicated. If the MIC is over 0.125 mg/L, treat with a third-generation cephalosporin and vancomycin.

Q: Martin looks puzzled as you explain this to him. 'I thought that *S. pneumoniae* was sensitive to penicillin when the MIC is under or equal to 1 mg/L, not under 0.125 mg/L.' Is Martin right or are you?

A: Actually, you both are. Martin is referring to the MIC of *S. pneumoniae* in community-acquired pneumonia. The reason the same organism has different MICs for 2 different conditions is related to the penetration of antibiotics across the blood–brain barrier.

The MIC for *S. pneumoniae* turns out to be < 0.125 mg/L. Therefore, Sachin continues on 10 days of IV benzylpenicillin monotherapy. He improves day by day, and is discharged after 11 days of IV antibiotics.

Q: Sachin has completely recovered from this bout of pneumococcal meningitis. Is everyone so lucky?

A: Beware the leading question! In truth, pneumococcal meningitis is a very nasty infection. It has case fatality rates of 16–37% during hospitalisation with 29–72% of survivors left with neurological sequelae (such as cranial nerve palsies [16–28%] and hearing loss [14–30%] or other focal deficits [22–44%]) (Weisfelt *et al.*, 2006).

Achievements

You now:
- know what blood tests should be performed in suspected acute meningitis
- understand why a head CT may need to be performed prior to an LP
- know why an LP is a useful test in suspected meningitis
- know what tests to order on CSF
- can detect white cell contamination of CSF using blood and CSF white/red cell ratios
- know the most common causes of viral and bacterial meningitis in Australia
- realise that you should get the lab to call you with initial CSF results
- know empirical antibiotic therapy for bacterial meningitis
- know the role of steroids in adults with bacterial meningitis

- know that invasive pneumococcal disease, *Listeria* and meningococcal meningitis are notifiable diseases
- understand how MICs dictate antibiotic therapy for *S. pneumoniae* infection
- appreciate what a dangerous infection pneumococcal meningitis is.

References

Antibiotic Expert Group (2014), *Therapeutic Guidelines: Antibiotic*, Version 15, Therapeutic Guidelines Ltd, Melbourne.

Beaman, M.H. and Wesselingh, S.L. (2002), '4: Acute community-acquired meningitis and encephalitis', *Medical Journal of Australia*, vol. 176, no. 8, pp. 389–396.

Hasbun, R. *et al.* (2001), 'Computed tomography of the head before lumbar puncture in adults with suspected meningitis', *New England Journal of Medicine*, vol. 345, no. 24, pp. 1727–1733.

Ostergaard, C., Konradsen, H.B. and Samuelsson, S. (2005), 'Clinical presentation and prognostic factors of Streptococcus pneumoniae meningitis according to the focus of infection', *BMC Infectious Diseases*, vol. 5, p. 93.

Tunkel, A.R., Hartman, B.J., Kaplan, S.L. *et al.* (2004), 'Practice guidelines for the management of bacterial meningitis', *Clinical Infectious Diseases*, vol. 39, no. 9, pp. 1267–1284.

Weisfelt, M., de Gans, J., van der Poll, T. *et al.* (2006), 'Pneumococcal meningitis in adults: New approaches to management and prevention,' *Lancet Neurology*, vol. 5, no. 4, pp. 332–342.

Chapter 24
Jean-Paul presents with fever and a rash

Scenario

You are near the end of a 15-hour shift. You pick up the final patient card for the day. It is a 30-year-old French tourist with a fever and rash.

Jean-Paul is an otherwise healthy schoolteacher from Paris. He takes no regular medications and has no known allergies. He arrived in Melbourne 2 weeks ago and is staying with a cousin and his family. His cousin has a wife and a 3-year-old son. Jean-Paul has not left Melbourne apart from 2 day trips outside the city.

He was well until 2 days ago, when he developed a sore throat. Yesterday he developed generalised muscle aches and lost his appetite. He slept poorly last night due to drenching sweats. Today, he has been feeling 'hot and cold'. About 3 hours ago, he developed pain in his left knee. It was then that he and his family decided to bring him to hospital. He denies all other focal symptoms of infection. He has not had sexual intercourse for 8 months and always practises safe sex.

On examination, Jean-Paul looks quite well. He is alert, but a bit flushed. His temperature is 38.6 °C and he is tachycardic at 110 regular beats/minute. The most striking abnormality, however, is a symmetrical rash on his lower limbs and lower abdominal wall. He also has a tender left knee with an effusion and a limited range of movement. The remainder of the cardiovascular, neurological, rheumatological and respiratory examination is normal.

The purpuric rash is typically seen with meningococcal infection (due to *Neisseria meningitidis*). It does not blanche with pressure, as would a viral rash.

Q: Amelia, one of the medical students allocated to the Emergency Department, looks at Jean-Paul and says: 'This can't be meningococcal infection. Sure, the rash is typical, but he doesn't look like he's about to die, which I would expect with meningococcal infection. And he doesn't have meningitis. It has to be something else'.
Do you agree with Amelia's statement?

A: No. However, these are common misconceptions among medical students.

Meningococcal infection is a serious disease. The mortality rate is approximately 9% in microbiologically confirmed disease in Australia. Even so, some patients with meningococcal disease may present to medical attention with only a very mild illness. The natural history of patients with mild meningococcal disease is either that it gradually resolves without antibiotic treatment, or it worsens. It is not easy to identify a mild case, but do not dismiss a diagnosis of meningococcal infection simply because a patient looks well when other clinical features would support this diagnosis.

The other common misconception Amelia has voiced is that meningococcal infection only causes meningitis. This is understandable given the name of the organism and its similarity to the word 'meningitis'. Again, however, there are a number of clinical presentations of meningococcal disease that do not involve meningitis. The most common meningococcal syndromes you are likely to encounter are:

- meningitis
- septicaemia with a rash
- septicaemia without a rash.

Even the characteristic rash of meningococcal infection does not have to be purpuric. In the early stages of infection it may simply be maculopapular. You should therefore keep an open mind when it comes to diagnosing meningococcal infection.

Q: Amelia again questions Jean-Paul's illness: 'Would you expect someone with meningococcal infection to develop a sore throat and an acute monoarthritis of the knee?'

A: Yes, it is quite possible. Remember that some people are chronic, asymptomatic carriers of *N. meningitidis*. These people can transmit the organism through respiratory droplets to the nasopharynx of close contacts. As a result, the primary site of invasion of *N. meningitidis* into the bloodstream is usually the nasopharynx. This is why patients with invasive meningococcal disease often complain of a sore throat.

Acute arthritis is also a well-recognised clinical feature of meningococcal infection. The 2 types are:

1. septic arthritis secondary to infection of the joint that occurs early in the infection
2. immune-complex-mediated arthritis that occurs later, in the convalescent phase of disease.

You convince Amelia that Jean-Paul's clinical presentation (fever, myalgias, sore throat, monoarthritis, purpuric rash) could be consistent with meningococcal disease, despite the fact that he looks quite well.

Q: How will you investigate Jean-Paul?

A:

1. Blood cultures (2 sets taken at different times from different sites)
2. aspirate of synovial fluid from the left knee
3. chest X-ray
4. midstream urine
5. full blood count, electrolytes, urea, creatinine and liver function tests.[1]

A polymerase chain reaction [PCR] assay is available for meningococcus. Munro (2002) notes that it is fairly sensitive and specific on cerebrospinal fluid (CSF) (89% and 100%, respectively) and blood (62–76% and 99–100%, respectively).

Q: Amelia has heard that there is a serological test for invasive meningococcal disease. Is there such a test?

A: Yes. An immunoglobulin M (IgM) directed against the outer membrane protein of the organism can be used to diagnose invasive meningococcal disease.

Diagnosis is based on:

- a rise in IgM titres between acute and convalescent samples OR
- a single IgM specimen with a significantly high titre.

In adults, and in children more than 4 years old, the test is very sensitive (97%) and specific (93%). In day-to-day practice, however, serology would rarely be ordered.

Q: What tests will you order on the synovial aspirate from the left knee?

A:

1. White cell count
2. Gram stain
3. culture
4. crystal examination (although Jean-Paul's whole presentation is unlikely to be due to gout or pseudogout, his overall acute illness may have precipitated gout or pseudogout in his left knee).

Q: Should you wait until you have microbiological confirmation of meningococcal disease before treating Jean-Paul?

A: In reality, it might take 48–72 hours for synovial fluid and blood cultures to become positive. If Jean-Paul does have invasive meningococcal disease, he could die if he remains untreated for this length of time, even

---

[1]You would order blood cultures, chest X-ray, midstream urine and full blood count, electrolytes, urea, creatinine and liver function tests in any febrile patient.

though he looks well now. He should therefore commence antibiotic therapy.

Q: What antibiotic therapy would you prescribe for Jean-Paul to specifically target meningococcus?

A: Five days of IV therapy with benzylpenicillin (1.8 g q4h) or a third-generation cephalosporin such as ceftriaxone (2 g q12h or 4 g daily) or cefotaxime (2 g q6h) would be fine for an adult. Ciprofloxacin can be used if there is a history of type 1 hypersensitivity to penicillin (Antibiotic Expert Group, 2014).

Q: The laboratory calls you 1 hour later: the Gram stain of the synovial fluid demonstrates numerous Gram-negative diplococci. What does this mean?

A: Meningococcus is a Gram-negative diplococcus, so it merely strengthens your diagnosis of meningococcal infection.

The other well-known Gram-negative diplococcus is *Neisseria gonorrhoeae*.

Q: Now that you are more confident of your diagnosis, you can treat Jean-Paul for meningococcal infection. What will you prescribe?

A: IV benzylpenicillin[2] or third-generation cephalosporins (cefotaxime/ceftriaxone) are the best choices. Penicillin, however, will treat only the invasive aspect of the infection. It will not eradicate nasopharyngeal carriage. Jean-Paul will need another antibiotic for that. On the other hand, cefotaxime or ceftriaxone will eradicate both the invasive disease and the nasopharyngeal disease.

Q: Is there anyone else you could consult about the acute monoarthritis in Jean-Paul's right knee?

A: You should consult the orthopaedic team about the need for surgical washout of the joint, as antibiotic therapy alone may not be adequate.

Q: You decide to commence Jean-Paul on IV ceftriaxone 1 g daily. The orthopaedic registrar takes him to theatre to wash out his left knee. Apart from hospital staff, who else needs to know about Jean-Paul's diagnosis and why?

A: In Australia, meningococcal infection is a notifiable disease. Therefore, the public health unit must be alerted. They will take on the responsibility of 'contact tracing'.

---

[2]Although we have meningococcal organisms in Australia with a reduced susceptibility to penicillin, they are *not* resistant to it.

Q: What does this mean?

A: Contact tracing involves trying to identify rapidly close contacts of the index case (here, Jean-Paul) because they may have been infected (or passed the infection on). The close contacts might have nasopharyngeal carriage of meningococcus. Two common examples of close contacts are household and sexual contacts. In fact, those at highest risk of infection are household contacts. Although the estimated risk to household contacts of meningococcal disease is only 0.4%, this is still up to 800 times higher than in the general population (Meningococcal Disease Surveillance Group, 1976).

Once close contacts have been identified, the public health team will administer antibiotic prophylaxis to them to eradicate nasopharyngeal carriage. It should be emphasised that prophylaxis will only eradicate nasopharyngeal carriage; it will not treat invasive disease. Post-exposure prophylaxis should be performed as soon as possible, preferably within 2 weeks of exposure, after which the risk of invasive disease becomes extremely low (Campsall *et al.*, 2013).

Q: Which antibiotics can be given as prophylaxis?

A: There are 3 choices:
- rifampicin (4 doses over 2 days)
- ciprofloxacin (1 dose)
- ceftriaxone (1 dose).

Q: Forty-eight hours later, the microbiology lab calls to say that Jean-Paul's blood cultures are growing Gram-negative diplococci. They have also confirmed that the Gram-negative diplococcus from his left knee is indeed *N. meningitidis*, serogroup C.

What are meningococcal serogroups?

A: There are approximately 13 serogroups, which are classified according to the capsular polysaccharide of the organism, of which five are responsible for most illnesses: A, B, C, W135 and Y.

In Australia, there has been a decline in notified cases with only 241 cases in 2011. Most are serogroup B (179/241) (Lahra and Enriquez, 2011); however, serogroup C appears to be associated with a higher mortality rate.

Q: Jean-Paul receives IV ceftriaxone and rapidly improves. He is shocked and asks how this could have happened to him. What are the risk factors for meningococcal disease?

A: There are host factors and environmental factors (Campsall *et al.*, 2013; Baccarini *et al.*, 2013).

Host factors include hyposplenism, HIV, late complement deficiencies and recent upper respiratory tract infection.

Environmental factors include smoking (active or passive) and crowded conditions (e.g. dormitories, nightclubs).

Q: Jean-Paul admits to going nightclubbing for a number of consecutive nights in Melbourne following his arrival. 'The air of the clubs was thick with smoke. Maybe that's how I got it. But I would have had to have met someone carrying the bug. It can't be that common?'

A: Actually, nasopharyngeal carriage of meningococcus is common. Overall, the figure is about 10% but it reaches as high as 24% in adolescence (Campsall *et al.*, 2013).

Q: One of the nurses asks if there is a vaccine for meningococcal disease. What do you tell him?

A: There are a number of conjugate and polysaccharide vaccines for meningococcus, which up until recently covered A, C, W135 and Y. Now, a fairly broad vaccine against the B serogroup (the dominant one in Australia) has been developed, which will target three-quarters of differing strains of the B serogroup in Australia (ATAGI, 2014; ATAGI, 2013).

Since invasive meningococcal infections don't induce immunity against subsequent infections with the same serogroup, it would be reasonable to offer Jean-Paul immunisation in the near future (ATAGI, 2013).

Achievements

You now:
- recognise the characteristic rash of invasive meningococcal disease
- understand that meningitis is only one of the presentations of invasive meningococcal disease
- realise that patients with invasive meningococcal disease do not have to look extremely sick, especially soon after infection
- know that septic arthritis can occur early in invasive meningococcal disease
- know that immune complex-mediated arthritis can occur in the convalescent phase
- can order the appropriate investigations for invasive meningococcal disease
- understand the role of serology in the diagnosis of invasive meningococcal disease

- know the investigations to order on synovial fluid in a suspected septic arthritis
- understand which antibiotics can be used to treat invasive meningococcal disease
- realise the limitation of penicillin in the eradication of nasopharyngeal carriage
- understand the important adjunctive role of orthopaedic surgery in septic arthritis
- know to inform the public health unit early on in cases of invasive meningococcal disease for the purposes of contact tracing
- know which medications can be used for prophylaxis against meningococcal carriage
- have a basic understanding of what serogroups of meningococcus are.

References

Antibiotic Expert Group (2014), *Therapeutic Guidelines: Antibiotic*, Version 15, Therapeutic Guidelines Ltd, Melbourne.

Australian Technical Advisory Group on Immunisation (ATAGI) (2014), 'Advice for immunisation providers regarding the use of Bexsero – a recombinant multicomponent meningococcal B vaccine (4CMenB)', Australian Government Department of Health, Canberra, at <www.immunise.health. gov.au/internet/immunise/publishing.nsf/Content/85A6879534C02B4DCA 257B640002F38E/$File/ATAGI-advice-bexsero.pdf>, accessed 23 November 2014.

Australian Technical Advisory Group on Immunisation (ATAGI), (2013), *The Australian Immunisation Handbook*, 10th ed., Australian Government Department of Health, Canberra.

Baccarini, C., Ternouth, A., Wieffer, H. and Vyse, A. (2013), 'The changing epidemiology of meningococcal disease in North America 1945–2010', *Human Vaccines & Immunotherapeutics*, vol. 9, no. 1, pp. 162–171.

Campsall, P.A., Laupland, K.B. and Niven, D.J. (2013), 'Severe meningococcal infection', *Critical Care Clinics*, vol. 29, no. 3, pp. 393–409.

Lahra, M.M. and Enriquez, R.P. (2011), 'Annual report of the Australian Meningococcal Surveillance Programme, 2011', *Communicable Disease Intelligence*, vol. 36, no. 3, pp. E251–E262.

Meningococcal Disease Surveillance Group (1976), 'Analysis of endemic meningococcal disease by serogroup and evaluation of chemoprophylaxis', *Journal of Infectious Diseases*, vol. 134, no. 2, pp. 201–204.

Munro, R. (2002), 'Meningococcal disease: Treatable but still terrifying', *Internal Medicine Journal*, vol. 32, no. 4, pp. 165–169.

Chapter 25
Ruby presents with fever and cough

Scenario

Ruby is a 54-year-old woman. She is sent to hospital by her local doctor with the following letter:

Dear Doctor,

Thank you for seeing Ruby, an Indigenous lady with fevers and a cough. I am concerned that she may have pneumonia. She has smoked a packet of cigarettes a day for 30 years. Ruby also has a poor record of complying with medications.

Regards,

Dr Verdi

You take a history from Ruby. She has been feeling unwell for the past 3 days. Initially she just felt tired, but then she started having sweats at night. Her appetite has disappeared. Yesterday she began to cough and last night she was producing small amounts of yellow sputum. She has been shivering the whole of today and producing more sputum. This afternoon she noticed left-sided chest pain. The pain is worse on inspiration and sharp in nature. Ruby has been in Canberra all her life and hasn't been away for years.

The fevers, constitutional symptoms, productive cough and pleuritic chest pain are consistent with community-acquired pneumonia (CAP).

Q: If Ruby does have CAP, what are the likely causes?
A: An Australian study by Johnson *et al.* (2002) examined the most common causes of CAP. These were:
- *Streptococcus pneumoniae* (42%)
- respiratory viruses (18%)
- *Haemophilus influenzae* (9%)
- *Mycoplasma pneumoniae* (8%)
- enteric Gram-negative bacteria (8%)
- *Chlamydia psittaci* (5%)
- *Staphylococcus aureus* (3%)

- *Legionella* (3%)
- *Mycobacterium tuberculosis* (3%).

In tropical Australia, other important causes of CAP include melioidosis (*Burkholderia pseudomallei*) and *Acinetobacter baumanii*. The consideration of these organisms will lead to a different antibiotic combination being used (e.g. ceftriaxone and gentamicin and doxycycline instead of benzylpenicillin and doxycycline) (Antibiotic Expert Group, 2014).

Q: What factors make *Legionella* or *C. psittaci* more likely causes of CAP in a patient?

A: Close contact with birds is a risk factor for psittacosis. The use of potting mixes is a risk factor (*Legionella longbeachae*, but not *Legionella pneumophila*). *Legionella* is also more likely in immunosuppressed hosts or those with underlying lung disease.

Q: You proceed to examine Ruby. She can talk freely but is tachypnoeic at 28 breaths/minute. She is tachycardic (110/minute and regular) with a blood pressure of 120/70. Her temperature is 38.8 °C. Her oxygen saturation is 93% on room air. She is not cyanosed. She has reduced chest expansion on the left with a dull percussion note at the left base. The breath sounds in the left base are of reduced intensity and are bronchial. Vocal resonance is increased over the left base. The remainder of the physical examination is normal.
What do you conclude from the examination?

A: Ruby has signs consistent with left lower lobe consolidation.

Q: Does Ruby have any risk factors that increase the risk for CAP?

A: The risk factors for CAP include:
- age over 50
- alcoholism
- Indigenous background
- smoking
- institutionalisation
- COPD
- asthma
- dementia
- heart failure
- immunosuppression
- seizures
- stroke.

Ruby has 3 risk factors: she is over 50, she smokes and she is an Indigenous Australian.

Q: How will you investigate Ruby's pneumonia?
A:

1. **Full blood count**. This will provide a baseline level. A raised neutrophil count will support a diagnosis of CAP, but its absence is not uncommon in CAP.

2. **Electrolytes, blood sugar level**. Hyponatraemia may be present in CAP as might be deranged blood sugar levels in diabetics and acute kidney injury.

3. **Liver function tests**. Abnormal liver function tests may be seen in CAP.

4. **Arterial blood gas**. This will tell you if Ruby has hypoxia or hypercapnia. It will also allow you to calculate the alveolar-arterial gradient (A–a gradient), which reflects any problems with gas exchange between the alveolus and blood vessels. You should learn the calculation, as it is useful for the wards and for exams. It is:
$$\text{A–a gradient} = P_AO_2 - P_aO_2$$
$$P_AO_2 = 150 - 1.25 \times P_aCO_2$$
(P_AO_2 = alveolar oxygen, P_aO_2 = arterial oxygen)
In practical terms, a normal A–a gradient suggests that hypoxaemia is probably due to hypoventilation rather than to damaged lung tissue (e.g. respiratory muscle weakness, heroin overdose). On the other hand, an abnormal (elevated) A–a gradient reflects underlying damage in the lung, although it does not differentiate between specific causes (e.g. pneumonia and fibrosing alveolitis). Hinds (1999) says that there are 3 pathological causes of a raised A–a gradient: diffusion defects, right-to-left shunts and ventilation-perfusion mismatches. Weinberger and Drazen (2002) note that the A–a gradient changes with age. In a young healthy person it should be less than 15 mm Hg; in elderly patients it may be as high as 30 mm Hg.

5. **Blood cultures**. Bacteraemia occurs in about 10% of patients.

6. **Sputum cultures**. Write 'sputum M/C/S' on the pathology form (M = microscopy, C = culture, S = sensitivities).
If you suspect tuberculosis, you will need 3 early morning sputum samples collected over 3 days and you should write on the form: 'Z–N stain, TB culture and PCR' (Z–N = Ziehl–Neelsen stain, PCR = polymerase chain reaction).

7. **ESR, C–reactive protein**. Both the ESR and CRP are likely to be elevated in acute infections, but are non-specific findings. They

can be useful, however, as markers of disease progression or improvement through the admission.

8. **Nasal flocked swabs for common respiratory viruses, including influenza.** This specimen can be used to test for viruses such as influenza, parainfluenza, respiratory syncytial virus and enterovirus. The tests that can be performed on an nasopharyngeal aspirate include immunofluorescence (influenza, RSV and parainfluenza) and culture.

9. **Chest X-ray.** Ask for posteroanterior (PA) and lateral views.

10. **Legionella urinary antigen.** This is a very sensitive and specific test for *L. pneumophila* serogroup 1 only. It does not identify *L. pneumophila* due to other serogroups. Nevertheless, only half the cases of *Legionella* pneumonia in Australia result from serogroup 1. Therefore, do not dismiss a diagnosis of *Legionella* pneumonia if the urinary antigen is negative.

11. **Pneumococcal urinary antigen.**

12. **Serology.** A serological diagnosis can be made if a four-fold rise in titre occurs between acute and convalescent samples. The disadvantage here is that a serological diagnosis cannot be made until the convalescent phase of the illness. Serology can be performed for *Mycoplasma*, *Legionella*, *Chlamydia*, influenza and parainfluenza.

Q: Surely, after all these investigations, you are likely to find the microbiological cause of Ruby's pneumonia?

A: Actually, a microbiological cause of CAP is discovered in only about 50% of patients. The results are as follows:

Test	Normal range	Ruby's result
Haematocrit	0.40–0.54	0.42
Haemoglobin	130–180 g/L	132
Mean cell volume	80–100 fL	82
White cell count	3.5–11 × 10^9/L	18* (neutrophilia)
Platelet count	150–450 × 10^9/L	182
Sodium	135–145 mmol/L	132*
Potassium	3.6–5.1 mmol/L	4.1
Chloride	95–107 mmol/L	98
Bicarbonate	22–32 mmol/L	25

Test	Normal range	Ruby's result
Urea	2.9–7.1 mmol/L	4
Creatinine	60–110 µmol/L	90
Glucose	3.0–5.8 mmol/L	5.0
CRP	<3 mg/L	120*
ESR	mm/hour	78*
Albumin	33–48 g/L	30*
Bilirubin	0–25 µmol/L	20
ALP	38–126 U/L	158*
GGT	0–30 U/L	60*
AST	<45 U/L	56*
ALT	<45 U/L	61*
pH	7.35–7.43	7.36
PaO₂ (room air)	—	65
PaCO₂ (room air)	—	40

* Abnormal results.

Q: How do you interpret these findings?

A: Ruby has a leukocytosis (apparently a neutrophilia), raised ESR, hyponatraemia and liver function abnormalities, which are all consistent with CAP. But these are all non-specific findings. She is also hypoxic with a normal arterial carbon dioxide.
The A–a gradient can be calculated as follows:
$$P_AO_2 = 150 - 1.25 \times 40$$
$$= 100$$
$$\text{A–a gradient} = P_AO_2 - P_aO_2$$
$$= 100 - 65$$
$$= 35 \text{ mm Hg}$$
An A–a gradient of 35 mm Hg in a 54-year-old woman is abnormally high. The chest X-ray is shown in Figure 25.1.

Q: What does it show?

A: The chest X-ray is consistent with left lower lobe pneumonia with a parapneumonic effusion.

Q: What empirical antibiotic treatment should be commenced?

A: There are various scores to assess the severity of community-acquired pneumonia that can be used as a guide to treatment. One of them is the SMART-COP scoring system, which is found in the *Therapeutic*

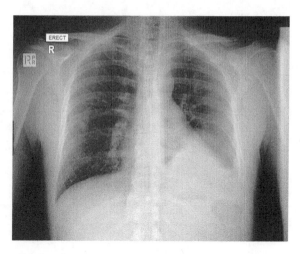

Figure 25.1 Ruby's chest X-ray

Guidelines: Antibiotic (Antibiotic Expert Group, 2014). This should be readily available from your hospital intranet.

Q: What is Ruby's SMART-COP score?

A: For people over 50 (Ruby is 54 years old):

S: systolic BP <90 – 2 points

M: multilobar involvement on CXR – 1 point

A: albumin <35 g/L – 1 point

R: respiratory rate ≥ 30/minute – 1 point

T: tachycardia of ≥ 125/minute – 1 point

C: confusion – 1 point

O: oxygen saturation ≤ 90%, PaO2 < 60 mm Hg or PaO2/FiO2 > 250 – 2 points

P: ph < 7.35 – 2 points)

Ruby's SMART-COP score is 1 (for her low albumin). This puts her at low risk of requiring intensive vasopressor or respiratory support (Antibiotic Expert Group, 2014), that is, she doesn't have a severe infection.

Q: Given Ruby's low SMART-COP score, she could be managed as an outpatient on oral antibiotics. You call the respiratory registrar to inform her. Is that reasonable?

A: It very well might be. But although the respiratory registrar will be impressed beyond words if an intern can tell her a patient's SMART-COP score, it is important to remember that such scores are only a guide.

They must be taken in the appropriate clinical context. For example, young people with pneumonia who are very hypoxic ($PaO_2 < 70$ mm Hg) should be considered for hospital admission irrespective of their score. You should therefore discuss the case with the respiratory registrar and see what she thinks.

Q: You call the respiratory registrar. As predicted, she is amazed by your knowledge of pneumonia severity scores. But the registrar is concerned about the comments Ruby's GP made about poor compliance with medications, and is worried that Ruby will not take her oral antibiotics at home. She would feel far more comfortable if Ruby were admitted to hospital and commenced on IV antibiotics, or alternatively admitted to the Hospital in the Home program for IV antibiotics. This would allow her to monitor Ruby's treatment and response to therapy. (This merely reinforces the fact that the SMART-COP score should be taken in the context of the clinical picture.) Ruby agrees to be admitted to hospital. What antibiotic regimen should you commence?

A: The Therapeutic Guidelines: Antibiotic (2014) recommend IV benzylpenicillin and oral doxycycline for non-severe CAP in hospitalised patients. The normal duration is about 7 days with the benzylpenicillin being switched to oral amoxycillin 1 g q8h when the patient improves.

Q: The respiratory registrar reviews Ruby and commences IV benzylpenicillin 1.2 g q6h and oral doxycycline 100 mg bd.
What other management strategies will you institute?

A:
1. Keep oxygen saturation above 95%, or 90% if she has hypercapnia.
2. Maintain hydration.
3. Give analgesia for pleuritic chest pain.
4. DVT prophylaxis.
5. A review by the ward physiotherapist for chest physiotherapy.

Q: Ruby is Aboriginal. Are there any services that the hospital can provide for Indigenous Australians?

A: If Ruby has identified herself as Aboriginal, she should be offered the services of the Aboriginal Liaison Officer (ALO). Most teaching hospitals employ an ALO, and this person is often an Indigenous Australian. The role of the ALO is to (ACT Health, 2014):
- assist with referrals to Aboriginal and Torres Strait Islander community organisations and other health, housing and external services

- arrange family meetings with medical and other health staff
- improve communication between hospital staff and patient and their family/carers, including talking on the patient's behalf
- offer emotional, social and cultural support
- provide information about the hospital and other health services.

This should help ensure a good relationship between Ruby and hospital staff and help avoid problems such as discharge against medical advice. However, do not assume that Ruby has identified herself as Aboriginal or that she wants to see the ALO. Find out these things before approaching the ALO.

Q: In 72 hours, Ruby is still experiencing high fevers and continues to feel unwell. She clinically has a persisting pleural effusion and is quite tender over that part of the chest wall. She has not improved clinically and her CRP has hardly moved. 3+ *Streptococcus pneumoniae* is isolated in the sputum. It is sensitive to benzylpenicillin, which is part of her current therapy. The oral doxycycline is ceased. Why isn't Ruby feeling any better?

A: At this stage, you would expect Ruby to be feeling a little better, particularly as she is on the correct antibiotic therapy. Generally, blood pressure and heart rate parameters should improve within 48 hours of starting therapy for CAP while respiratory rate, fever and oxygen saturations should improve within 72 hours. The CRP should ideally drop by 50% (Davies *et al.*, 2014). Although she may still have fevers, it is worrying that she has not improved at all.

A chest X-ray shows no radiological deterioration. The consolidation and pleural effusion persist.[1]

Q: What is the most likely reason for Ruby's lack of improvement?

A: A lack of improvement in parameters described above in patients with CAP and pleural effusion is most likely due to infection of the pleural fluid (empyema, which is frank pus in the pleural fluid, or a complicated parapneumonic effusion, where the pleural fluid is not frankly purulent but has features of infection). Although you must investigate for other causes of fever (e.g. peripheral catheter infections, pulmonary emboli), one of your first steps should be to exclude pleural infection.

---

[1] The radiographical appearance of pneumonia is slow to resolve. It may take 4–6 weeks for the X-ray to become normal, so do not be concerned that there is no improvement after 3 days. The reason for performing a chest X-ray is to look for any deterioration.

Q: How do you diagnose pleural infections?

A: Clinically, the presence of tenderness when lightly punching the area overlying the effusion may indicate infected pleural fluid. Ruby has this sign. Radiological investigations can also support a diagnosis of complicated parapneumonic effusion or empyema. The investigation of choice, however, is diagnostic sampling of the pleural fluid. About 14% of patients with infected pleural fluid will be bacteraemic; therefore, collect a blood culture (Davies *et al.*, 2010).

Q: How can radiological investigations support a diagnosis of pleural fluid infection?

A:

1. **Chest X-ray.** It is difficult to diagnose an empyema on a chest X-ray alone. However, a chest X-ray can be helpful in distinguishing between loculated pleural fluid (more common in empyema) and free pleural fluid. Free pleural fluid will change with posture and has a meniscus sign. Loculated pleural fluid moves far less with changes in posture.

   Loculated pleural fluid can be confused with a lung abscess. Some distinguishing features are that loculated fluid has a different appearance on frontal and lateral X-rays. Loculated pleural fluid may also have a lenticular shape.

2. **Ultrasound.** An ultrasound may demonstrate multiple septae in a loculated effusion. Also, different locules of fluid may have varying degrees of echogenicity, representing varying degrees of purulence.

3. **CT scan.** A CT scan can differentiate between a pleural effusion and lung abscess. In comparison to lung abscesses, empyemas have a lenticular shape and compress adjacent lung tissue. The 'split pleura' sign demonstrates the separation and enhancement of visceral and parietal pleural surfaces, and is characteristic of a pleural collection of fluid. In addition, the absence of pleural thickening on CT makes empyema and complicated parapneumonic effusion less likely.

Q: The respiratory registrar agrees that Ruby needs a diagnostic pleural fluid tap. Is there any test that you should organise before removing the fluid?

A: You should organise an ultrasound of the pleural space. The reason for this is that infected pleural fluid will often occur in distinct locules. Therefore, aspirating 'blindly' could result in a 'dry tap', precipitate a pneumothorax, or result in trauma to lung parenchyma.

The radiographers will easily see the pleural fluid on ultrasound. They will then use a black marker pen to mark the spot through which you should aspirate.

Q: Ruby returns from the ultrasound with reports that there are multiple locules within the collection of pleural fluid. The radiographers have marked the appropriate spot on her back for aspiration. You use an aseptic technique to aspirate 30 mL of cloudy fluid rather than frank pus. The macroscopic appearance alone suggests a complicated parapneumonic effusion.

What other precautionary test would you order after completing the diagnostic tap?

A: Order a chest X-ray to exclude a pneumothorax. This is a potential complication of aspirating pleural fluid.

Q: The chest X-ray demonstrates no pneumothorax. You call the laboratory in an hour to get the results of the fluid, which are as follows:
- Gram stain: positive for Gram-positive cocci and Gram-negative bacilli
- polymorphonuclear cells: 1+
- pH: 7.19
- pleural fluid glucose: 2.0 mmol/L
- LDH: 1500 IU/L.

Although this isn't an empyema because there wasn't frank pus, the loculated appearance on ultrasound and the preliminary results from the fluid analysis confirm that this is a complicated parapneumonic effusion.

How can you treat the infected pleural fluid?

A: There are a number of management options (in addition to IV antibiotics) (Koegelenberg *et al.* 2008). However, the first question to be asked is whether the effusion needs drainage or not. Immediate drainage is recommended when there is:
1. frank pus present
2. the effusion involves more than half the hemithorax
3. loculated effusion
4. positive Gram stain or culture of pleural fluid
5. pleural fluid pH < 7.20
6. pleural fluid glucose < 3.4 mmol/L.

Ruby's pleural fluid meets a number of the above criteria and therefore warrants immediate drainage or she risks an adverse outcome. There are a number of available methods to drain a complicated parapneumonic effusion (most of these begin with 't', which might make them easier to remember!).

1. Therapeutic thoracentesis—a one-off drainage of the effusion (not recommended if there is an empyema, pleural fluid pH < 7.20 or if the effusion involves more than half the hemithorax).
2. Tube thoracostomy (insertion of an intercostal catheter, ICC).
3. Thorascopy (video-assisted thorascopic surgery, or VATS, is commonly used in Australia).
4. Thoracotomy.

And note ...

Always order a chest X-ray after inserting an ICC to exclude pneumothorax and ensure that the ICC is in a good position.

Q: Your registrar performs tube thoracostomy, inserting an ICC into the effusion. The cultures return with a growth of *S. pneumoniae* but also mixed anaerobes. You therefore add metronidazole to the IV benzylpenicillin. What organisms are most commonly grown from infected pleural fluid?

A: This varies according to whether it is a community-acquired or hospital-acquired infection. It is worth noting that about 50% of infected pleural fluid will remain culture-negative but of those that are positive the most common organisms are as follows (Davies *et al.* 2010; Koegelenberg *et al.*, 2008).

For community-acquired infection:
- Streptococci (52%): *S. milleri, S. pneumoniae, S. intermedius*
- Anaerobes (20%)
- *Staphylococcus aureus* (11%)
- Gram-negative aerobic organisms (9%).

For nosocomial infection:
- *Staphylococcus aureus* (35%) (Methicillin-resistant *S. aureus* [MRSA] > methicillin-sensitive *S. aureus*)
- Gram-negative aerobic organisms (17%)
- Anaerobes (8%).

Q: Initially, there is good drainage through the ICC. However, it slows down, then stops after 24 hours. What can you do next?

A:

1. Flush the ICC with saline to make sure it is not blocked.

2. If the drainage does not improve, repeat the chest X-ray to make sure that the ICC is in a useful position. A contrast chest CT will provide better anatomical information, but is more difficult to organise.

Q: A 50 mL saline flush does not improve the drainage. Ruby still doesn't look well and is febrile. A chest X-ray confirms that the drain is in a good position. What about thrombolytic agents?

A: Free drainage of empyema fluid through the ICC may be difficult due to high pleural viscosity or the presence of numerous fibrinous septae and a visceral fibrinous rind (Davies *et al.* 2003). Thrombolytics have been used to address this problem since 1949 (e.g. streptokinase, urokinase) but currently, their routine use is not recommended for patients with pleural infection (Davies *et al.*, 2010).

Q: What is your next option?

A: It is now appropriate to consult the cardiothoracic surgery team regarding surgical treatment of Ruby's infected pleural effusion. VATS is a minimally invasive surgical technique that is available in most teaching hospitals in Australia.

The cardiothoracic surgeon agrees that Ruby requires surgery. Ruby consents to this and undergoes a VATS procedure 2 days later, with a good outcome.

Achievements

You now:
- know the most common microbiological causes of CAP
- know the factors that increase the risk of CAP
- can order appropriate investigations for CAP
- can calculate the A–a gradient and know that it increases with age
- can order appropriate empirical antibiotic therapy for CAP
- know how to manage patients with CAP
- know to consider empyema or complicated parapneumonic effusion in patients with CAP and persisting fever
- can diagnose empyema or complicated parapneumonic effusion using a pleural fluid aspirate
- appreciate how radiological investigations can support a diagnosis of infected pleural fluid
- know the steps in managing empyema and complicated parapneumonic effusion
- know that ALOs are available to Indigenous people who want to see them.

References

ACT Health (2014), 'Aboriginal and Torres Strait Islander Health Portal: Health liaison officers', at <www.health.act.gov.au/health-services/aboriginal-torres-strait-islander/information/act-health-liaison-officers>, accessed 24 November 2014.

Antibiotic Expert Group (2014), *Therapeutic Guidelines: Antibiotic*, Version 15, Therapeutic Guidelines Ltd, Melbourne.

Davies, C.W. *et al.* (2003), 'BTS guidelines for the management of pleural infection', *Thorax*, vol. 58 (suppl. 2), pp. ii18–28.

Davies, H.E., Davies, R.J.O. and Davies C.W.H, on behalf of the BTS Pleural Disease Guidelines Group (2010), 'Management of pleural infection in adults: British Thoracic Society pleural disease guidelines', *Thorax*, vol. 65 (suppl. 2), pp. ii41–53.

Hinds, C.J. (1999), 'Intensive care medicine', in P. Kumar and M. Clark (eds), *Clinical Medicine*, Harcourt, London, pp. 829–861.

Johnson, P.D., Irving, L.B. and Turnidge, J.D. (2002), '3: Community-acquired pneumonia', *Medical Journal of Australia*, vol. 176, no. 7, pp. 341–347.

King, S. and Thomson, A. (2002), 'Radiological perspectives in empyema', *British Medical Bulletin*, vol. 61, pp. 203–214.

Koegelenberg, C.F., Diaconi, A.H. and Bolligeri, C.T. (2008), 'Parapneumonic pleural effusion and empyema', *Respiration*, vol. 75, no. 3, pp. 241–250.

Weinberger, S.E. and Drazen, J.M. (2002), 'Disturbances of respiratory function', in E. Braunwald, A.S. Fauci, D.L. Kasper, S.L. Hauser, D.L. Longo and J.L. Jameson (eds), *Harrison's Principles of Internal Medicine*, McGraw-Hill, New York, pp. 1446–1453.

Chapter 26
Mr Edison's case of antibiotics and anaphylaxis

Scenario

It is the start of a Saturday day shift on the medical wards. You are receiving a handover of the previous night's events from the night intern. Nothing out of the ordinary occurred. There are a few APTTs to repeat and an ECG to check.

Then your colleague mentions Mr Edison, who is one of your patients from during the week who is recovering from a motor vehicle accident. Apparently, about 2 hours ago, the night intern reviewed him for possible cellulitis and commenced him on IV cephalothin.

You look surprised, 'Isn't Mr Edison allergic to penicillin?'

Your colleague replies, 'Yes, I know. That's why I charted cephalothin, a cephalosporin.'

Q: What are your views on the matter of penicillin and cephalosporin allergies?

A: Cephalosporins and penicillins both have beta-lactam rings. This structural similarity can lead to cross-reactivity between the 2 groups of antibiotics. Individuals with a history of penicillin allergy are 8 times more likely to have an allergic reaction to cephalosporins. However, serious reactions to cephalosporins are rare.

Q: How do you classify penicillin allergies?

A: Gell and Coombs (1975) classified them according to mechanism, as follows.

1. **Type I.** This involves immunoglobulin E-mediated activation and degranulation of mast cells and/or basophils. The immunoglobulin E (IgE) is bound to mast cells and circulating basophils. On re-exposure to an antigen, cross-linking of the IgE molecules occur, resulting in degranulation of these cells. The degranulation results in the release of mediators such as histamine and tryptase. Arachidonic acid derivatives such as

prostaglandins and leukotrienes also play a role. Anaphylaxis results from type I reactions.

2. **Type II.** This is mediated by immunoglobulin G (IgG) or immunoglobulin M (IgM) and results in complement-mediated or cell-mediated death of cells with beta-lactam antigens.

3. **Type III.** In this reaction, IgM or IgG form complexes with beta-lactam antigens and complement and deposit in tissues. Serum sickness and drug fevers can occur through this mechanism.

4. **Type IV.** This is a T-cell-mediated reaction.

Another way to classify allergies is according to time of onset (Levine, 1966).

Reaction type	Onset (hours)	Clinical reactions	Mechanism
Immediate	0–1	Anaphylaxis	Type I
		Hypotension	Type I
		Laryngeal oedema	Type I
		Urticaria/angioedema	Type I
Accelerated	0–72	Urticaria/angioedema	Type I
		Laryngeal oedema	Type I
		Wheezing bronchospasm	Type I
Late	>72	Morbiliform rash	
		Interstitial nephritis	Type II
		Haemolytic anaemia	Type II
		Neutropaenia	Type II
		Thrombocytopaenia	Type II
		Serum sickness	Type III
		Antibiotic drug fever	Type III
		Stevens–Johnson syndrome	
		Exfoliative dermatitis	

Source: Adapted from Weiss and Adkinson (2000).

One of the most important aspects of penicillin allergy is to take a detailed history to ensure that the reaction is indeed a true penicillin allergy. Some 80–90% of patients who report a penicillin allergy are not allergic on skin testing.

A detailed history may reveal that the reaction attributed to allergy was atypical (e.g. tingling in the right hand), or that it occurred in the setting of an illness or other medications that can cause the same reaction (e.g. a rash from an anticonvulsant or a viral illness).

The consequences of labelling an individual as allergic to penicillin include increased health care costs and even suboptimal treatment when penicillin is the drug of choice. As interns and residents, it is critical that you take a good history regarding drug allergies. Doing so could make a difference to the patient's outcome.

Scenario

Of course, you did take a thorough history from Mr Edison when he was first admitted. You recall that 10 years ago he received benzylpenicillin for cellulitis. Apparently, within the first hour of taking the penicillin, he developed wheezing and a rash and his blood pressure dropped. He was told never to take penicillin again.

This sounds like a type I anaphylactic 'immediate' reaction. You tell your colleague that Mr Edison is 8 times more likely to get a reaction to cephalosporins than individuals who do not have a penicillin allergy. Given the severity of the reaction to penicillin, it would have been advisable not to give Mr Edison cephalothin at all. You decide to check up on Mr Edison, just in case. Your colleague is grateful for being enlightened on this topic and heads home.

Q: On arriving in Mr Edison's ward, his nurse tells you that he received the cephalothin dose about 20 minutes ago. You rush into the room, and Mr Edison tells you that he began to feel unwell about 3 minutes ago. His oxygen saturation on room air is 91% (it has normally been 98%). His heart rate is 100/minute and his blood pressure is 80/60 (it has normally been 130/70).

His tongue and uvula seem swollen. There is diffuse wheeze throughout the lungs. His trunk and limbs are covered in wheals consistent with urticaria. He seems somewhat sluggish and it is clear that he has been incontinent of urine. What is most likely happening?

A: He is having an anaphylactic reaction to the cephalothin!

Q: Is it surprising that he has been incontinent of urine if this is anaphylaxis?

A: No. The hypotension alone can lead to a variety of symptoms such as nausea, vomiting, collapse, dizziness and urinary incontinence. Although certain features of anaphylaxis are instantly recognisable (such as hypotension, bronchospasm and angio-oedema), it is worth remembering that anaphylaxis is a multi-system disorder that can also manifest with symptoms such as abdominal or pelvic pain and a vascular-type headache (Brown *et al.*, 2006).

Q: What do you do?

A: There are a number of steps (Brown *et al.*, 2006).

1. **Call a Code Blue or MET call.** This will bring the arrest team to the scene very quickly. You will have the benefit of the experience and expertise of the intensive care staff, medical registrars and critical care nurses. Although you should not call Code Blues unless you really feel it is warranted, anaphylactic shock is a condition that you should not have to deal with alone as an intern.
2. **Place the patient in the supine position (or lateral decubitus position if vomiting)** (Brown *et al.*, 2006).
3. **Support the airway and breathing.**
4. **Give adrenaline (most important medication).**
5. **Gain IV access.**
6. **Give supplemental oxygen.**
7. **If hypotensive, IV fluid resuscitation is important.** This may require another IV cannula (a large-bore 14 or 16 gauge) to administer a normal saline bolus 20 mL/kg over as fast as 1–2 minutes under pressure.

Q: How does adrenaline work in anaphylaxis?
A: Austen (2002) states that adrenaline acts at 3 levels in anaphylaxis:
1. vasoconstriction (alpha-agonist activity) counters hypotension in anaphylaxis
2. bronchial smooth muscle relaxation (beta-agonist activity) counters bronchospasm in anaphylaxis
3. reduction of vascular permeability counters angio-oedema.

Q: By what route do you administer the adrenaline?
A: It should be first given intramuscularly (Brown *et al.*, 2006).

Q: Where should you give it?
A: Site is important! Simons *et al.* (2001) found that intramuscular administration in the thigh leads to higher peak plasma levels of adrenaline than intramuscular or subcutaneous injection in the upper arm.

Q: What dose should you give?
A: You will encounter vials of adrenaline being referred to as '1 in 1000' (1:1000) or '1 in 10 000' (1:10 000). The first, '1 in 1000', refers to 1 mg of adrenaline in 1 mL. The second, '1 in 10 000', refers to 1 mg of adrenaline in 10 mL.

Give 0.01 mg/kg up to a maximum dose of 0.5 mg IMI into the lateral thigh (Brown *et al.*, 2006).

Q: What can be done if Mr Edison doesn't respond well to this single dose of IM adrenaline?

A: If there is a poor response, the options are (Brown *et al.*, 2006):
- commence an IV adrenaline infusion OR
- repeat the IM adrenaline dose every 3–5 minutes as necessary (Brown *et al.*, 2006).

As an intern, you wouldn't be used to prescribing IV adrenaline infusions; however, by now the Code Blue team would have arrived and a more senior colleague could do this if necessary.

Q: What other interventions and medications may be helpful?

A: Interventions and medications could include:
- nebulised beta-2-agonists to help reduce bronchospasm
- nebulised adrenaline to treat persisting stridor.

Q: What should you recommend for patients who do not respond to repeated intramuscular or subcutaneous adrenaline and who are persistently hypotensive despite the adrenaline and IV fluids?

A:
1. IV adrenaline or noradrenaline (need close monitoring because of side effects).
2. Parenteral glucagon, which works by increasing both the heart rate and cardiac output.
3. Vasopressors such as vasopressin may play a role but have their own side effects.

Q: You give Mr Edison 0.5 mg intramuscular adrenaline in the thigh. The nurses commence IV normal saline through his cannula and administer nebulised salbutamol. Although the Code Blue team arrives quickly, it is apparent even by this stage that the adrenaline is working and that Mr Edison is improving. IV hydrocortisone (a steroid) is commenced at 100 mg every 6 hours, as are IV antihistamines. Are antihistamines and corticosteroids useful in reversing the immediate life-threatening effects of anaphylaxis?

A: No. Adrenaline is the cornerstone of treating the immediate life-threatening side effects of anaphylaxis; however, medications such as antihistamines and corticosteroids might improve mild allergic reactions of the skin (Brown *et al.*, 2006).

Q: The cardiac arrest team takes over the resuscitation, but thanks you for a job well done. Mr Edison will live to fight another day, but he should never have beta-lactam antibiotics again. Is Mr Edison out of danger now?

A: Possibly not. Ellis and Day (2003) note that anaphylactic reactions follow a biphasic course in 20% of cases. This means that there is a 20% chance that Mr Edison will suffer another anaphylactic reaction. The timeframe for the second reaction is variable, but studies have suggested anywhere from 1–38 hours (but mainly 1–8 hours) after the first reaction.

Ellis and Day (2003) found that, compared to first-phase reactions, one-third of second-phase reactions were more severe, one-third were similar and one-third were milder. Therefore, in patients with anaphylaxis it is important to observe them for at least 4–6 hours after resolution of symptoms (Brown *et al.*, 2006). If they are discharged within 38 hours of presentation (which they often will be), inform them of the possibility of a second-phase reaction. Ensure that they live near a hospital and that they have easy phone access to emergency services.

Q: For individuals who have previously developed anaphylaxis to an allergen commonly found in the community (e.g. bee stings, peanuts), is there any way of initiating treatment before an ambulance arrives or before they reach a hospital?

A: Yes. These people can carry auto-injectable adrenaline devices. If they are exposed to an allergen and believe that they will suffer an allergic reaction, they can quickly administer a dose of adrenaline. This may terminate the episode or minimise the symptoms until paramedics arrive. These devices are available in Australia.

Achievements

You now:

- know that cephalosporins and penicillins share a beta-lactam ring
- know that there is increased risk of cephalsporin allergy in patients with a penicillin allergy
- can classify allergic reactions to antibiotics according to time and immunological mechanism
- appreciate the importance of taking a detailed history of an antibiotic allergy to see if it is genuine
- know how to manage anaphylaxis
- know that adrenaline is the most important medication for treating anaphylaxis
- know the best route and site for administering adrenaline
- understand the terminology '1 in 1000' and '1 in 10 000' with reference to adrenaline

- realise that, as an intern, you should ask for assistance when dealing with anaphylaxis
- know that there are auto-injectable adrenaline devices that people at risk of an anaphylaxis reaction can carry.

References

Austen, K.F. (2002), 'Allergies, anaphylaxis, and systemic mastocytosis', in E. Braunwald, A.S. Fauci, D.L. Kasper, S.L. Hauser, D.L. Longo and J.L. Jameson (eds), *Harrison's Principles of Internal Medicine*, McGraw-Hill, New York, pp. 1913–1922.

Brown, S.G., Mullins R.J. and Gold, M.S. (2006), 'Anaphylaxis: Diagnosis and management', *Medical Journal of Australia*, vol. 185, no. 5, pp 283–289.

Ellis, A.K. and Day, J.H. (2003), 'Diagnosis and management of anaphylaxis', *Canadian Medical Association Journal*, vol. 169, no. 4, pp. 307–312.

Gell, P.G.H. and Coombs, R.R.A. (1975), 'Classification of allergic reactions responsible for clinical hypersensitivity and disease', in P.G.H. Gell, R.R.A. Coombs and P.J. Lachmann (eds), *Clinical Aspects of Immunology*, Blackwell Science Publications, Oxford, pp. 761–781.

Kelkar, P.S. and Li, J.T. (2001), 'Cephalosporin allergy', *New England Journal of Medicine*, vol. 345, no. 11, pp. 804–809.

Levine, B.B. (1966), 'Immunologic mechanisms of penicillin allergy: A haptenic model system for the study of allergic diseases of man', *New England Journal of Medicine*, vol. 275, no. 20, pp. 1115–1125.

Rusznak, C. and Peebles, R.S. Jr (2002), 'Anaphylaxis and anaphylactoid reactions: A guide to prevention, recognition, and emergent treatment', *Postgraduate Medicine*, vol. 111, no. 5, pp. 101–104, 107–108, 111–114.

Salkind, A.R., Cuddy, P.G. and Foxworth, J.W. (2001), 'The rational clinical examination. Is this patient allergic to penicillin? An evidence-based analysis of the likelihood of penicillin allergy', *Journal of the American Medical Association*, vol. 285, no. 19, pp. 2498–2505.

Simons, F.E., Gu, X. and Simons, K.J. (2001), 'Epinephrine absorption in adults: Intramuscular versus subcutaneous injection', *Journal of Allergy and Clinical Immunology*, vol. 108, no. 5, pp. 871–873.

Weiss, M.A. and Adkinson, N.F. Jr (2000), 'Beta-lactam allergy', in G.L. Mandell, J.E. Bennett and R. Dolin (eds), *Principles and Practice of Infectious Diseases*, Churchill Livingstone, Philadelphia, pp. 299–305.

Chapter 27
Mr Darcy presents with anaemia

Scenario

It is your first week as the haematology intern. You are asked to attend the outpatients clinic. The first patient you see is a 74-year-old obese man referred by his local doctor with anaemia. According to the referral letter, Mr Darcy went to his general practitioner to get a check-up 3 weeks ago. Apart from his obesity, the only abnormality is a mild anaemia. You have been asked to find the source of the anaemia.

First you take a history. Mr Darcy leads a full, independent life. He admits that he doesn't exercise enough and probably eats too much. But he is not symptomatic from his anaemia and has no constitutional symptoms. Indeed, he was surprised to learn of the abnormality. He cannot recall any melaena, bright red rectal bleeding, haematuria, haematemesis or epistaxis. There is no history of peptic ulcer disease and he does not take any ulcerogenic medications.

Physical examination yields no findings apart from conjunctival pallor. He has no organomegaly in the abdomen, no masses or blood on rectal examination and no lymphadenopathy. The neurologic, respiratory and cardiology examination is unremarkable.

You now look over the blood results from the investigations his GP ordered:

Haemoglobin	130–180 g/L	105*
Mean cell volume	80–100 fL	69*
Mean cell haemoglobin concentration	310–360 g/L	298*
White cell count	3.5–11 × 10⁹/L	5.5
Platelets	150–450 × 10⁹/L	200
Electrolytes		Normal
Urea, creatinine		Normal
Liver function tests		Normal

* Abnormal results.

Q: How do you interpret these tests?

A: The low haemoglobin, mean cell volume (MCV) and mean cell haemoglobin concentration (MCHC) all support the presence of a microcytic anaemia.

Q: The blood film demonstrates hypochromic, microcytic red cells. What are the likely causes of the microcytic, hypochromic anaemia?

A: The 2 most common causes of anaemia in the elderly are anaemia of chronic disease (30–45%) and iron deficiency anaemia (15–30%). Both can cause a microcytic picture although anaemia of chronic disease often causes a normochromic normocytic anaemia.

Thalassaemia and sideroblastic anaemia are other causes of a microcytic, hypochromic picture that you would consider. However, you would expect these disorders to have been discovered at a younger age.

In each of these 4 conditions, there is a distinctive cause responsible for the microcytic anaemia (DeLoughery *et al.*, 2014):
- limited iron delivery to the haem group (anaemia of inflammation)
- no iron delivered to the haem group (iron deficiency anaemia)
- defective haem synthesis (sideroblastic anaemia)
- missing globin product (thalassaemia).

Q: Is there likely to be folate or vitamin B12 deficiency?

A: Typically, deficiencies of B12 and folate result in a macrocytic anaemia (mean cell volume over 100 fL), unlike Mr Darcy's microcytic anaemia. Nevertheless, given that malabsorption or malnutrition can lead to a combination of iron, B12 and folate deficiencies that can result in a normocytic or microcytic anaemia, it is possible.

Q: Mr Darcy says he hates blood tests. Will he need to have a lot of blood taken today?

A: No. Although you could order a huge number of tests to investigate every cause of anaemia, it is reasonable to order a few basic screening tests before pursuing further investigations.

Q: What preliminary tests would you order?

A: Initially, you should check:
- iron studies
- vitamin B12
- folate levels.

If these do not suggest iron deficiency you can order further investigations to find a cause for the anaemia.

Q: What tests do you order to assess iron, vitamin B12 and folate levels?

A: The obvious answer would be iron studies, serum folate and serum B12 levels. However, there is more to this than meets the eye! Iron studies are sufficient to screen for iron deficiency. But serum folate does not always accurately reflect the presence of folate deficiency. Here, red cell folate is more reliable. Serum vitamin B12 levels should be ordered. However, Smith (2000) cites Stabler (1998) and notes that up to 30% of patients with low to normal serum B12 levels have neurologic disease and anaemia.

Q: You decide to order iron studies, vitamin B12 and red cell folate, and review Mr Darcy in the clinic next week.

When Mr Darcy returns to the clinic, he is anxious to hear the results. He is accompanied by his wife. Although the vitamin B12 and red cell folate levels are both at the upper limit of normal, the iron studies are abnormal.

Do the iron studies represent anaemia of chronic disease or iron deficiency anaemia?

Test	Range	Result
Iron	5–30 μmol/L	3.4*
Transferrin	1.9–2.8 g/L	3*
Iron saturation	16–51%	15*
Ferritin	15–200 μg/L	14*

* Abnormal results.

A: This pattern is consistent with iron deficiency anaemia. The differences between iron deficiency anaemia and anaemia of chronic disease are highlighted below.

	Iron deficiency anaemia	Anaemia of chronic disease
Iron	Low	Low
Transferrin	High	Low
TIBC	High	Low
Iron saturation	Low	Low or normal
Ferritin	Low	Normal or high

TIBC = total iron binding capacity
Source: Adapted from Smith (2000).

A ferritin level below 15 μg/L is an extremely strong indicator of iron deficiency. A level above 100 μg/L makes iron deficiency very unlikely.

A ferritin level between 15 μg/L and 100 μg/L could be due to either chronic disease or iron deficiency. However, ferritin is an acute phase reactant and may be elevated in the presence of iron deficiency if there is an acute inflammatory process present.

An elevated TIBC is specific for iron deficiency but not sensitive as it can be reduced by other factors such as ageing, malnutrition and inflammation (DeLoughery *et al.*, 2014).

Q: Is there a 'gold standard' diagnostic test to differentiate between iron deficiency and anaemia of chronic disease?

A: Yes. A bone marrow biopsy would demonstrate absent iron stores in iron deficiency. In anaemia of chronic disease, iron stores would be present.

Q: Why does anaemia of chronic disease result in abnormal iron studies?

A: Iron stores in the reticuloendothelial system are normal or high in anaemia of chronic disease, but, for reasons unknown, there is a fundamental inability to use them.

Q: Mrs Darcy asks you why her husband would be iron deficient. What is your response?

A: Chronic gastrointestinal blood loss is the most common cause of iron deficiency anaemia in the elderly. The source is upper gastrointestinal bleeding in 20–40% of cases and colonic in 15–30% of cases. In 10–40% of cases, the source is not found.

Mr Darcy has no other features to suggest malabsorption as a cause of his iron deficiency, and his dietary history suggests that inadequate dietary intake of iron is not the cause. Therefore, you tell him that gastrointestinal bleeding is the most likely cause.

Q: Mrs Darcy asks, 'Are you sure it couldn't be something to do with his weight? I've been telling him for years that being so big would harm his health'. Is she right?

A: She could be right. Obesity alone is associated with iron deficiency. The reason for this may be elevated serum hepcidin levels and reduced iron absorption (Aigner *et al.*, 2014). However, it is still important to exclude gastrointestinal blood loss in Mr Darcy.

Q: Mrs Darcy shakes her head at Mr Darcy. 'If only you'd been fit like my brother, none of this would have happened to you. He was a top footy player, you know'. What is the irony here?

A: Surprisingly, athletes are also at increased risk of iron deficiency. Like obese people, they can have elevated hepcidin levels and reduced iron absorption. In addition, there are gastrointestinal tract blood losses and even urinary losses due to haemolysis following exercise (DeLoughery *et al.*, 2014).

Q: Mr Darcy asks, 'Do I have to worry about a peptic ulcer, Doc?'

A: It could well be peptic ulcer disease. The sources of upper gastrointestinal blood loss in the elderly include peptic ulcer disease, gastric cancer, gastritis and oesophagitis. The sources of colonic blood loss include colon cancer, polyps, colitis and angiodysplasia.

Q: What do you advise next?

A: You should talk to the consultant haematologist about arranging a gastroscopy and colonoscopy for Mr Darcy.

Iron replacement therapy should be commenced. You prescribe ferrous sulphate 325 mg tds. You warn Mr Darcy of the side effects of the iron replacement, which are nausea and diarrhoea or constipation. You tell him to expect a rise in haemoglobin of 1 g/L/day.

Q: Mrs Darcy asks, 'Can I give the iron with his cup of tea in the morning and afternoon?'

A: No. Tea, calcium, fibre and possibly coffee can reduce the absorption of oral iron. On the other hand, meat, protein and vitamin C can enhance absorption.

Q: Your consultant agrees with your management plan and the Darcys are keen for a diagnosis to be made. How would you obtain consent from Mr Darcy for the colonoscopy?

A: There are 2 aspects to a colonoscopy: the dietary preparation and the procedure itself.

A typical dietary preparation would begin 4 days before the colonoscopy. This would involve 2 days of a low-residue diet followed by a day of clear fluids only. On the same day as Mr Darcy takes clear fluids, he needs to drink a bowel aperient such as 'fleet' or 'glycoprep'. This is to empty the bowel so the endoscopist has an unobscured view of the colon. Mr Darcy also needs to be nil by mouth on the day of the procedure.

The major risks arising from the procedure are bowel perforation and haemorrhage. Haemorrhage is more likely to occur after biopsies have been taken. Therefore, advise Mr Darcy to attend the Emergency Department if he develops abdominal pain or bleeding after the colonoscopy.

Q: A week later Mr Darcy undergoes the gastroscopy and colonoscopy. The gastroscopy is normal, but unfortunately a mass lesion is seen in the ascending colon. A biopsy confirms that this is a colorectal carcinoma. Naturally, Mr and Mrs Darcy are upset. 'If only I had taken aspirin! I've heard that it prevents colon cancer', Mr Darcy declares. Is he right?

A: Various studies appear to show that both aspirin and nonsteroidal anti-inflammatory drugs (NSAIDs) are protective against colorectal cancer. But there is enough uncertainty about their role and their side effects that they aren't firmly recommended as primary prevention agents (GSA, 2009).

Q: What happens now?

A: At a minimum, Mr Darcy needs a chest X-ray and liver function tests to look for metastatic disease. Although an abdominal CT scan can be considered, the pick-up rate in an asymptomatic individual is quite low. After the X-ray and tests, Mr Darcy will need to undergo a laparotomy for therapeutic and staging purposes.

Q: How do you stage colorectal cancer?

A: A number of staging systems exist, but the TNM system appears to be popular in Australia.

1. **Primary tumour (T)**
    TX: Primary tumour cannot be assessed
    T0: No evidence of primary tumour
    T1: Invades submucosa
    T2: Invades muscularis propria
    T3: Invades through muscularis propria into subserosa, or into non-peritonealised pericolic or perirectal tissues
    T4: Tumour directly invades other organs or structures, and/or perforates visceral peritoneum
2. **Regional lymph nodes (N)**
    NX: Nodes cannot be assessed
    N0: No nodal metastasis
    N1: Metastasis in 1–3 regional nodes
    N2: Metastasis in 4 or more regional nodes
3. **Distant metastasis (M)**
    MX: Metastasis cannot be assessed
    M0: No distant metastasis
    M1: Distant metastasis.[1]

Q: Mr Darcy undergoes a right hemicolectomy. Thankfully, the abdominal CT and chest X-ray are normal. You are also pleased to learn that the tumour is only T2N0M0 on histological examination. Does Mr Darcy need chemotherapy?

---

[1]Adapted from Greene *et al.* (2002).

A: No. Only patients with regional lymph-node-positive disease (and certain advanced T stage, negative lymph node stage patients) are eligible for adjuvant chemotherapy.

Common agents used in combination include 5-fluorouracil, but newer combinations are likely to replace these in the near future.

Q: Mr Darcy wants to know what sort of follow-up he will need. What do you tell him?

A: He should be reviewed by his surgeon every 3 months for 2 years. Then an annual review will suffice. He should have a colonoscopy every 3–5 years to detect any metachronous tumour.

Carcinoembryonic antigen (CEA) blood testing performed at regular intervals and possibly periodic abdominal CTs are also reasonable standards of care in patients who can undergo surgical intervention.

Q: This whole experience has traumatised Mrs Darcy. She tells you that she wants to be screened for colorectal cancer but wonders whether she is being over-anxious as she is only 50 years old, is otherwise quite healthy and has no family history of colorectal cancer. Is she too young to be screened for colorectal cancer?

A: Not at all. In fact, Australia's bowel cancer screening program offers screening from the age of 50 years. The 5-year risk of colorectal cancer for a 50-year-old is 1 in 300, which is a 4-fold increase compared to a 40-year-old (ACNCCGRC, 2005).

Q: What screening tests would you perform?

A: A reasonable approach in someone of average risk of colorectal cancer would be faecal occult blood testing every 2 years using an immunochemical test. If a test is positive, then one would proceed to a colonoscopy.

Achievements

You now:

- can classify anaemia on the basis of the full blood count and film
- know the causes of hypochromic and microcytic anaemia
- appreciate the limitations of serum folate and serum B12 in diagnosing their respective deficiencies
- know the best investigations to order to identify iron, B12 and folate deficiency
- know how to use iron studies to differentiate between anaemia of chronic disease and iron deficiency anaemia

- know the common causes of iron deficiency in the elderly
- know how to initiate iron replacement therapy and explain its side effects
- know how to obtain consent from patients for a colonoscopy
- understand some of the epidemiological risks for colorectal carcinoma
- know how to stage colorectal cancer
- understand basic approaches to management of colorectal cancer
- can recommend appropriate screening methods for colorectal cancer in asymptomatic patients over 50 years old
- understand the appropriate use of faecal occult blood as a screening tool for colorectal cancer.

References

Aigner, E., Feldman, A. and Datz, C. (2014), 'Obesity as an emerging risk factor for iron deficiency', *Nutrients*, vol. 6, no. 9, pp. 3587–3600.

Australian Cancer Network Colorectal Cancer Guidelines Revision Committee (ACNCCGRC) (2005), *Guidelines for the Prevention, Early Detection and Management of Colorectal Cancer*, Cancer Council Australia and Australian Cancer Network, Sydney, at <www.cancer.org.au/health-professionals/clinical-guidelines/colorectal-cancer.html>, accessed 20 July 2009.

DeLoughery, T.G. (2014), 'Microcytic anemia', *New England Journal of Medicine*, vol. 371, no. 14, pp. 1324–1331.

Frewin, R., Henson, A. and Provan, D. (1997), 'ABC of clinical haematology: Iron deficiency anaemia', *British Medical Journal*, vol. 314, no. 7077, pp. 360–363.

Gastroenterological Society of Australia (GSA) (2009), 'Early detection, screening and surveillance for bowel cancer', Gastroenterological Society of Australia, at <www.gesa.org.au/files/editor_upload/File/Professional/Bowel%20Cancer.pdf>, accessed 30 November 2014.

Greene, F.L., Page, D.L., Fleming, I.D., Fritz, A.G., Balch, C.M., Haller, D.G. and Morrow, M. (eds) (2002), *AJCC Cancer Staging Handbook*, Springer, New York.

Smith, D.L. (2000), 'Anemia in the elderly', *American Family Physician*, vol. 62, no. 7, pp. 1565–1572.

Teixeira, M.C., Braghiroli, M.I., Sabbaga, J. and Hoff, P.M. (2014), 'Primary prevention of colorectal cancer: Myth or reality?', *World Journal of Gastroenterology*, vol. 20, no. 41, pp. 15060–15069.

US Preventive Services Task Force (2007), 'Routine aspirin or nonsteroidal anti-inflammatory drugs for the primary prevention of colorectal cancer: US Preventive Services Task Force recommendation statement', *Annals of Internal Medicine*, vol. 146, no. 5, pp. 361–364.

Chapter 28
Mr Wayne develops fever during blood transfusion

Scenario

You are the haematology intern. You are rewriting some of your patients' medication charts when a nurse interrupts you to tell you that Mr Wayne wants to talk to you. Mr Wayne is a 60-year-old man with newly diagnosed myelodysplasia, who has come in for the day to receive a blood transfusion. In fact, you wrote him up for 3 units of packed cells not 10 minutes ago. You wonder what the problem is.

'Doc, I was sitting in front of the television just about to get my blood. Then on the news they showed some poor lady who got HIV 25 years ago from a blood transfusion. I don't want to get HIV. Is there a big risk that I'll get it from this transfusion?'

You inform Mr Wayne that although blood in Australia was not screened for HIV 25 years ago, all blood donors are now screened and so the risk is very low.[1]

You quote the latest figures from the Australian Red Cross Blood Service (2014) regarding the risk of acquiring certain bloodborne infections per unit of blood transfusion:

HIV (antibody and nucleic acid testing): <1 in 1 million
Hepatitis C (antibody and nucleic acid testing): <1 in 1 million
Hepatitis B (HBsAg): 1 in 468 000
HTLV I and II (antibody): <1 in 1 million
Variant CJD: possible but not yet reported in Australia
Malaria (antibody): <1 in 1 million
You say that although the risk is not zero, it is extremely low.

Q: Mr Wayne is relieved to hear that the risk is so low and is happy to proceed with the transfusion. You return to the excitement of rewriting

---

[1]In Australia, blood has been screened for hepatitis B since 1972, for HIV since 1985 (in 1984, just before the introduction of HIV testing kits, hepatitis B cAb was used as a screening marker of possible infection with HIV), for hepatitis C since 1990 and for human T-lymphotropic virus I/II since 1993.

medication charts. About half an hour later, however, the nurse returns to tell you that Mr Wayne is febrile at 38 °C.

What do you do?

A: You have to decide whether Mr Wayne's fever is due to a 'haemolytic transfusion reaction' or a 'febrile non-haemolytic transfusion reaction' (FNHTR). FNHTR is relatively mild and harmless, but haemolysis is fatal! (The third, unlikely alternative is bacterial contamination of the blood products.)

Febrile and non-febrile reactions during blood transfusions can be divided as follows:

- acute (under 24 hours)—immunologic
- acute (under 24 hours)—non-immunologic
- delayed (over 24 hours)—immunologic
- delayed (over 24 hours)—non-immunologic.

You can see from the following table that both haemolytic transfusion reactions and FNHTR are acute immunologic reactions.

Acute immunologic	Acute non-immunologic	Delayed immunologic	Delayed non-immunologic
Haemolytic	Hypotension/ACE	Alloimmunisation	Iron overload
Febrile non-	Transfusion- related	Haemolytic	
haemolytic	acute lung injury	Graft vs host	
Urticaria	Circulatory overload	Post-transfusion	
Anaphylaxis	Non-immune	purpura	
	haemolysis	Immuno-	
	Air embolus	modulation	
	Hypocalcaemia		
	Hypothermia		
	Bacterial contamination		

Source: Adapted from Brecher (2002).

You do not need to learn this whole list! Just be aware that transfusion reactions can be divided in this manner.

Q: How do you clinically tell the difference between haemolytic reactions and FNHTR?

A: This can be difficult and there are different approaches to the problem.

Symptom	Haemolytic reaction	FNHTR
Temperature rise 1–2 °C and barely symptomatic	+ / −	+
Temperature rise ≥2 °C	+	−

Rigors/chills	+	−
Hypotension	+	−
Blood oozing from IV site*	+	−
Back, chest or abdominal pain	+	−
Respiratory symptoms	+	−
Feeling unwell†	+	−

*Oozing at the IV site may represent the development of a coagulopathy.
†When rigors/chills, hypotension, blood oozing from IV site, respiratory symptoms and an unwell feeling occur, consider haemolysis irrespective of the temperature.

As you can see from the above table, only consider an FNHTR if the temperature rise is between 1 °C and 2 °C and the patient is asymptomatic or has minimal symptoms. Even then, however, do not dismiss the possibility of haemolysis. Also note that this is a guide; protocols may vary from hospital to hospital.

Q: You speak to Mr Wayne. He feels well, apart from being slightly hot. The nurse has been checking his temperature as a matter of routine, and it has come as a surprise to Mr Wayne that he has a fever. He denies feeling unwell, denies back, flank or chest pain, as well as rigors or chills.

The nurse tells you his baseline temperature was 37 °C and is now 38 °C. His heart rate and blood pressure are stable. There is no oozing from the IV site.

What do you think?

A: Mr Wayne has had a 1 °C temperature rise and is feeling well. On examination, he has no hypotension and no oozing from the IV site. You feel this is likely to be an FNHTR.

Q: How do you manage an FNHTR?

A: Ask the nurse to:

- administer paracetamol (acetaminophen) to bring down the fever
- slow the transfusion rate down.

If Mr Wayne deteriorates despite these measures, you will have to consider haemolysis as a strong possibility and stop the transfusion.

Q: Mr Wayne's temperature falls below 38 °C not long after administering the paracetamol. The transfusion continues without further incident.

What is the pathogenesis of haemolytic reactions and FNHTR?

A: Haemolytic transfusion reactions occur from interaction of the recipient's antibodies and tranfused red cells. FNHTR occurs from interaction of the recipient's antibodies and transfused white cells, platelets and cytokines. In fact, one method to prevent further episodes of FNHTR is to avoid transfusing white cells by measures such as using a filter.

Q: If you had been concerned that Mr Wayne was suffering from a haemolytic reaction, how would you have managed him?

A: This would be a life-threatening emergency. You would have to:
- cease the blood transfusion immediately
- inform the medical registrar
- keep the IV line in situ and run IV fluids to maintain the blood pressure
- have the nurses double-check the compatibility of the patient's blood group to the donor blood units
- repeat the cross-match to ensure that an error wasn't made with either the donor's or recipient's blood grouping
- have an urgent Gram stain and culture performed on the blood products to exclude bacterial contamination
- take blood cultures from the recipient
- aim for a urine output of 100 mL/hour in the first 24 hours to maintain adequate renal perfusion; you may require diuretics to assist you with this
- treat any coagulopathy that is present
- perform a 'haemolytic screen' to confirm your diagnosis of haemolysis
- give empirical broad-spectrum antibiotic treatment in case of bacterial contamination.

Q: During your career, you will be asked to perform haemolytic screens to investigate anaemic patients. Unfortunately, you cannot write 'haemolytic screen' on the pathology form! The laboratory will want to know exactly what tests you wish to order. What will you write on the form?

A: You should ask for:
- full blood count (low haemoglobin)
- blood film
- bilirubin (increased unconjugated or indirect bilirubin)
- Coombs test (direct antiglobulin test)
- reticulocyte count (raised) and blood film
- haptoglobin (reduced or absent)
- lactate dehydrogenase (raised but non-specific)
- urine specimen may detect haemoglobinuria (only in severe intravascular haemolysis such as a haemolytic transfusion reaction).

Q: Can blood products become contaminated with bacteria?

A: Yes. Transfusion-associated sepsis can occur with any blood product but is most strongly associated with platelets that are stored at room temperature. The citrate and iron content of red cells makes *Yersinia enterocolitica* the most common bacterial contaminant in packed red cells. Platelets, on the other hand, can have a wide range of bacteria, especially from the skin (e.g. *Staphylococcus aureus*, streptococci, *Salmonella*, *Klebsiella*, *Bacillus*) (Osterman and Arora, 2014).

Q: Mr Wayne wants to talk to you before he leaves. He says that the patient next to him was talking about getting 'iron overload'. Mr Wayne recalls the haematologist mentioning this, too, but he wasn't paying much attention at the time. He asks you what iron overload is.

A: Iron overload is a long-term consequence of multiple blood transfusions. It occurs when a non-bleeding patient has received 50–100 units of red cells. The iron deposits in various organs, in particular the liver, heart and endocrine glands. The heart and liver effects account for most of the morbidity and mortality of iron overload. Iron chelation with agents such as desferoxamine are used to remove iron from the patient's system without worsening their anaemia.

Q: Are you aware of any genetic conditions that are associated with abnormal accumulation of iron in the body?

A: Yes, haemochromatosis.

Q: But this is an uncommon condition that you are not likely to encounter anyway—right?

A: Wrong! Yapp *et al.* (2001) note that the most common inherited disorder in Caucasian populations is haemochromatosis associated with mutations in the HFE gene. It is definitely worth learning about.

Q: Just as you've finished seeing Mr Wayne, the nurse says that she has two more patients for you to see. The first is a 63-year-old man, Mr Warne, receiving his first unit of packed cells following blood loss from a total hip replacement 2 days ago. He is otherwise healthy and has never been transfused before. While receiving the first unit of blood, he became generally itchy and the nurse just noticed a widespread urticarial rash. What is happening and what should you do?

A: He is almost certainly having an allergic reaction to the blood products. This is quite common, occurring in about 1% of all transfusions. However, the spectrum can vary widely, from a mild skin reaction to full-blown anaphylaxis. Sometimes the anaphylactic reaction can be associated with fever, making it difficult to distinguish it from a febrile haemolytic transfusion reaction (Wu *et al.*, 2008). Therefore, the first priority is to:

1. cease the transfusion immediately (which the experienced nurse has already done)
2. assess Mr Warne for signs of life-threatening anaphylaxis (e.g. hypotension, bronchospasm, airway compromise, fever).

Q: Mr Warne feels well apart from the itchy rash. There are no signs of haemodynamic instability, bronchospasm or airway compromise. Now that you are convinced that Mr Warne isn't having anaphylaxis, what would a reasonable approach be at this point?

A: A reasonable approach would include the following (Wu *et al.*, 2008):

- Administer an antihistamine (e.g. 25–50 mg diphenhydramine or promethazine).
- If the rash settles within a short time, you can recommence the transfusion and closely observe him (do not recommence the transfusion if there was evidence of life-threatening anaphylaxis).
- Premedicate Mr Warne with antihistamines prior to future transfusions.
- Of course, if you are at all unsure, speak to the on-duty medical registrar.

(Washed cells can be used for people who experience severe allergic reactions during a transfusion or continue to develop mild reactions despite being premedicated with antihistamines.)

Q: The nurse takes you to the second patient, an elderly woman named Miss Rook. She had an unsuccessful attempt at taking blood from Miss Rook to check her platelet count and wonders if you could have a go. Apparently, Miss Rook developed thrombocytopaenia about a week following her transfusion. Can transfusion reactions occur so much later?

A: They certainly can, although these delayed reactions are not common. Two examples of delayed transfusion reactions are post-transfusion purpura (which Miss Rook probably has) and delayed haemolytic reactions (Wu *et al.*, 2008).

1. Post-transfusion purpura occurs with 1/7000 transfusions and typically affects middle-aged or elderly women. It is a serious disorder with thrombocytopaenia lasting up to 120 days and case fatality rates as high as 10%. The major treatment is intravenous immunoglobulin.
2. Delayed haemolytic reactions typically occur 3–10 days after the transfusion but tend to be milder than the acute haemolytic

reactions. Like the acute haemolytic reactions, the haemolysis can extravascular or intravascular (Wu *et al.*, 2008).

Q: A few hours later, your registrar calls you to take bloods urgently from Mr Wayne, who has become acutely short of breath. Your registrar says, 'I think he's got TRALI'. What is she talking about?

A: TRALI stands for transfusion-related acute lung injury. It typically presents as acute respiratory distress within 6 hours of a transfusion. It is due to non-cardiogenic pulmonary oedema probably generated by a reaction of the donor's HLA/granulocyte-specific antibodies to the recipient's white cells. There is a broad differential diagnosis including cardiogenic pulmonary oedema, sepsis and anaphylaxis. TRALI tends to respond fairly quickly to ventilatory, and, if necessary, haemodynamic support. Naturally, the transfusion must be immediately stopped if it was still continuing at the time of the reaction (Wu *et al.*, 2008).

Q: A medical student standing nearby listens to your conversation and then asks, 'What about taco?' Why is the medical student thinking of Mexican food when a patient is so unwell?

A: He most likely is referring to TACO or transfusion-associated circulatory overload. It presents in a similar way to TRALI but is cardiogenic rather than noncardiogenic in aetiology. The combination of transfusion and reduced cardiac function leads to cardiogenic pulmonary oedema. TACO is treated with diuretics (unlike TRALI, where diuretic use is controversial) and noninvasive or invasive ventilation (Osterman and Arora, 2014). Your patient has no known cardiac history so you suspect TRALI over TACO.

Achievements

You now:

- know the risk of transmitting hepatitis B, hepatitis C and HIV through blood transfusions in Australia
- know how to approach the febrile patient during a blood transfusion
- can tell the difference between haemolysis and FNHTRs
- are familiar with some of the other early and delayed reactions to blood transfusions
- know that repeated blood transfusions and haemochromatosis can cause iron overload.

References

Australian Red Cross Blood Service (2014), Transfusion Medicine Services, 'Residual risk estimates for transfusion-transmissible infections', at <www.transfusion.com.au/adverse_events/risks/estimates>, accessed 30 November 2014.

Brecher, M.E. (ed.) (2002), *AABB Technical Manual*, American Association of Blood Banks, Bethesda.

Bussel, J. and Cines, D.B. (2008), 'Immune thrombocytopenic purpura, neonatal alloimmune thrombocytopenia, and posttransfusion purpura', in R. Hoffman, E.J. Benz Jr, S.J. Shattil, B. Furie, L.E. Silberstein, P. McGlave and H.E. Heslop (eds), *Hematology: Basic Principles and Practice*, Churchill Livingstone, Philadelphia, Chapter 138.

Osterman, J.L. and Arora, S. (2014), 'Blood product transfusions and reactions', *Emergency Medicine Clinics of North America*, vol. 32, no. 3, pp. 727–738.

Wu, Y.Y., Mantha, S. and Snyder, E.L. (2008), 'Transfusion reactions', in R. Hoffman, E.J. Benz Jr, S.J. Shattil, B. Furie, L.E. Silberstein, P. McGlave and H.E. Heslop (eds), *Hematology: Basic Principles and Practice*, Churchill Livingstone, Philadelphia, Chapter 153.

Yapp, T.R., Eijkelkamp, E.J. and Powell, L.W. (2001), 'Population screening for HFE-associated haemochromatosis: Should we have to pay for our genes?', *Internal Medicine Journal*, vol. 31, no. 1, pp. 48–52.

Chapter 29
Mr Papadopoulos is assessed for low sodium

Scenario

Mr Papadopoulos is referred to the Emergency Department by his GP, Dr Spock, who writes:

> Thank you for seeing Mr Papadopoulos, a 65-year-old man with hypo-natraemia. He has been feeling generally unwell for the past 4 or 5 days. In particular he has felt lethargic, anorexic and nauseated, although he hasn't been vomiting.
>
> Apart from Mylanta occasionally for some heartburn, he is on no regular medications and has no serious medical problems.
>
> He has smoked a packet of cigarettes a day for 20 years. I did a basic blood work-up for him. The results are enclosed. The only thing of note was a plasma Na^+ level of 125 mmol/L. His serum osmolality is 269 mosm/kg. Do you think that the hyponatraemia is the culprit? Could you please investigate and treat him further?
>
> Live long and prosper,
>
> Dr Spock

You review the blood tests, which were taken yesterday. A full blood count, electrolytes and liver function tests have been performed. As Dr Spock asserted, the only abnormalities are the hyponatraemia, which is Na^+ 125 mmol/L (the normal range is 135–145 mmol/L) and the serum osmolality of 269 mosm/kg (normal, 280–300 mosm/kg).

Q: But surely a sodium of 125 mmol/L is not that low? It couldn't be responsible for Mr Papadopoulos's symptoms, could it?

A: Beware the leading question! Such a low plasma sodium level could indeed be solely responsible for Mr Papadopoulos's illness.

The following table gives an idea of the relationship between plasma sodium levels and various clinical features. Remember, however, that these are not concrete rules. There can be a large variation between individuals. In addition, the rapidity of the drop in plasma sodium, and not only the absolute sodium level, can determine the severity of symptoms.

Plasma sodium (mmol/L)	130–135	125–129	115–124	<115
No symptoms	Yes	No	No	No
Anorexia	No	Yes	Yes	Yes
Nausea and vomiting	No	Yes	Yes	Yes
Abdominal cramps	No	Yes	Yes	Yes
Agitation	No	No	Yes	Yes
Confusion	No	No	Yes	Yes
Hallucinations	No	No	Yes	Yes
Impaired mental function	No	No	Yes	Yes
Incontinence	No	No	Yes	Yes
Seizures	No	No	No	Yes
Coma	No	No	No	Yes

Source: Smith *et al.* (2000).

According to this table, all of Mr Papadopoulos's symptoms could be attributed to his low plasma sodium. He has been unwell for 4–5 days, so assume that his hyponatraemia is chronic (>48 hours) (Sahay and Sahay, 2014).

Q: What is your approach to the hyponatraemic patient?

A: The 2 aims are to correct the hyponatraemia and identify the underlying cause.

Q: How do you try to find the underlying cause of Mr Papadopoulos's hyponatraemia?

A: There are many causes of hyponatraemia. However, a systematic method for evaluating the cause of hyponatraemia is based on the patient's fluid status.

1. **Hypovolaemic** (deficit in both total body water and sodium):
   a. thiazide diuretics (the most common cause of hypovolaemic hyponatraemia; usually occurs within 2 weeks of commencing treatment)
   b. Addison's disease
   c. cerebral salt wasting syndrome
   d. gastrointestinal losses (vomiting and diarrhoea)
   e. pancreatitis (third space losses)
   f. burns (mucosal losses).

Hypovolaemic causes can be further classified according to urinary Na^+ concentration:

- urinary $[Na^+] > 40$ mmol/L: causes a, b, c
- urinary $[Na^+] < 20$ mmol/L: causes d, e, f

2. **Hypervolaemic** (excess of total body sodium with relative excess of water):
   a. cirrhosis
   b. congestive cardiac failure
   c. chronic renal failure (nephrotic syndrome).

3. **Euvolaemic:***
   a. syndrome of inappropriate antidiuretic hormone (SIADH)
   b. hypothyroidism
   c. hypopituitarism
   d. postoperative (often due to excessive hypotonic fluid).

Q: Does a low serum sodium automatically mean true hyponatraemia?

A: Not necessarily. The key to working out whether or not the hyponatraemia is real is the serum osmolality. Ideally, true hyponatraemia is present when the low serum sodium is associated with a low serum osmolality, as with Mr Papadopoulos. But a low serum sodium can occur with a normal serum osmolality ('pseudohyponatraemia') due to the presence of hypertriglyceridaemia or hyperproteinaemia (e.g. multiple myeloma). Or a low serum sodium can occur with an elevated serum osmolality ('translocational hyponatraemia') due to the presence of osmotically active substances/states (e.g. hyperglycaemia and mannitol). In such cases, the true serum sodium can be determined by correcting for the level of elevation of these substances (e.g. glucose, protein, triglycerides) (Sahay and Sahay, 2014).

Q: What is SIADH?

A: It is worth knowing the basics about SIADH, as you will inevitably encounter patients with hyponatraemia due to this condition. It is a disorder characterised by decreased body sodium and an increase in total body water. These changes are precipitated by increased concentrations of plasma ADH (also known as vasopressin).

Q: SIADH is a complication of a number of different conditions. What are some of the causes?

---

*Euvolaemic hyponatraemia is the most common cause of hyponatraemia, accounting for 60% of cases (Sahay and Sahay, 2014).

A: In broad terms, the 4 most common causes are:
1. malignancy (the most common cause)
2. pulmonary infections
3. central nervous system disorders (infections and haemorrhages)
4. medications (selective serotonin reuptake inhibitors, carbamazepine, cyclophosphamide, tricyclic antidepressants and phenothiazines).

Q: What are the diagnostic criteria for SIADH?

A: The main criteria are:
- euvolaemic patient
- plasma osmolality under 270 mosmol/kg
- inappropriate urinary concentration (urinary osmolality over 100 mosmol/kg)
- urinary sodium usually over 40 mmol/L
- exclude hypothyroidism and glucocorticoid deficiency.

In addition, there are some supplemental criteria.

Q: Armed with your knowledge of hyponatraemia, you proceed to examine Mr Papadopoulos. You find that he is euvolaemic. There is no postural hypotension, tachycardia, reduced turgor or dry mucous membranes to suggest hypovolaemia. There is no raised JVP, pulmonary oedema, ascites, sacral or pedal oedema to suggest hypovolaemia. The remainder of his examination is also unremarkable.

You conclude that Mr Papadopoulos has euvolaemic hyponatraemia. What investigations will you order?

A: You should order:
- urinary osmolality and sodium (a 24-hour urinary sodium is preferable to a spot urinary sodium)
- urine:serum electrolyte ratio*
- plasma sodium and osmolality
- formal blood glucose
- thyroid function tests
- serum cortisol (0800–0900 hours)
- chest X-ray
- possible CT brain, chest and abdomen.

---

*The 'urine:serum electrolyte ratio' is mathematically represented by (urinary sodium concentration + urinary potassium concentration)/serum sodium concentration. If the ratio is <0.5 in euvolaemic hyponatraemia, the use of fluid restriction alone may be enough to correct the hyponatraemia. If the ratio is >1.0 in euvolaemic hyponatraemia, then fluid restriction alone is unlikely to correct the hyponatraemia (Sahay and Sahay, 2014).

Q: The serum cortisol and thyroid function tests return as normal. The urinary and plasma sodium and osmolality results are consistent with SIADH. The urine:serum electrolyte ratio is 0.45. You are satisfied that Mr Papadopoulos's symptoms are due to hyponatraemia and that the hyponatraemia is due to SIADH. Now you wait to see if the imaging reveals a possible source of the SIADH. The CT brain is unremarkable. What does Mr Papadopoulos's chest X-ray demonstrate?

A: Mr Papadopoulos has a prominent right-sided apical opacity. This needs to be further investigated. However, given his long history of smoking, lung carcinoma would be high on the list of possible causes of both the abnormal chest X-ray and the SIADH.

Q: Your priority now is to treat the SIADH and correct the hyponatraemia. Of course, removal or treatment of the underlying cause of the SIADH (in this case, the lung opacity) is essential. However, what additional measures should you use to treat Mr Papadopoulos's SIADH?

A: For SIADH, a daily fluid restriction of 1 litre/day should be adequate, especially given his urine:serum electrolyte ratio of 0.45. If it is inadequate, other options include demeclocycline or IV isotonic saline.

Q: What is demeclocycline?

A: Surprisingly, this is an antibiotic. Nevertheless, it inhibits the effects of vasopressin on the kidney and so is therapeutic in SIADH (Smith *et al.*, 2000). However, it only starts working after 3 or 4 days, doesn't

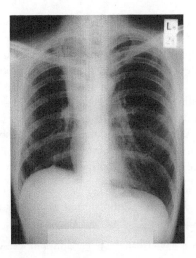

Figure 29.1 Mr Papadopoulos's chest X-ray

reach its maximal efficacy for 3 weeks and can cause nephrotoxicity (Patel and Balk, 2007).

Q: Have other medications been used to correct hyponatraemia?

A: Yes. Lithium and even phenytoin (an anticonvulsant which can have a suppressive effect on vasopressin) have been used but are both prone to serious side effects. A new class of drugs that antagonise vasopressin receptors are the vaptans (such as conivaptan, lixivaptan, tolvaptan). They can be administered both orally or parenterally and are showing promise as therapy for hyponatraemia (Sahay and Sahay, 2014; Patel and Balk, 2007).

Q: Kenji, one of the medical students, has been looking on with interest. 'If his symptoms are due to low sodium, why don't you quickly fix it with lots of hypertonic saline?'

Do you agree with him?

A: No. What Kenji says should make sense (i.e. returning the plasma sodium level to normal as soon as possible will make the symptoms from the hyponatraemia disappear quickly), but correcting the plasma sodium level too rapidly can lead to osmotic demyelination syndrome (ODS) (previously known as central pontine myelinolysis [CPM]).

Smith *et al.* (2000) note that ODS is a clinically devastating disorder, typically characterised by spastic quadraparesis and pseudobulbar palsy occurring 2–3 days after correcting the low plasma sodium. As well as the clinical features, MRI and electrophysiologic features can assist in diagnosis.

The patients at most risk of ODS include those with chronic symptomatic hyponatraemia, those who are malnourished, alcoholics, those with severe hypokalaemia and a subset of patients after liver transplantation. In those at low risk of ODS, aim to increase the plasma sodium concentration by no more than 4–8 mmol/day. In those at high risk of ODS, raise the plasma sodium concentration by no more than 4–6 mmol/day (Sahay and Sahay, 2014; Endocrinology Expert Group, 2014).

Hypertonic saline (e.g. IV sodium chloride 3%) should be used with great caution in the hyponatraemic patient. Often it will be used only in the presence of severe hyponatraemia with neurological symptoms.

Q: Can ODS be treated?

A: Relowering sodium and administering desmopressin can potentially reverse ODS (Sahay and Sahay , 2014).

Q: How would you have treated Mr Papadopoulos's hyponatraemia if it were due to hypovolaemia or hypervolaemia?

A: In hypovolaemic hyponatraemia (e.g. dehydration), IV fluid replacement with normal saline is a reasonable therapeutic measure. In hypervolaemic patients (e.g. congestive cardiac failure), a combination of fluid restriction and diuretics may be required to correct the hyponatraemia. Assessing the fluid status in hyponatraemic patients is extremely important, as it will direct your management strategy.

Q: Mr Papadopoulos is admitted under the endocrine team. His hyponatraemia and symptoms improve with fluid restriction alone. You later learn that the respiratory team was consulted about the apical lung opacity. Unfortunately, your suspicions are confirmed: Mr Papadopoulos has small-cell cancer of the lung. The last thing you hear is that he is referred to the oncology team for chemotherapy.

A few weeks pass and you are once again working in the Emergency Department. Who should you see in Bed 1 but Mr Papadopoulos! The triage nurse tells you that he is febrile after finishing chemotherapy about 9 or 10 days ago.

Based on the limited information the triage nurse has given you, what do you think could be wrong with Mr Papadopoulos?

A: Febrile neutropenia is a likely cause. Certain chemotherapeutic regimens are highly myelosuppressive. This results in neutropenia, which makes patients more susceptible to infection. The primary manifestations of these infections are fever, hence the term 'febrile neutropenia'. Furthermore, febrile neutropenia will often occur 10–14 days after chemotherapy. It is a common occurrence with chemotherapy for both solid organ (10–50%) and haematological malignancies (>80%) (Freifeld et al., 2011). The timing of Mr Papadopoulos's febrile illness would also be consistent with febrile neutropenia.

Q: At what level of neutropenia is a patient at significant risk of infection?

A: Patients with a neutrophil count of less than 1.0×10^9/L are more susceptible to infection. But the risk significantly increases at neutrophil counts below 0.5×10^9/L.

Q: Mr Papadopoulos is pleased to see you again. He gives you his oncology clinic card, which shows that he is now day 10 post-etoposide and cisplatin.

Is this combination of chemotherapeutic agents potentially myelosuppressive?

A: It certainly is. Yesterday, Mr Papadopoulos became lethargic and started shivering and sweating. His daughter checked his temperature and found him to be febrile (39 °C). He has no focal symptoms of infection.

Q: In oncology patients, what iatrogenic source of sepsis must be excluded?

A: Vascular access for oncology patients can be a long-term difficulty. As a result, many of these patients will have Hickman lines and portacaths, which are tunnelled or surgically implanted intravascular catheters. Peripherally inserted central venous catheters (PICCs) are also used in this setting.

Q: Do these forms of intravascular access carry a higher risk of infection than peripheral venous catheters and central venous catheters?

A: The daily infection risk of Hickman lines, portacaths and PICC lines as a group is 5 times higher than that of peripheral venous catheters, but a quarter of that associated with central venous catheters.

Q: Mr Papadopoulos has no form of long-term intravascular access. Apart from tachycardia and fever, his physical examination is normal.

Does the lack of localising signs and symptoms surprise you in a patient with febrile neutropenia?

A: Not really. The lack of neutrophils results in an ability to mount a suitable pyogenic response. This may result in:

- an absence of urinary white cells in a UTI
- minimal inflammation in bacterial cellulitis
- normal chest X-ray despite the presence of a chest infection
- absent pleocytosis in bacterial meningitis.

Q: What broad group of bacteria accounts for most cases of febrile neutropenia in which the organism is identified?

A: Hughes *et al.* (2002) note that some 60–70% of micro-biologically documented cases are due to Gram-positive bacteria. In fact, coagulase-negative staphylococci are the most common blood culture isolates in febrile neutropenia, which reflects the increased use of long-term intravenous lines (Freifeld *et al.*, 2011). Gram-negative organisms also account for a significant proportion of disease, however.

Q: What investigations will you order?

A: You should order the following:

- full blood count (this will provide a neutrophil count)
- electrolytes, urea, creatinine (these will provide a baseline and allow antibiotic dosage adjustments in the presence of renal impairment)
- liver function tests (these will provide a baseline)
- 2 sets of blood cultures taken at different times from different sites (if a permanent form of IV access is present, blood cultures

should be taken simultaneously from each lumen of the device as well as from a peripheral vein)
- midstream urine specimen (possible source of infection)
- chest X-ray (possible source of infection).

Q: Are you confident that your thorough investigations and clinical evaluation will find the cause of Mr Papadopoulos's presumed febrile neutropenia?

A: You should not be too confident. In only 20–30% of cases of febrile neutropenia is a clinically documented infection identified, while only 10–25% of cases have positive blood cultures (Freifeld *et al.*, 2011).

Q: The laboratory phones to confirm what you suspected: Mr Papadopoulos is extremely neutropenic (0.1×10^9/L).

The electrolytes, renal and liver function tests are unremarkable. Microscopy of the midstream urine is normal with no cells or organisms seen, and the chest X-ray is normal. You now will have to wait for the results from the blood and urine cultures.

What empirical antibiotic therapy will you commence?

A: There are many different protocols for febrile neutropenia. Nevertheless, a common empirical regimen would be single therapy with an IV anti-pseudomonal beta-lactam agent. The reason for an anti-pseudomonal agent despite coagulase-negative staphylococci being the commonest cause of bacteraemia is that pseudomonal infections are associated with a bad outcome. Options for an adult with normal renal function include (Antibiotic Expert Group, 2014):
- piperacillin/tazobactam 4g/0.5g q6h OR
- ceftazidime 2g q8h OR
- cefepime 2g q8h.

Q: Should you add vancomycin to the empirical regimen?

A: Vancomycin is not recommended for the initial regimen of antibiotics except in specific circumstances (e.g. severe sepsis, high suspicion of methicillin-resistant *Staphylococcus aureus* infection) (Antibiotic Expert Group, 2014; Freifeld *et al.*, 2011). Pizzo (2000) cites studies that have demonstrated no survival benefit in doing so.

Q: What is the role of colony-stimulating factors in febrile neutropenia?

A: Colony-stimulating factors such as granulocyte colony-stimulating factor (G–CSF) and granulocyte-macrophage colony-stimulating factor (GM–CSF) are used as prophylaxis when there is a significant risk of febrile neutropenia; however, their use in the treatment of febrile neu-tropenia is not recommended (Freifeld at el., 2011). These shorten the duration of neutropenia, but do not affect many of the other measures of morbidity in febrile illnesses.

Once again, the role of these agents in febrile neutropenia will vary between institutions, and sometimes even between specialists within the same unit.

Q: What is the major side effect of G–CSF?

A: Bone pain is the most common side effect.

Q: Mr Papadopoulos receives empirical IV therapy with piperacillin-tazobactam. Over the next 5 days his neutrophil count returns to normal and he becomes afebrile. His antibiotics are ceased without any of the investigations identifying the cause.

Before being discharged, he asks you a question: 'Doc, if this "febrile neutro-thing" happens again, do I have to come to hospital? All you hospital people are nice but I hate being in here'.

What do you tell him?

A: Patients with febrile neutropenia can be classified as being at 'low risk' or 'high risk' for severe infection. Patients who are low risk can often be managed as an outpatient with broad-spectrum oral antibiotics such as ciprofloxacin and amoxycillin-clavulanic acid. Some factors for low-risk infection include (Freifeld *et al.*, 2011):

- duration of neutropenia anticipated to be 7 days or less
- being clinically stable
- having no comorbid medical conditions.

You do not need to memorise this list. Nevertheless, it is worth noting that patients with low-risk infection may be suitable for outpatient therapy with oral antibiotics (e.g. ciprofloxacin, amoxycillin-clavulanic acid). Not all patients with febrile neutropenia will be admitted to hospital.

Achievements

You now:

- know that the lower the plasma sodium, the worse the symptoms that can occur
- know how to approach the problem of hyponatraemia using the patient's fluid status
- know how to diagnose and treat SIADH
- realise that too-rapid correction of plasma sodium can be dangerous
- recognise the timing of febrile neutropenia in relation to chemotherapy

- know the neutrophil count at which people are at risk of febrile neutropenia
- realise that, despite extensive investigation, a cause of febrile neutropenia may not be found
- are aware of the empirical antibiotic treatment of febrile neutropenia
- realise that the empirical antibiotic combination may vary between institutions
- know the role of G–CSF in the management of febrile neutropenia.

References

Antibiotic Expert Group (2014), *Therapeutic Guidelines: Antibiotic*, Version 15, Therapeutic Guidelines Ltd, Melbourne.

Endocrinology Expert Group (2014), *Therapeutic Guidelines: Endocrinology*, Version 5, Therapeutic Guidelines Ltd, Melbourne.

Freifeld, A.G., Bow, E.J., Sepkowitz, K.A., *et al.* (2011), 'Clinical practice guideline for the use of antimicrobial agents in neutropenic patients with cancer: 2010 update by the Infectious Diseases Society of America', *Clinical Infectious Diseases*, vol. 52, no. 4, e56–e93.

Horvarth, R. and Collignon, P. (2003), 'Controlling intravascular catheter infections', *Australian Prescriber*, vol. 26, no. 2, pp. 41–43.

Hughes, W.T. *et al.* (2002), '2002 guidelines for the use of antimicrobial agents in neutropenic patients with cancer', *Clinical Infectious Diseases*, vol. 34, no. 6, pp. 730–751.

Patel, G.P. and Balk, R.A. (2007), 'Recognition and treatment of hyponatraemia in acutely ill hospitalized patients', *Clinical Therapeutics*, vol. 29, no. 2, pp. 211–229.

Pizzo, P.A. (2000), 'Empirical therapy and prevention of infection in the immunocompromised host', in G.L. Mandell, J.E. Bennett and R. Dolin (eds), *Principles and Practice of Infectious Diseases*, Churchill Livingstone, Philadelphia, pp. 3102–3112.

Sahay, M. and Sahay, R. (2014), 'Hyponatremia: A practical approach', *Indian Journal of Endocrinology and Metabolism*, vol. 18, no. 6, pp. 760–761.

Smith, D.M., McKenna, K. and Thompson, C.J. (2000), 'Hyponatraemia', *Clinical Endocrinology*, vol. 52, no. 6, pp. 667–678.

Chapter 30
Mr Caesar presents with confusion

Scenario

It is a beautiful summer's day. With a wistful sigh, you enter the Emergency Department for another 10-hour shift. Your first patient is a 75-year-old man, Mr Caesar. He is accompanied by his wife, who looks very worried. She tells you that her husband has been very confused for the past 3 days, and that he is seeing weird things around the house.

Mr Caesar is not attentive enough to provide a history. Nevertheless, his wife is very helpful. She says her husband is overall very healthy. The only medication he takes is a thiazide diuretic for mild hypertension. He drinks 1 glass of red wine every evening. He has been increasingly forgetful over the past year, which his GP has attributed to early dementia. He is due to see a geriatrician for this next month.

Mr Caesar's forgetfulness was mild and he functioned normally. But 3 days ago, he deteriorated rapidly. He became very confused and disoriented. His attention span dropped and he has been extremely lethargic. Mrs Caesar can't cope with him in this state any longer. And although he was much more lucid this morning, his confusion returned after 2 hours.

Q: What is wrong with Mr Caesar?
A: He is almost certainly suffering from delirium.

Q: What is delirium?
A: This is a disorder characterised by:
- reduced attention span
- cognitive disturbance (e.g. memory, speech, disorientation)
- perceptual disturbances (e.g. illusions and hallucinations)
- mood and sleep disorders
- fluctuation in severity
- development over days to weeks.
The DSM-5 has specific definitions for delirium (Kalish *et al.*, 2014).

And note ...

It is important to remember that this disturbance fluctuates. Delirium in hospitalised patients is sometimes missed because a person who is confused in the evening may be lucid in the morning. The morning staff may assume that the problem has resolved when what they are actually witnessing is the natural fluctuation of delirium.

Q: Mrs Caesar asks if the illness is due to his dementia. What do you think?

A: This is a good question. Dementia is one of the main differential diagnoses of delirium. Indeed, in a patient with advanced dementia, a superimposed delirium can be very difficult to diagnose. The other main differential diagnoses of delirium are psychosis and depression.

The following table demonstrates some of the differences between delirium and dementia.

	Delirium	Dementia
Onset	Acute or subacute	Slow
Course	Fluctuates	Progresses
Conscious level	Often impaired	Clear
Cognitive defects	Poor attention/short-term memory	Poor short-term memory but attention normal
Hallucinations	Common	Uncommon
Delusions	Fleeting	Uncommon
Psychomotor activity	Variable	Can be normal

Source: Adapted from Brown and Boyle (2002).

According to this table, Mr Caesar's illness fits with delirium. Patients with a functional psychosis often have no cognitive impairment and are less likely to experience visual hallucinations than those with delirium.

Patients with depression tend to be unhappy and have no interest in activities that they previously found pleasurable. They may also have difficulty sleeping and a reduced appetite. Suicidal ideation and low self-esteem may be apparent.

Q: Sim Wai, one of the medical students in the Emergency Department, has accompanied you to see this patient. However, he doesn't look very excited. 'So he has delirium—big deal. It's just a bit of confusion. Does it really matter?'

A: It does matter actually. Delirium is associated with longer hospital admissions and higher mortality rates (14.5–37%). Also, delirium can persist in over 40% of patients for as long as 1 year following discharge, which can be distressing and difficult for both patients and their friends and family. These issues are particularly important since delirium is such a common problem, affecting anywhere from 10–30% of patients on admission to hospital (Attard *et al.*, 2008). If not identified and addressed, delirium can result in poor long-term outcomes and a functional decline in people (Kalish *et al.*, 2014).

Q: Although anyone can develop delirium, some groups are at increased risk of delirium if exposed to certain precipitants. Who are some of these groups?

A: Some of these susceptible groups include those with (Attard *et al.*, 2008):
- visual impairment
- cognitive impairment (e.g. dementia)
- male sex
- increasing age
- depression
- severe medical illness.

Q: What precipitates delirium?

A: Unfortunately, almost anything can cause delirium and often there'll be more than 1 cause! Some of the more common causes are:
- acute infections
- prescribed drugs[1]
- drug withdrawal (alcohol, opiate analgesics, benzodiazepines, anticholinergics)
- hypoxia
- recreational drugs
- stroke/transient ischaemic attacks
- cerebral haemorrhage (intracerebral, subdural, epidural)
- cardiovascular disorders (MI, PE, heart failure)
- endocrine disorders (thyroid disease, Cushing's syndrome, parathyroid disease, hypopituitarism, hyperglycaemia or hypoglycaemia)
- epilepsy
- cancer
- acute severe pain

---

[1] Acute infections and prescribed drugs are 2 of the most common causes of delirium. Specifically, the addition of ≥3 medications in the previous 24 hours is a risk factor for delirium (Attard *et al.*, 2008).

- metabolic disturbances (acidosis, renal or hepatic failure, electrolyte abnormalities, alkalosis)
- vitamin B12, niacin and thiamine deficiencies
- heavy metals.

Q: Sim Wai says, 'I can't remember that long list! Give me a mnemonic!'

A: Medical students and their mnemonics! Fortunately, you can give Sim Wai a mnemonic to help him remember the causes of delirium. It is the rather morbid I WATCH DEATH.

I: Infection
W: Withdrawal
A: Acute metabolic
T: Trauma
C: Central nervous system pathology
H: Hypoxia
D: Deficiencies
E: Endocrinopathies
A: Acute vascular
T: Toxins and drugs
H: Heavy metals
  (If this is too morbid for you, try switching the letters around: WHAT I'D TEACH!)

Q: Sim Wai looks at the lethargic figure that is Mr Caesar and says, 'The last person I saw with delirium was singing and yelling and trying to fight with anybody who came near him. Mr Caesar is completely the opposite. Is that a different kind of delirium?'

A: Yes, there are three types of delirium: hypoactive, hyperactive and mixed. There are specific criteria for the hypoactive and hyperactive types: in essence, people with hypoactive delirium are slow and lethargic while those with hyperactive delirium are loud, hypervigilant and combative. The mixed subtype, however, is the most commonly diagnosed (Kalish *et al.*, 2014).

Q: You explain to Sim Wai that Mr Caesar probably has a hypoactive delirium. He shrugs his shoulders. 'Hyperactive, hypoactive: does it really matter?'

A: In terms of prognosis, a hypoactive delirium is associated with a worse outcome (Kalish *et al.*, 2014).

Q: How can you confirm this is a delirium?

A: An effective way of identifying a delirium is by using the Confusion Assessment Method, which has a sensitivity of 94–100%. The tool

itself can easily be found online. According to CAM, delirium can be diagnosed when there is ((Kalish *et al.*, 2014):
- Acute onset and fluctuating course AND Inattention
  AND EITHER
- Disorganised thinking OR Altered level of consciousness

Q: You examine Mr Caesar thoroughly but unfortunately, you don't find any clues. He is afebrile with a heart rate of 95 regular beats/minute. The blood pressure is 130/80 and his oxygen saturation on room air is 97%. He is too inattentive to complete the MMSE. His speech is normal and not slurred. There is no obvious weakness in his face or limbs. The cardiovascular, respiratory and gastrointestinal examinations are normal.

Mrs Caesar says, 'He doesn't have a fever so I guess it can't be an infection'. What is your response to this?

A: It is very important to remember that a proportion of elderly people with a serious infection will not mount a febrile response. During your medical career you will assess a large number of sick elderly people. Do not dismiss a diagnosis of infection in the elderly simply because there is no fever.

Q: What investigations will you order?

A:

1. **Full blood count**. A raised white cell count is evidence of infection, but its absence should not make you dismiss this diagnosis. An elevated mean cell volume may represent alcoholism, and anaemia may represent underlying malignancy or B12 deficiency (particularly if it is macrocytic).

2. **Electrolytes, calcium, magnesium, phosphate and blood sugar**. Any number of abnormalities here can result in delirium.

3. **Liver function tests**. Abnormalities here may support a diagnosis of cholangitis or other sources of sepsis, drug toxicity, metastatic disease or chronic alcohol use.

4. **Blood cultures**. You should take 2 sets at different times from different sites.

5. **Urinalysis**. If this is abnormal, proceed to a midstream urine specimen.

6. **Arterial blood gas**. This may demonstrate hypoxia or hypercapnia.

7. **CRP and ESR**. If elevated, these are a sign of an ongoing inflammatory process, but are very non-specific.

8. **12-lead ECG and serial troponins**. These tests are used to look for an acute coronary syndrome.

9. **Chest X-ray**. Any infiltrate, whether due to pneumonia, heart failure, cancer or other causes, may be significant.
10. **CT brain scan**. This will identify intracerebral, subdural, epidural and subarachnoid bleeding. Thromboembolic strokes more than 48 hours old should be visible (Mr Caesar has had symptoms for 3 days). Neoplastic lesions may be visible.
11. **Lumbar puncture**. Consider a lumbar puncture if you are concerned about encephalitis or meningitis.

Q: How will you treat Mr Caesar's delirium?
A:

1. **Treat the underlying cause**. Your investigations should reveal the underlying cause of the delirium, which can then be addressed.
2. **Environment**. Mr Caesar should be in a room with adequate lighting, and family members and friends should visit regularly. If possible, the same nurses should look after him to promote trust and recognition. It is also a good idea to provide aids such as clocks to promote orientation. Likewise, if Mr Caesar wears glasses or uses a hearing aid, he should be using them. Familiar objects from home might also help reassure him.
3. **Look for sources of discomfort** that he might not be able to communicate to you (e.g. constipation, dehydration, pain).
4. **Sleep**. Try to ensure that he has undisturbed sleep at a regular time.
5. **Pharmacotherapy**. You should only prescribe medications to treat delirium if the patient is (Inouye, 2006):
   - a danger to themselves
   - a danger to others
   - unable to receive essential treatment.

Also, use 1 medication at a time, ensure that the medications are reviewed daily and that they have been discontinued within 7–10 days of the delirium resolving (Attard *et al.*, 2008).

Q: Sim Wai asks, 'What medications should we use?'
A: Antipsychotics are the mainstay of pharmacological therapy for delirium. The most commonly used antipsychotic for the treatment of delirium in Australian hospitals is probably haloperidol but other antipsychotics such as risperidone and olanzapine are also commonly used. A Cochrane review found that low-dose haloperidol (<3.5 mg/day) was comparable to risperidone and olanzapine with regard to both efficacy and adverse effects. Higher doses of haloperidol (>4.5 mg/day),

however, were more likely to cause Parkinsonian side effects (Lonergan *et al.*, 2007).

The use of these medications in delirium is a complex affair; therefore, it would be best as an intern to speak to a registrar or even a consultant before initiating an antipsychotic for delirium.

Although interns shouldn't initiate antipsychotics for delirium, the table opposite gives an approach for the use of the routes, dosages, monitoring required and adverse effects of these medications.

But again, speak to a more senior doctor before initiating these medications for delirium.

Drug	Route	Dose	Maximum daily dose	Peak effect	Monitoring	Adverse effects
Haloperidol (these haloperidol doses have been reduced for the elderly)	po	0.5–1 mg every 2–4 hours	5 mg/day	4–6 hours	ECG monitoring*	Most commonly extrapyramidal side effects but more common over 4.5 mg/day
	IM/IV	0.25–0.5 mg every 30–60 minutes	2.5 mg/day	20–40 minutes	ECG monitoring*	Lower risk of extrapyramidal side effects but higher risk of prolonged QTc and torsades de pointes
Risperidone	po	0.5 mg bd (every 4 hours)	4 mg/day			Extrapyramidal and anticholinergic side effects
Olanzapine	po	2.5–5 mg/day	20 mg/day			Extrapyramidal and anticholinergic side effects

* Although the risk of QTc and torsades de pointes are thought to be less with oral haloperidol, some guidelines still recommend ECG monitoring of patients receiving haloperidol by the oral route (Attard *et al.*, 2008). Certainly, prolonged QTc and torsades have been documented after oral haloperidol (LLerena *et al.*, 2002; Jackson *et al.*, 1997). Having said that, many Australian hospitals don't advocate ECG monitoring for even IV or IM haloperidol.

Source: Adapted from Attard *et al.*, 2008.

Q: The results of Mr Caesar's investigations are ready. The 12-lead ECG, chest X-ray and CT brain scan are normal, and the blood gas and urinalysis are unremarkable. How do you interpret the following blood results?

Test	Normal range	Result
Haemoglobin	130–180 g/L	110*
Mean cell volume	80–100 fL	82
White cell count	3.5–11 × 10⁹/L	4.5
Platelet count	150–450 × 10⁹/L	182
Sodium	135–145 mmol/L	137
Potassium	3.6–5.1 mmol/L	4.1
Chloride	95–107 mmol/L	98
Bicarbonate	22–32 mmol/L	25
Urea	2.9–7.1 mmol/L	4
Creatinine	60–110 umol/L	90
Calcium	2.25–2.58 mmol/L	2.90*
Albumin	33–48 g/L	30*
Bilirubin	0–25 μmol/L	20
Alkaline phosphate	38–126 U/L	90
GGT	0–30 U/L	23
Aspartate aminotransferase	<45 U/L	12
Alanine aminotransferase	<45 U/L	12
ESR	mm/hour	78*
CRP	<3 mg/L	3

* Abnormal results.

A: Mr Caesar has hypercalcaemia.

Q: The hypercalcaemia is associated with a normochromic normocytic anaemia and a raised ESR. Could hypercalcaemia account for Mr Caesar's delirium?

A: Yes, hypercalcaemia is a recognised cause of delirium.

Q: Is Mr Caesar's calcium level really 2.90 mmol/L?

A: No. Calcium in the blood is found in ionised and protein-bound forms. It is the ionised component, not the protein-bound component, which can diffuse across membranes.

Approximately 90% of the protein-bound calcium is bound to albumin. As a result, any change in serum albumin will require an adjustment in the measured plasma calcium level.

The formula to work out the correct calcium level is:

$$[(40 - \text{serum albumin}) \times 0.02] + \text{measured calcium}$$

This is one formula that you will need to know as an intern! In Mr Caesar's case:

$$
\begin{aligned}
\text{corrected calcium} &= [(40 - 30) \times 0.02] + 2.90 \\
&= 0.20 + 2.90 \\
&= 3.10 \text{ mmol/L}
\end{aligned}
$$

Having said that you need to know this formula, many clinical chemistry labs will, however, provide a corrected calcium result.

Q: You explain to Mrs Caesar that her husband is most likely delirious secondary to hypercalcaemia with subsequent dehydration. You reassure her that this can be treated, but it is just as important to find the underlying cause. What are some clinical features of hypercalcaemia?

A: These include:
- nausea and vomiting
- anorexia
- constipation
- polyuria and polydipsia (with dehydration if not corrected)
- depression
- confusion
- coma
- seizures.

Q: What are some complications of hypercalcaemia?

A: Complications include:
- nephrolithiasis
- arrhythmias (shortened QT interval)
- peptic ulcer disease
- pancreatitis.

Q: What are the possible mechanisms of hypercalcaemia?

A:

1. **Bone resorption** is the most common mechanism. However, bone resorption can be induced in a number of ways. Primary hyperparathyroidism is usually caused by an adenoma. In this case, there is excessive production of para-thyroid hormone

(PTH). This results in elevated or inappropriately normal PTH levels, hypercalcaemia and reduced plasma phosphate levels. Malignancies can produce agents that stimulate bone resorption. The best known example here is parathyroid hormone-related protein (PTHrP). Malignancies can also cause bone resorption by skeletal metastases.

2. **Increased GIT absorption of calcium.** This can be seen in lymphoma and granulomatous diseases such as sarcoidosis. The increased absorption of calcium is usually mediated by increased production of 1,25-dihydroxy-vitamin D.

3. **Decreased renal excretion of calcium.** Drugs such as lithium and diuretics have been implicated here.

    Note: in general, primary hyperparathyroidism and malignancy are the most common causes of hypercalcaemia (Blackburn and Diamond, 2007).

Q: What blood tests will you order to find the cause of Mr Caesar's hypercalcaemia?
A:

1. PTH (elevated or inappropriately normal in primary hyperparathyroidism, generally low in other causes)
2. PTHrP (elevated in malignancy)
3. serum angiotensin converting enzyme (ACE, often elevated in granulomatous disease, especially sarcoidosis)
4. tests for multiple myeloma (discussed below)
5. 25-OH Vitamin D.

Q: What other investigations would you order?
A:

1. Chest X-ray (looking for malignancy)
2. whole body bone scan (may detect skeletal metastases but usually won't pick up metastases from myeloma).[2]

Q: How would you treat the hypercalcaemia?
A: A reasonable approach would be (Lumachi *et al.*, 2008):

1. **Vigorous rehydration with normal saline.**
    - This is because patients with symptomatic hypercalcaemia are often dehydrated due to nausea, vomiting and inhibition of water reabsorption in the distal renal tubules.

---

[2] In multiple myeloma there is activation of osteoclasts rather than osteoblasts. Therefore, the bone scan classically shows no uptake.

- Initially 500 mL/hour in the first few hours; however, this has to be titrated with the individual's cardiovascular/hepatic/renal status.

2. **Loop diuretics (e.g. frusemide).**
   - Only use diuretics once adequately hydrated.
   - Loop diuretics promote urinary calcium excretion.
   - Don't use thiazide diuretics as these paradoxically increase calcium reabsorption.

3. **IV bisphosphonates (e.g. pamidronate or zoledronate).**
   - These inhibit bone resorption, therefore they are not so useful in conditions like sarcoidosis where bone resorption isn't the main mechanism of hypercalcaemia.
   - Clinically relevant adverse effects include self-limiting fever (due to cytokine release by macrophages), renal toxicity (acute tubular necrosis) and radionecrosis of the jaw. This last complication is often seen with myeloma patients receiving long courses of bisphosphonates or in those who have had recent invasive procedures on the jaw or maxilla.

4. **Corticosteroids.**
   - For hypercalcaemia in general, corticosteroids aren't very useful. They work by reducing both calcium absorption in the intestine and hypercalcaemia-induced nausea. On the other hand, hypercalcaemia due to specific causes such as sarcoidosis responds well to corticosteroids.

5. **Treat the underlying disease.**
   It takes 3–5 days after treatment for the plasma calcium level to return to normal. In fact, it might rise in the first 48 hours, before decreasing. The confusion could take a similar period to resolve. In other words, don't expect immediate clinical and biochemical improvement.

Q: How long does it take for bisphosphonates to work?
A: A sustained reduction in plasma calcium is usually seen after 12–48 hours. This effect will continue for 2–4 weeks (Wagner and Arora, 2014).

Q: Mr Caesar responds well to your therapy and is back to his normal self within 3 days. His corrected plasma calcium is now 2.60 mmol/L.

By this stage, you have the results of your investigations for hypercalcaemia. The PTHrP and serum ACE are normal while the serum PTH is low. The bone scan is unremarkable. However, your registrar tells you that the lab called him to say that the multiple myeloma 'blood tests' are strongly suggestive of a diagnosis of multiple myeloma.

What is multiple myeloma?

A: Multiple myeloma is a disease in which malignant plasma cells produce a monoclonal protein and accumulate in the bone marrow. The monoclonal protein is usually IgG (70%) or IgA (20%). The diagnosis is based on the following (Rajkumar, 2009):

- >10% clonal plasma cells in bone marrow (or biopsy-proven plasmacytoma) AND
- M (monoclonal) protein in the serum and/or urine (except in the 1–2% of myeloma patients with non-secretory myeloma) AND
- evidence of end-organ damage (anaemia, bone lesions, hypercalcaemia, renal insufficiency).

Q: What are likely to be the 'blood tests' for multiple myeloma that your registrar is talking about?

A: A combination of blood tests can strongly support a diagnosis of multiple myeloma. These are (Rajkumar, 2009):

1. Serum protein electrophoresis (serum EPP)—this will identify an M protein.
2. Serum immunofixation—determines the heavy- and light-chain class of the M protein; more sensitive than serum EPP at detecting low levels of M protein.
3. Serum-free light-chain assay—can quantify free kappa and lambda light chains as a ratio and determine which light chain is responsible for the M protein.

   It would be very reasonable to ask for all these tests if considering a diagnosis of multiple myeloma.

Q: Indeed, the serum EPP, immunofixation and serum-free light-chain assay together identify an M protein due to IgG kappa. A bone marrow biopsy is performed. It shows that the marrow consists of 15% of monoclonal plasma cells. These findings, in addition to the evidence of end-organ damage (hypercalcaemia and normochromic normocytic anaemia in the initial blood tests) are sufficient to make a diagnosis of multiple myeloma. Now that multiple myeloma has been confirmed, what other simple tests can be performed?

A: It would be reasonable to perform the following blood tests for staging and prognosis (Rajkumar, 2009):

- beta-2-microglobulin
- lactate dehydrogenase
- albumin.

   Haemoglobin, serum calcium, creatinine and C-reactive protein are other important blood tests for multiple myeloma, but they have already been performed as part of Mr Caesar's delirium work-up on admission.

Q: Apart from blood tests, what radiological test should be performed?

A: A skeletal survey should be ordered to identify lytic bone lesions. This typically involves plain radiographs of the lateral skull, spine, pelvis and both humeri and femora. If the skeletal survey is negative in a patient in whom multiple myeloma is still suspected, then an MRI STIR (short-tau inversion recovery) can be ordered, which is more sensitive than a skeletal survey (Eslick and Talalulikar, 2014).

Q: What are the major clinical features of multiple myeloma?

A: The major features relate to:
- recurrent bacterial infections due to hypogammaglobulinaemia
- renal insufficiency
- osteolytic lesions (causing pathological fractures, pain and spinal cord compression)
- hypercalcaemia
- anaemia
- hyperviscosity syndrome.

Q: What is the cause of renal insufficiency in multiple myeloma?

A: This is multifactorial. Two of the common causes are deposition of light-chain tubular casts and hypercalcaemia.

Q: Mr Caesar's skeletal survey demonstrates multiple lytic lesions in the humeri and thoracolumbar spine.

The Caesars are devastated by the diagnosis of multiple myeloma. 'Doctor, is there any treatment for this?'

A: Although there is treatment for myeloma, the overall prognosis is poor, with a median survival of 4 years after conventional therapy (Rajkumar, 2009).

Factors that modify this figure include:
- the degree of anaemia
- presence of hypercalcaemia
- level of serum paraprotein
- presence of renal insufficiency
- presence of multiple lytic lesions
- beta-2-microglobulin levels.

Although you shouldn't need to know all the therapeutic regimens for treating multiple myeloma, it is worth knowing that therapy can be divided into (Rajkumar, 2009):

- those who are suitable for autologous stem cell transplantation (ASCT)
- those who are not suitable for ASCT.

Both groups receive different chemotherapy regimens. The ASCT group receives combinations without melphalan such as lanlidomide/dexamethasone, thalidomide/dexamethasone, bortezomib/dexamethasone. The non-ASCT candidates usually receive combinations containing melphalan/prednisone.

In addition to treatment of the multiple myeloma itself, the complications of the disease will need to be addressed, for example bisphosphonates for hypercalcaemia and bone disease.

Q: Because of Mr Caesar's age, the haematologist decides he is not suitable for ASCT and therefore treats him with thalidomide/melphalan/prednisone. Some months pass by and you find yourself working as the haematology intern. In your second week on the job there is a direct admission to the ward. You immediately recognise Mr Caesar.

Mr Caesar has not had chemotherapy for 6 weeks. Unfortunately, the response was poor. His anaemia and renal failure are worse, and the bony disease has become more widespread. In the past 2 days, Mr Caesar has noticed increasing thoracic back pain.

What is the most serious cause of back pain to consider in Mr Caesar?

A: In patients with cancer and back pain, you must consider epidural spinal cord compression (ESCC) secondary to bony metastases. ESCC is a medical emergency.

Q: What are the clinical features of ESCC?

A: These include:

- pain (often the first symptom, as in Mr Caesar's case)
- weakness (upper motor neurone weakness if the lesion occurs at the level of the conus or above)
- sensory deficits (sensory level on examination tends to be 1–5 segments below the true level of the ESCC)
- bowel and bladder dysfunction.

And note ...

It is vital for you to realise that once a patient has neurological features of ESCC (e.g. paraplegia, urinary retention), the chances of recovery are extremely poor. You must diagnose this condition early (e.g. with the onset of back pain) to avoid a bad outcome.

Q: What do you do now?

A: Mr Caesar has cancer with bony metastases and acute onset of back pain, so you must exclude cord compression.

You take a history and examine Mr Caesar. He does not have any neurological symptoms and signs of cord compression. Therefore, if this is cord compression you have identified it early and so increased your chances of a good outcome.

You must now call the radiation oncology and/or the neurosurgery teams urgently. As well as needing to know about the cord compression early, their influence will help in getting tests, such as an MRI, done promptly.

Q: How do you confirm your clinical diagnosis?

A: In the majority of cases, an urgent MRI of the whole spine is sufficient. It is important to request that the whole spine be imaged, rather than the area of back pain alone, in order to identify any early asymptomatic spinal metastases. If the patient is unable to have an MRI, CT myelography can be performed. The disadvantage of the latter is that it is an invasive test that can occasionally worsen the neurological deficit. In fact, modern CT machines may be good enough to identify the cord compression without the need for invasive myelography (Walji *et al.*, 2008).

Q: How would you treat Mr Caesar?

A: The following approach is reasonable (Khan *et al.*, 2014; Walji *et al.*, 2008; Schiff, 2003):

- **Direct decompressive surgical resection in combination with radiotherapy**. There is increasing evidence that a combined approach will lead to better functional outcomes.

OR

- **Radiotherapy alone**. Tumours such as myeloma, lymphoma, breast, small-cell lung and prostate cancer are radiosensitive and respond well. Even radiotherapy on radio-resistant tumours such as renal cell carcinoma and melanoma will have a palliative benefit. Stereotactic beam radiation therapy may be less toxic to the spinal cord than external beam radiation therapy (Khan *et al.*, 2014).

Important adjunctive therapy to surgery/radiotherapy or radiotherapy alone include:

- **Corticosteroids**. They may improve functional outcome and alleviate symptoms due to reducing peri-tumour oedema. Dexamethasone is the steroid most commonly used. The

recommended dose is variable (up to 96 mg/day), but use at least 16 mg/day (8 mg bd or 4 mg qid).
- **Supportive measures**. These include urinary catheterisation if in urinary retention, relief of constipation, DVT prophylaxis, measures to prevent the development of bed sores, etc.

Q: While on dexamethasone, is there a particular blood level that should be checked?

A: Corticosteroids can lead to hyperglycaemia. Therefore, Mr Caesar should have his blood sugar level taken once a day. A pinprick glucose test of his finger should be adequate.

An urgent MRI of the whole spine reveals cord compression at T9. After commencing dexamethasone and receiving urgent radiotherapy, Mr Caesar's back pain resolves. Your prompt actions have saved him from becoming a paraplegic. Thanks to you, he can walk out of the hospital on his own two feet.

Achievements

You now:
- can recognise the clinical features of delirium
- know the major differential diagnoses of delirium
- realise that there are many causes of delirium
- realise that elderly people with an infection may not have a fever
- can investigate delirium
- can treat delirium
- know how to calculate the corrected blood calcium using the serum albumin
- know the causes of hypercalcaemia
- can investigate and treat a patient with hypercalcaemia
- can diagnose multiple myeloma
- know the clinical features and complications of multiple myeloma
- understand the principles of treating multiple myeloma
- recognise the clinical features of spinal cord compression
- realise that cord compression is a medical emergency
- know how to investigate and treat cord compression.

References

Attard, A., Ranjith, G. and Taylor, D. (2008), 'Delirium and its treatment', *CNS Drugs*, vol. 22, no. 8, pp. 631–644.

Bataille, R. and Harousseau, J.L. (1997), 'Multiple myeloma', *New England Journal of Medicine*, vol. 336, no. 23, pp. 1657–1664.

Blackburn, M. and Diamond, T. (2007), 'Primary hyperparathyroidism and familial hyperparathyroid syndromes', *Australian Family Physician*, vol. 36, no. 12, pp. 1029–1033.

Brown, T.M. and Boyle, M.F. (2002), 'Delirium', *British Medical Journal*, vol. 325, no. 7365, pp. 644–647.

Deftos, L.J. (2002), 'Hypercalcemia in malignant and inflammatory diseases', *Endocrinology and Metabolism Clinics of North America*, vol. 31, no. 1, pp. 141–158.

Eslick, R. and Talaulikar, D. (2013), 'Multiple myeloma: From diagnosis to treatment', *Australian Family Physician*, vol. 42, no. 10, pp. 684–688.

Falk, S. and Fallon, M. (1997), 'ABC of palliative care: Emergencies', *British Medical Journal*, vol. 315, no. 7121, pp. 1525–1528.

Gleason, O.C. (2003), 'Delirium', *American Family Physician*, vol. 67, no. 5, pp. 1027–1034.

Hauser, S.L. (2002), 'Diseases of the spinal cord', in E. Braunwald, A.S. Fauci, D.L. Kasper, S.L. Hauser, D.L. Longo and J.L. Jameson (eds), *Harrison's Principles of Internal Medicine*, McGraw-Hill, New York, pp. 2426–2434.

Inouye, S.K. (2006), 'Delirium in older persons', *New England Journal of Medicine*, vol. 354, no. 11, pp. 1157–1165.

Jackson, T., Ditmanson, L. and Phibbs, B. (1997), 'Torsade de pointes and low-dose oral haloperidol', *Archives of Internal Medicine*, vol. 157, no. 17, pp. 2013–2015.

Kalish, V.B., Gillham, J.E. and Unwin, B.K. (2014), 'Delirium in older persons: Evaluation and management', *American Family Physician*, vol. 90, no. 3, pp. 150–158.

Khan, U.A., Shanholtz, C.B. and McCurdy, M.T. (2014), 'Oncologic mechanical emergencies', *Emergency Medicine Clinics of North America*, vol. 32, no. 3, pp. 495–508.

LLerena, A., Berecz, R., de la Rubia, A. and Dorado, P. (2002), 'QTc interval lengthening and debrisoquine metabolic ratio in psychiatric patients treated with oral haloperidol monotherapy', *European Journal of Clinical Pharmacology*, vol. 58, no. 3, pp. 223–224.

Lonergan, E., Britton, A.M., Luxenberg, J. and Wyller, T. (2007), 'Antipsychotics for delirium', *Cochrane Database of Systematic Reviews*, 2, CD005594.

Lumachi, F., Brunello, A., Roma, A. and Basso, U. (2008), 'Medical treatment of malignancy-associated hypercalcaemia', *Current Medicinal Chemistry*, vol. 15, no. 4, pp. 415–421.

Norman, D.C. and Toledo, S.D. (1992), 'Infections in elderly persons: An altered clinical presentation', *Clinics in Geriatric Medicine*, vol. 8, no. 4, pp. 713–719.

Podczaski, E. and Cain, J. (2002), 'Multiple myeloma', *Clinical Obstetrics and Gynecology*, vol. 45, no. 3, pp. 928–938.

Rajkumar, S.V. (2009), 'Multiple myeloma', *Current Problems in Cancer*, vol. 33, no. 1, pp 7–64.

Schiff, D. (2003), 'Spinal cord compression', *Neurologic Clinics of North America*, vol. 21, no. 1, pp. 67–86, viii.

Wagner, J. and Arora, S. (2014), 'Oncologic metabolic emergencies', *Emergency Medicine Clinics of North America*, vol. 32, no. 3, pp. 509–525.

Walji, N., Chan, A.K. and Peake, D.R. (2008), 'Common acute oncological emergencies: Diagnosis, investigation and management', *Postgraduate Medical Journal*, vol. 84, no. 994, pp. 418–427.

Chapter 31
Cases of hype and hypertension on the wards

Scenario

You are halfway through a 15-hour shift. It has been fairly busy, with the usual barrage of fluid and medication charts, APTTs and IV cannulae. You return to Ward 3A, which you left only 30 minutes ago, to find that the board is again full of tasks for you to do! The first item reads, 'Bed 10.1—BP 179/105 mm Hg'.

Q: Do you urgently arrange a bed in the coronary care unit and order a sodium nitroprusside infusion?

A: No, definitely not at this stage! One of the most common tasks that junior doctors must perform during overtime shifts is reviewing patients with high blood pressure. You may occasionally feel pressured by nursing staff to lower a patient's blood pressure rapidly. However, this may not be appropriate in all situations and, in fact, it may be quite dangerous.

As a doctor on an overtime shift, the following checklist can be useful in assessing a hypertensive patient.

1. **Before you see the patient:**
   a. Look at the current and old patient notes, specifically to see if a history of hypertension and antihypertensive medications has been documented.[1]
   b. Look at the observation ('obs') chart, specifically the patient's blood pressure readings throughout this admission, to see if there has been a pattern to the hypertension over the past few days.
   c. Look at the medication chart to find out whether any antihypertensive medications have been charted.
2. **When you see the patient:**
   a. Measure the blood pressure yourself to see if it is truly elevated.

---

[1]Normally, when patients are admitted to hospital, their old medical records, which document previous admissions, are sent along with them.

b. Ensure that the blood pressure cuff size is appropriate since false elevations of blood pressure have occurred in obese people using a cuff that was too small (Marik and Varon, 2007).

c. Clinically assess the patient to find out whether there are acute symptoms and signs related to the hypertension.

d. Try to identify an acute reversible precipitant for the elevated blood pressure (e.g. urinary retention, pain).

3. **Conclusion:**

You must now decide if this is a 'hypertensive emergency' (see below). If it is, the blood pressure must be lowered rapidly. If not, the blood pressure can be lowered more slowly.

Q: What blood pressure measurement defines a 'hypertensive emergency'?

A: A 'hypertensive crisis' is usually defined as occurring in patients with a systolic BP > 179. Or they may have a diastolic BP > 109 or >120 (Johnson *et al.*, 2012; Marik and Varon, 2007). This is further subdivided into:

- **'Hypertensive urgency'**—this is a hypertensive crisis without evidence of acute end-organ damage. The blood pressure should be lowered over 1–2 days, usually with oral medication.

- **'Hypertensive emergency'**—this is a hypertensive crisis with evidence of acute end-organ damage where the blood pressure should be lowered immediately, often with parenteral medication; however, the blood pressure doesn't have to be lowered to normal levels.

Having given the above BP thresholds for a hypertensive crisis, it is worth noting that a hypertensive emergency can sometimes occur below these levels. Kitiyakara and Guzman (1998) note that the blood pressure can range from 150–290 (systolic) or from 100–180 (diastolic) in hypertensive emergencies. Therefore, there is no universal level of blood pressure at which acute target organ damage occurs.

Q: Why shouldn't you rapidly lower the blood pressure all the time?

A: The risk that clinicians face in rapidly lowering a patient's blood pressure is hypoperfusion to target organs (e.g. the heart, brain and kidneys), leading to stroke, acute coronary syndromes (ACSs) and acute renal failure. Many clinicians have seen patients develop strokes and ACSs after being given sublingual nifedipine (no longer available in Australia). Chan (2001) also notes that there is no proven benefit in acute reduction in blood pressure in patients with blood pressure over 180/110 in the absence of target organ damage. You should therefore restrict rapid lowering of blood pressure to those with hypertensive emergencies.

Q: What can be the clinical manifestations of a 'hypertensive emergency'?

A: Such hypertensive emergencies include:
- hypertensive encephalopathy[2]
- intracranial haemorrhage
- pulmonary oedema/left ventricular failure (LVF)
- ACSs
- dissecting aortic aneurysm
- acute renal failure
- eclampsia.

One study found that the most common presentations with hypertensive emergencies were chest pain (27%), dyspnoea (22%) and neurological deficits (21%) (Zampaglione *et al.*, 1996).

Q: Then how do you assess for acute target organ damage in a hypertensive patient?

A: Simply take a history, examine the patient and order a 12-lead ECG. When taking a history, ask about:
- neurological symptoms (e.g. headache, blurred vision, nausea, vomiting, seizures, confusion, dizziness, focal neurological deficits)
- cardiac symptoms (e.g. chest and back pain, shortness of breath)
- with regard to precipitants of the crisis, compliance with antihypertensives and the use of any new medications, be they over-the-counter, recreational or prescription medications.

When examining the patient, make sure you perform a:
- fundoscopy (grade III, for retinal haemorrhages, and grade IV, for papilloedema changes, are important features of malignant hypertension)
- neurological examination (to exclude focal deficits)
- cardiovascular examination (to exclude aortic dissection—including measurement of blood pressure in both arms—angina/infarction and pulmonary oedema).

On the 12-lead ECG, you should look for acute ischaemic changes.[3] Test the serum electrolytes to assess renal function.

---

[2]Hypertensive encephalopathy refers to a syndrome characterised by features such as seizures, headache, nausea, vomiting and impaired cognition. It probably reflects a loss of cerebral autoregulation, resulting in cerebral oedema.

[3]Left ventricular hypertrophy may be seen on the ECG, but this represents chronic rather than acute target organ damage from the hypertension.

You should also assess the patient for chronic target organ damage, although this would not change your acute management of the hypertension. It would simply involve:
- auscultation for carotid bruits
- palpation for an abdominal aortic aneurysm and auscultation for abdominal bruits
- palpation of the peripheral pulses
- urinalysis.

Once again, remember that you should ask the duty medical registrar if you do not know what to do.

Q: Now, returning to our hypertensive patient on Ward 3A. You find the nurse looking after the patient in 10.1. She tells you that Mr Al Furblocher was admitted 3 days ago for investigation of diarrhoea. He has been quite well and is awaiting a colonoscopy sometime next week. Al also has a history of prostatism and is due for surgery next month. While doing routine observations, the nurse found that his blood pressure was 179/105.

What do you do?

A: Go through the steps outlined above.

Scenario

You look at the observations ('obs') chart (see Fig. 31.1 overleaf) and see that Al only became hypertensive this afternoon. His medication chart lists no antihypertensive medications. You measure his blood pressure yourself, and agree with the nurse's finding of 179/105.

Al denies any symptoms related to the hypertension and has no signs of hypertensive emergency, and he has a normal ECG. He also denies a history of hypertension. Nevertheless, he looks very restless and is grimacing with pain.

On closer questioning about acute precipitants, Al comments on gradually worsening lower abdominal pain. He did not want to tell the nursing staff about the pain because they looked too busy. Your examination reveals a distended bladder halfway up to the umbilicus.

It is likely that Al's episode of hypertension may be either in part or totally related to urinary retention. You insert a urethral indwelling catheter (IDC) and watch the wave of relief spread across his face.

One hour later, with the IDC draining freely, you check Al's blood pressure again, and are pleased to see that it is 135/75. It appears that the pain from acute urinary retention was, in fact, the cause of the hypertension.

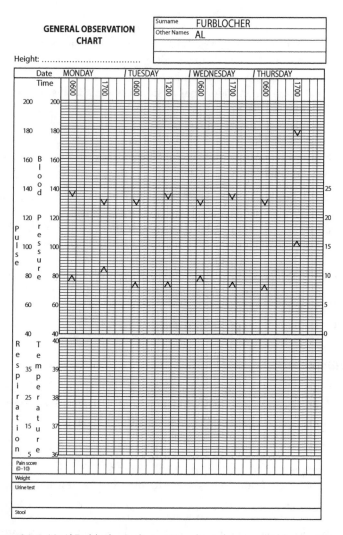

Figure 31.1 Mr Al Furblocher's observation chart, showing his blood pressure readings

You finish your jobs in 3 West and head off to 4 North. You look at the board—you have another hypertensive patient to see!

The nurse tells you that Mr Petrovich was admitted 4 days ago with a chest infection. She measured his blood pressure this afternoon and found it to be 180/107.

Q: What do you do?

A: Go through your checklist once again:

1. The 'obs' chart (see Fig. 31.2 overleaf) shows a blood pressure of 135/80 on admission. However, over the past 2 days it has been gradually climbing.

2. There are no antihypertensive medications listed on the medication chart.

3. You measure Mr Petrovich's blood pressure and confirm that it is 180/107.

4. The clinical assessment and 12-lead ECG are normal in relation to the raised BP.

Scenario

Mr Petrovich tells you that he does have a history of hypertension and is normally on atenolol. You tell him that the atenolol has not been charted. He is puzzled by this.

You go through the notes and find that no reason is given for stopping the atenolol. You phone the specialist to see if he wanted the atenolol ceased. He certainly did not, and is more than happy for you to recommence the medication. The admitting intern probably forgot to write it on the medication chart (this happens in real life).

You chart the atenolol and reassure the nurse that Mr Petrovich's blood pressure should improve in the next few hours. She thanks you and then tells you about another hypertensive patient in the next room.

Mrs Hill is a 56-year-old woman admitted with acute gout 6 days ago. Although she is now doing well on paracetamol alone, her blood pressure is high, at 180/100.

You go through the familiar checklist:

1. The chart (see Fig. 31.3 on page 337) shows a consistently elevated BP since admission 6 days ago, varying between 160/85 and 185/105.

2. According to the medication charts, Mrs Hill takes no antihypertensive medications.

3. You measure her blood pressure and find that it is 180/105.

4. Mrs Hill is completely asymptomatic from the hypertension. There are no signs of acute target organ damage and the 12-lead ECG is normal.

5. Mrs Hill denies a history of hypertension, but adds that her blood pressure was last checked more than 4 years ago.

6. There is no acute precipitant; in particular, the pain from the gout is well under control.

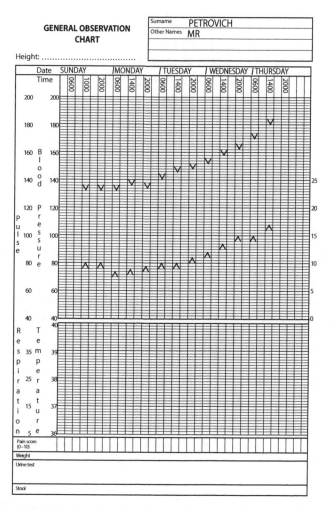

Figure 31.2 Mr Petrovich's observation chart, showing his blood pressure readings

7. From the preceding information, Mrs Hill does not have a hypertensive emergency.

8. As her systolic blood pressure is >179 mm Hg but with no evidence of acute end-organ damage, she meets the criteria for a hypertensive urgency. Thus, her blood pressure does not have to be lowered immediately but should be lowered over 24–48 hours.

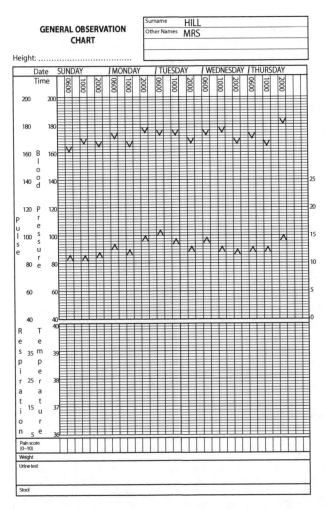

Figure 31.3 Mrs Hill's observation chart, showing her blood pressure readings

Q: What should you do now?

A: Commence an oral antihypertensive medication now.

Deciding which antihypertensive medication to commence is not easy, especially during a busy overtime shift. You need to consider which antihypertensive medication will be of most benefit to Mrs Hill without adversely affecting any of her other medical conditions. If you are uncertain about what to do, page the overtime medical registrar for advice.

Also make a note in the patient's file for the team informing them of your assessment of her hypertension and your management plan.

It is also always worth personally contacting the team the next day, just in case they failed to read your entry and notice that you have started an antihypertensive agent.

The table opposite lists some of the things you must take into consideration when deciding on an antihypertensive medication. For example, according to this table, Mrs Hill's gout makes a thiazide diuretic a bad choice as an antihypertensive agent.

Q: You tell the nurse that there is no need to lower Mrs Hill's blood pressure rapidly. She will need long-term treatment of her hypertension; you speak to the Medical Registrar and commence her on an ACE inhibitor, after discussing the risks and benefits with her.

The table opposite details antihypertensive medications and their interactions with medical conditions.

Drug class	ACEI	ARA	Beta-blockers	Calcium channel blockers	Thiazide diuretics
Heart failure	Good	Good	Good*	Bad	Good
Asthma			Bad**		
Diabetes	Good†	Good†	Bad		Bad***
MI	Good	Good	Good (most)		
Peripheral vascular disease			Bad		
Renovascular disease (bilateral renal artery stenosis)	Bad	Bad			
Gout					Bad
Bradycardia	Bad		Bad (verapamil, diltiazem)		
Stroke	Good	Good			

ACEI—ACE inhibitor; ARA—angiotensin II receptor antagonist.

* Some beta-blockers can be very useful in patients with heart failure (e.g. bisoprolol, metoprolol CR, carvedilol), but they can worsen heart failure if used incorrectly; therefore, only an experienced registrar or a specialist should start beta-blockers in such patients.

** Cardioselective beta-blockers can be used with caution in mild–moderate asthma (e.g. metoprolol, atenolol).

*** A thiazide and ACE inhibitor combination may be useful in type 2 diabetes.

† ACEI and ARA are particularly useful in diabetic patients with proteinuria or microalbuminuria.

Source: Adapted from Heart Foundation (2008, updated 2010).

The nurse is satisfied with your explanation; however, she wants to ask you a quick question about hypertension: 'I know you are busy, but I need to know something. Our GP started my mother on an ACE inhibitor last week. I thought you had to have a renal artery Doppler before starting ACE inhibitors. Is this right?'
What is your response?

A: The nurse has raised an interesting issue. As the table above demonstrates, the use of ACEIs or ARAs in renovascular disease can be disastrous. Certainly, if there is a known history of renal artery stenosis or a serum potassium >5.0 mmol/L, you should avoid these agents. If you do start them, however, check the EUCs within a few days. If the creatinine rises >30% above baseline, then cease them. A rise of 30% or less is quite common and acceptable but continue to monitor it closely (Heart Foundation, 2008, updated 2010).

Scenario

The next 3 hours of your shift are characterised by a number of minor tasks. You make your way to 6 South. When you arrive there, one of the nurses rushes up to you and says, 'I'm glad you're here. Could you please take a look at Mr Potter? His blood pressure is 190/120. He doesn't look at all well'.

The nurse tells you that Mr Potter is 55 years old and was admitted yesterday for the insertion of pectoral implants. He has a history of hypertension for which he takes medication. About 30 minutes ago, he began to complain of a terrible headache. It was then that the nurse measured his blood pressure and found it to be elevated.

Q: What is your approach?
A: Go through the checklist:
1. The 'obs' chart (see Fig. 31.4 overleaf) shows that Mr Potter's blood pressure averages around 160/90, but in the past 6 hours it has been climbing to its current levels.
2. Mr Potter has been charted for 'lisinopril 10 mg/day' in the medication chart.
3. Your blood pressure readings are consistent with the nurse's finding of 190/120.
4. Mr Potter is alert, but obviously distressed. The headache started 30 minutes ago and is severe. He is quite dizzy and his vision is blurred. Physical examination is unremarkable. Although there may be retinal haemorrhages, you do not have much confidence in your fundoscopic skills. The 12-lead ECG demonstrates left

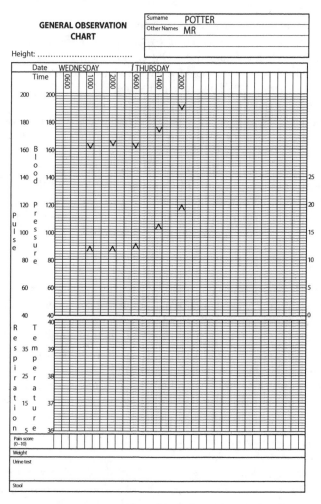

Figure 31.4 Mr Potter's observation chart, showing his blood pressure readings

ventricular hypertrophy consistent with chronic hypertensive damage, but no acute ischaemic changes.

5. Mr Potter confirms that he normally only takes lisinopril for his hypertension. He also confirms that 10 mg/day is the correct dose and that he has been receiving it in hospital.
6. You can identify no acute precipitant for the elevated BP.
7. You conclude that Mr Potter's acute neurological symptoms in the presence of this markedly elevated blood pressure (190/120) is consistent with a hypertensive emergency.

8. His blood pressure must therefore be lowered rapidly and you must alert the medical registrar.

Q: The medical registrar runs up 6 flights of stairs and assesses Mr Potter. She agrees with your assessment and is certain that retinal haemorrhages are present on fundoscopy. Mr Potter will need a brain CT scan to exclude intracranial haemorrhage. But his blood pressure will have to be lowered rapidly.

The medical registrar addresses you: 'I don't expect interns to know the intricacies of treating a hypertensive emergency, but tell me the principles of managing it and the medications that can be used'.

What do you tell her?

A: In such a case, you need to:

- admit the patient to an intensive care unit
- insert an arterial line for close monitoring of blood pressure
- take baseline blood for full blood count, electrolytes and renal function
- initiate IV antihypertensive treatment (be aware that a combination of drugs, not only monotherapy, may be used to treat a hypertensive emergency; e.g. sodium nitroprusside and labetalol in aortic dissection)
- in hypertensive encephalopathy, reduce the mean arterial pressure by 20% or the diastolic BP to 100 mm Hg within the first hour. In aortic dissection, the systolic BP should be reduced to 100–110 mm Hg as soon as possible (Vaughan and Delanty, 2000)
- specifically treat the acute target organ damage associated with the hypertensive emergency (e.g. MI, LVF).

A number of medications can be used to reduce the blood pressure in hypertensive emergencies. These are typically given parenterally. They all have their advantages and disadvantages; therefore, the choice of antihypertensive will vary according to the patient's comorbidities and the nature of the hypertensive emergency. For example, patients with a history of asthma should avoid beta-blockers or at least use them with caution. But on the other hand, patients with acute aortic dissection as their hypertensive emergency ideally should have a beta-blocker combined with a vasodilator (e.g. sodium nitroprusside) (Marik and Varon, 2007). In other words, there is no single antihypertensive of choice for a hypertensive emergency—pick the most appropriate drug for each situation.

As to the choice of drugs available, here are some common ones:

1. Labetalol (IV rather than oral for hypertensive emergencies). Labetalol has both alpha- and beta-blocking ability and is relatively contraindicated in LVF.

2. **Beta-blockers** (e.g. propranolol and esmolol). Beta-blockers are relatively contraindicated in LVF.
3. **IV GTN.** This is often the first-line agent used in hypertensive emergencies with myocardial ischaemia because it improves coronary perfusion to a greater degree than sodium nitroprusside—but sodium nitroprusside is still effective in this situation.
4. **Sodium nitroprusside** (also known as SNIP). It is administered as a continuous IV infusion.
   This should be immediate onset and of short duration. Adverse effects include nausea and vomiting. It produces toxic metabolites if given for a period of days (e.g. thiocyanate, cyanate). SNIP can be affected by light, which is why you will often see it wrapped in foil or some other opaque material.
5. **Hydralazine.** This vasodilator is relatively contraindicated in myocardial ischaemia and aortic dissection because it can cause reflex tachycardia. Another problem with hydralazine is its prolonged antihypertensive effect, for example it has a circulating half-life of 3 hours but the half-time of its antihypertensive effect is 10 hours (Marik and Varon, 2007).

And note ...

There are a number of increasingly popular newer agents to treat hypertensive emergencies but they aren't currently all available in Australia (this may change in the future). These agents include two calcium channel blockers, nicardipine (not available in Australia) and clevidipine (available in Australia) as well as fenoldopam (a vasodilator that acts on peripheral dopamine receptors) (Marik and Varon, 2007).

The medical registrar is impressed with your knowledge! She urgently arranges transfer to the intensive care unit where a SNIP infusion is commenced and an arterial line inserted. Within 45 minutes, Mr Potter's blood pressure has been lowered to 160/95 and he has begun to feel better.

You hear that the renal team used the opportunity to adjust his oral antihypertensive therapy and he was weaned off SNIP within 36 hours. Thankfully, a brain CT scan demonstrated no intracerebral bleeding.

Achievements

You now:
- can use the checklist provided to assess any hypertensive ward patient
- know what a hypertensive emergency is

- are familiar with the syndromes associated with a hypertensive emergency
- realise that rapid lowering of blood pressure is dangerous and should only be used for a hypertensive emergency
- understand the basic management principles for a hypertensive emergency
- know the commonly used medications for a hypertensive emergency and their relative contraindications
- know that SNIP can be used safely for almost any hypertensive emergency.

References

Chan, S.S.W. (2001), 'The management of hypertension in the acute setting', *The Hong Kong Practitioner*, vol. 23, pp. 92–98.

Heart Foundation (National Blood Pressure and Vascular Disease Advisory Committee) (2008) (updated December 2010), *Guide to Management of Hypertension 2008*, at <www.heartfoundation.org.au/ SiteCollectionDocuments/HypertensionGuidelines2008to2010Update.pdf>, accessed 10 December 2014.

Johnson, W., Nguyen, ML. and Patel, R. (2012), 'Hypertension crisis in the emergency department', *Cardiology Clinics*, vol. 30, no. 4, pp. 533–543.

Kitiyakara, C. and Guzman, N.J. (1998), 'Malignant hypertension and hypertensive emergencies', *Journal of the American Society of Nephrology*, vol. 9, no. 1, pp. 133–142.

Marik, P.E. and Varon, J. (2007), 'Hypertensive crises: Challenges and management', *Chest*, vol. 131, no. 6, pp. 1949–1962.

Vaughan, C.J. and Delanty, N. (2000), 'Hypertensive emergencies', *Lancet*, vol. 356, no. 9227, pp. 411–417.

Zampaglione, B., Pascale, C., Marchisio, L. *et al.* (1996), 'Hypertensive urgencies and emergencies: Prevalence and clinical presentation', *Hypertension*, vol. 27, no. 1, pp. 144–147.

Chapter 32
A case of clots

Scenario

You have the pleasure of being the medical ward intern for 15 hours on a Saturday as part of your overtime roster. On the morning handover with the overnight doctors, you are told to check the result of a CT pulmonary angiogram (CTPA).

It turns out that the scan is to be performed on a patient you looked after during the week. The 55-year-old man, Hajinder, was admitted 4 days ago with sepsis due to a nasty case of olecranon bursitis, which has responded fairly well to antibiotics; however, 1 hour ago he developed pleuritic chest pain and shortness of breath despite receiving prophylactic subcutaneous unfractionated heparin. But he is haemodynamically stable with an oxygen saturation of 97% on room air.

Naturally, the major concern is pulmonary embolism (PE). The on-call radiology registrar has agreed to perform the CTPA. This should happen at any moment. The night intern asks you to pass the result of the scan on to Hajinder's specialist.

The next hour flies by as you insert numerous cannulae and write up many fluid and medication charts. You then receive a call from the radiology registrar. He informs you that Hajinder's CTPA is positive for PE.

Q: What do you do now?

A: Contact the specialist looking after the patient. Most specialists want to know about any major developments in their patients, as they are ultimately responsible for their patients' care. The new diagnosis of PE in Hajinder is certainly a new development; indeed, it is a life-threatening one.

Q: The infectious diseases physician is grateful that you have phoned. She ends the call by saying, 'Well, I guess you better anticoagulate him if he has a pulmonary embolus'.

How do you anticoagulate Hajinder?

A: In broad terms, this patient requires parenteral heparin followed by the introduction of warfarin.

Q: How long should Hajinder be anticoagulated for?

A: In general, the following is a useful guide for duration of treating venous thromboembolism (VTE) (Chapman *et al.*, 2009):
- First episode of VTE secondary to reversible risk factors: 3–6 months.
- First episode of idiopathic VTE: 6 months plus.
- Recurrent episode of VTE secondary to reversible risk factors: 6 months.
- Recurrent episode of idiopathic VTE: 12 months plus.
- First episode in patients with cancer: until cancer resolves.
- First episode provoked distal DVT: 6 weeks.
- First episode unprovoked distal DVT: 3 months.

Q: How does heparin work?

A: One-third of an administered dose of heparin binds to antithrombin (also known as antithrombin III). This heparin–antithrombin complex inactivates various coagulation enzymes and is responsible for the majority of heparin's anticoagulant effect. The remainder of the administered heparin acts on heparin cofactor II, which has an antithrombin effect.

Q: How can you give the heparin?

A: In general terms, it can be given as IV unfractionated heparin or subcutaneous low molecular weight heparin (e.g. enoxaparin). The ID physician suggests unfractionated heparin for now as Hajinder still has acute kidney injury secondary to his sepsis.

Q: Hajinder has been receiving (unfractionated) heparin 5000 units subcutaneously bd as DVT prophylaxis for the past 4 days. Does this mean you have to reduce the dose of unfractionated heparin you are going to use?

A: No, but you must cease the old prophylactic heparin order on his medication chart before charting the new one.

Q: How would you chart IV unfractionated heparin?

A: Check the hospital's protocol for commencing IV heparin. Probably every teaching hospital in Australia will have an easily accessible protocol which gives simple steps for the dosing and monitoring of IV heparin. They are generally weight based as weight-based dosing of IV heparin is associated with significantly lower recurrences of VTE

(Hirsh *et al.*, 2008). An example of a weight-based protocol is given below (Haematology and Pharmacy Departments, 2005):

- IV loading dose of 5000 units of heparin (if 60–80 kg weight) or 80 units/kg if outside the 60–80 kg weight range.
- Then an IV infusion of 1250 units/hour (if 60–80 kg weight) or 18 units/kg/hour if outside the 60–80 kg weight range.

And note ...

One of your first jobs as an intern must be to familiarise yourself with your hospital's IV heparin guidelines as you will be dealing with heparin issues all the time as an intern.

For the infusion, the heparin is mixed with normal saline, for example 25 000 units of heparin in 500 mL normal saline.

Q: What tests would you use to monitor the level of anti-coagulation with IV heparin?

A: APTT or APTT ratio.

Q: What therapeutic APTT or APTT ratio would you aim for?

A: The figure may vary between hospitals and depend on variables such as reagents used, but an APTT ratio of 1.5–2.5 or an APTT of 40–70 seconds are commonly used therapeutic targets (Hirsh *et al.*, 2008; Haematology and Pharmacy Departments, 2005).

Q: When would you check the APTT?

A: After 6 hours. If the APTT is therapeutic after this time, it would only be necessary to check the APTT on a daily basis. However, if any changes whatsoever are made to the rate of the heparin infusion, the APTT must be repeated 6 hours afterward.

Use the hospital guideline to adjust the heparin dose if the APTT/ APTT ratio is too high or low—this is usually charted in a simple table that is easy to follow. In broad terms, if the anticoagulation is subtherapeutic (APTT < 40s or APTT ratio < 1.5), then give another IV bolus and increase the infusion rate. If the APTT/APTT ratio is too high, then the infusion rate will have to be decreased with or without ceasing the infusion for a brief period.

After 2 changes to the infusion rate followed by checking the APTT/ APTT ratio 6 hours later, you have finally achieved a therapeutic APTT at an infusion rate of 12 mL/hour. Therefore, continue at the current rate and put a pathology request in for an APTT/APTT ratio tomorrow morning.

Q: Are there any other blood tests that need to be performed regularly (especially within the first 2 weeks) of starting heparin?

A: The full blood count must be checked every 48 hours or 3 times per week while a patient is receiving heparin. This is done to check for the development of heparin-induced thrombocytopaenia (HIT). HIT is an immune-complex-mediated phenomenon. The HIT antigen is a complex between heparin and platelet factor 4 (PF4).

HIT usually occurs 4–14 days after commencing heparin; the diagnosis is still possible even if the patient is no longer on heparin at the time the diagnosis is suspected. HIT can occur even earlier than 4 days after starting heparin if the patient had been exposed to heparin in the preceding 100 days. Although thrombocytopaenia is not technically required for a diagnosis (see definition below), in practice haematologists would be sceptical of a diagnosis of HIT without marked thrombocytopaenia.

A diagnosis of HIT should be suspected if any of the following occur within 4–14 days (usually) of starting heparin (Warkentin *et al.*, 2008):

1. arterial or venous thrombosis OR
2. necrotising skin lesions at heparin injection sites OR
3. anaphylactoid (severe systemic reactions) after IV bolus administration OR
4. a fall in platelet count of ≥50% from an earlier peak platelet count.

If any of these phenomena occur, then assays to detect the heparin-dependent antibody should be performed to confirm the diagnosis of HIT. Once confirmed, the heparin must be stopped.

Q: If Hajinder develops HIT while on unfractionated heparin, can you use a low molecular weight heparin (like enoxaparin) instead?

A: No—do not use low molecular weight heparin in HIT. HIT is definitely less likely to occur with low molecular weight heparins because they bind less to platelets and PF4 than unfractionated heparin (Hirsh *et al.*, 2008); however, the risk is there.

In Australia, alternatives to unfractionated heparin and low molecular weight heparin in the setting of HIT include lepirudin (recombinant hirudin), fondaparinux (synthetic pentasaccharide), bivalirudin and danaparoid sodium.

Q: On Monday you return to your usual job as the infectious diseases intern. You are pleased to see that Hajinder's APTT has continued to be therapeutic. You commence warfarin.

What blood test will you use to monitor the warfarin level?

A: You should use the International Normalised Ratio (INR).

Q: Should you cease heparin now?

A: No. Hajinder should remain on IV heparin till the INR has been therapeutic for 48 hours. Warfarin works by depleting vitamin K-dependent factors ('Australian TV channel' factors—II, VII, IX, X; unfortunately the advent of the SBS channel and cable TV has spoilt this somewhat!). Some of these clotting factors take a long time to degrade (factor VII has a half-life of 60 hours). Consequently, you need to continue the heparin to allow the warfarin time to break them down.

Even so, some specialists will commence warfarin without heparin in their private rooms in patients with a 'non-urgent' need for anticoagulation. An example here would be chronic AF. There have been concerns that patients with an underlying protein C deficiency could develop a hypercoagulable state after commencing warfarin, but Ansell *et al.* (2001) have remarked that these have not been substantiated.

Q: How would you go about commencing warfarin?

A: Most hospitals will have their own protocol for prescribing warfarin and checking the INR. As with the IV heparin guidelines, you should familiarise yourself with the warfarin guidelines. As you will discover, finding the correct warfarin dose is more of a guessing game than an exact science. However, a reasonable approach would be the following (Ansell *et al.*, 2008):

- Check the baseline INR.
- On days 1 and 2 in elderly patients and those with severe underlying illnesses (e.g. liver disease and heart failure), give ≤5 mg/day.
- On days 1 and 2 in other patients, give between 5 and 10 mg/day.
- Check the INR on the third day and then daily until the INR is therapeutic.
- Once a therapeutic INR has been consistently achieved, less frequent INR testing can be performed, for example every 2 weeks but no less than once a month.

Q: What is the therapeutic INR that you are aiming for in Hajinder?

A: For most conditions, an INR of 2–3 is accepted (Ansell *et al.*, 2008). One exception is mechanical heart valves where higher INRs are sought after (2.5–3.5) (Salem *et al.*, 2008).

Q: If anticoagulation were contraindicated in Hajinder or if he suffered from recurrent VTE despite therapeutic anticoagulation with warfarin, how else could you treat him?

A: An inferior vena caval filter (IVCF) is an alternative in these situations (discussed more fully in Chapter 5).

Q: After 7 days Hajinder reaches and maintains a therapeutic INR on a warfarin dose of 4 mg/day. He is now ready to be discharged from hospital. He asks whether there is anything important he needs to know about being on warfarin. What do you tell him?

A:

1. He will need continual monitoring of his INR by his local doctor. He will not require daily testing once a steady therapeutic INR level has been achieved; at this point, once a week or once every 2 weeks should be adequate.
2. He should avoid aspirin unless specifically prescribed by a doctor.
3. He should drink alcohol only in moderation.
4. Any new medication could interfere with warfarin metabolism and therefore the INR. The most common culprits here are antibiotics; therefore, the prescribing doctor must check to see whether a new medication will interfere with warfarin metabolism. Hajinder's INR should be monitored more frequently until the new medication is ceased or the INR is stable.
5. Avoid any activities involving heavy contact (e.g. boxing, touch football) because of the increased tendency to bleed.
6. He should have heightened awareness of signs of bleeding (e.g. headache, abdominal pain).
7. He should not continually change his dietary habits. A number of foods contain vitamin K, and changing his diet might reduce or increase the amount of vitamin K he consumes. This will affect his INR.

Many hospitals give patients a small information booklet about warfarin before they are discharged. You should find out if your hospital supplies these. They contain much of the information covered here.

Q: Jamie, one of the medical students, asks you if warfarin acts on the extrinsic or intrinsic coagulation pathway. What do you tell him?

A: Jamie probably knows that this is a popular question in medical students' examinations!

Think of the mnemonic, WET HIT:

WET: Warfarin ExTrinsic pathway

HIT: Heparin InTrinsic pathway.

Q: Three weeks later, Hajinder returns to clinic. He is frustrated with having to check his INR. 'Look, I hate blood tests. Isn't there something else that I can use?' Is there an oral alternative to warfarin for Hajinder?

349

A: Yes. In Australia, rivaroxaban has been approved for treatment of DVT and PE in the absence of cancer or antiphospholipid syndrome. Rivaroxaban is a factor Xa inhibitor that doesn't require therapeutic dose monitoring, which would address Hajinder's concern. The usual dose is 15 mg bd for 3 weeks followed by 20 mg/day. The other new oral anticoagulants, dabigatran and apixaban, may also eventually be approved for use in DVT/PE treatment in Australia, but they currently are not (Brieger and Curnow, 2014).

Scenario

One month later you are working an overtime shift in the Emergency Department. The first patient you see is a 52-year-old woman on warfarin for a DVT. This is her second month of therapy.

Her local doctor referred her because her INR is 8.4. She recently developed an upper respiratory tract infection. Without telling her GP, she self-medicated with some clarithromycin that she had in the cupboard at home. When she presented for her weekly INR test, he discovered what had happened.

Q: What would you do?

A: It is important to tell her to stop taking the clarithromycin for the moment, as it is almost certainly responsible for her precipitously high INR. Next, you must determine if she is actively bleeding. Take a history focusing on:
- symptoms of anaemia
- overt bleeding (i.e. haematuria, melaena, epistaxis)
- neurological symptoms suggestive of an intracerebral haemorrhage and abdominal pain suggestive of a retro-peritoneal bleed.

Examine her, looking for evidence of bleeding:
- tachycardia and postural hypotension
- neurological signs
- abdominal tenderness or abdominal wall bruising.

The most important blood test is a haemoglobin.

Q: The woman, Melanie, is asymptomatic and has a normal examination. An INR repeated in the hospital confirms the local doctor's result of 8.4. Melanie's haemoglobin is normal. You are confident that she is not bleeding, but what do you do about such a high INR?

A: Once again, it is worth emphasising that your hospital's warfarin guide-line is likely to provide a step-by-step approach to managing an elevated

INR with or without active bleeding. In general, if the INR is elevated without active bleeding, ceasing warfarin is enough. But if the INR is >10, even without bleeding, then it is reasonable to give vitamin K 5–10 mg IV (Tran *et al.*, 2013).

Q: A few days later, you unfortunately encounter another warfarin complication. A 75-year-old man is brought to the resuscitation room with a reduced level of consciousness. He takes warfarin for atrial fibrillation. A CT scan confirms a large intracerebral haemorrhage. His INR is 4.6. What should you do to address his anticoagulation?

A: This man has suffered life-threatening bleeding with an elevated INR while on warfarin. He requires (Tran *et al.*, 2013):

- vitamin K 5–10 mg IV
- Prothrombinex-VF 50 IU/kg IV (Prothrombinex-VF contains factors II, IX, X and low levels of factor VII)
- fresh frozen plasma (FFP) 150–300 mL (if the bleeding was significant but not life-threatening, the FFP wouldn't have to be given).

And note ...

Avoid giving intramuscular vitamin K as it might cause a large haematoma at the injection site and delay a return to a therapeutic INR if warfarin is recommenced.

Q: It is said that bad things happen in threes. Before your shift ends, you are asked by the Emergency Department registrar to help resuscitate a man with a large retroperitoneal bleed who takes dabigatran for atrial fibrillation. How do you reverse the dabigatran?

A: While the new oral anticoagulants (NOACs) (e.g. rivaroxaban, apixaban, dabigatran) are convenient because they don't require blood tests to monitor levels, they can be difficult to address if bleeding occurs. Apart from standard resuscitation measure for bleeding, it is reasonable to do the following for those bleeding from dabigatran (Tran *et al.*, 2014):

- Discontinue the NOAC at least temporarily.
- Check APTT, thrombin time, dabigatran level (anti-Xa level if rivaroxaban or apixaban).
- Give activated charcoal if the patient has presented within 2 hours of his last dose of NOAC.
- Dialysis is an option in certain circumstances (it is *not* an option with apixaban and rivaroxaban, which have limited renal excretion).

- If life-threatening bleeding, consider using procoagulants such as Prothrombinex-VF, FEIBA or tranexamic acid (speak with a haematologist about this first).

Scenario

You are now asked to see another patient with a newly diagnosed DVT in her right femoral vein. Leena has no contraindications to anticoagulation. The haematologist wants to anticoagulate her at home under the 'hospital in the home' program. However, the nurses cannot run an IV heparin infusion at home and will have to use subcutaneous enoxaparin.

Q: You are asked by the haematologist to chart the enoxaparin. What dose will you use?

A: Once daily subcutaneously, 1.5 mg/kg/day, or twice daily subcutaneously, 1 mg/kg/bd. Even obese patients should have a weight-based dose (Hirsh *et al.*, 2008).

Q: The nurse who is caring for the patient is curious to know whether unfractionated heparin can be given subcutaneously as therapeutic anticoagulation. What do you tell her?

A: Although IV unfractionated heparin and subcutaneous low molecular weight heparins account for the vast majority of regimens to treat VTE, subcutaneous unfractionated heparin can also be used. Two regimens for therapeutic subcutaneous unfractionated heparin include (Hirsh *et al.*, 2008):

- initial IV bolus of 5000 units followed by subcutaneous heparin 250 units/kg bd OR
- initial subcutaneous bolus of 333 units/kg followed by subcutaneous heparin 250 units/kg bd.

Q: What blood test, other than coagulation studies, must you check before commencing enoxaparin?

A: It is important to know the patient's creatinine clearance (CrCl), which reflects renal function. Patients with marked renal impairment (CrCl < 30 mL/min) should only use 50% of the normal dose of enoxaparin or avoid enoxaparin altogether (Hirsh *et al.*, 2008). (This is why the ID physician suggested IV heparin to anticoagulate Hajinder above; i.e. he had acute kidney injury with his sepsis.)

Q: How often should you check the APTT to monitor the level of anticoagulation with enoxaparin?

A: Trick question! The APTT is not a useful marker of enoxaparin activity. Anti-Xa levels can be used to follow enoxaparin activity. However, apart from patients with severe renal failure or those who are at high risk of bleeding, patients on enoxaparin will not need monitoring with coagulation studies. This is one advantage of enoxaparin over IV heparin.

Q: Protamine sulfate can be used to reverse the effects of unfractionated heparin completely if required (e.g. if serious bleeding has occurred). Does protamine reverse the effects of low molecular weight heparins such as enoxaparin?

A: Yes, but it only partially reverses the effects of enoxaparin.

The following table demonstrates some of the differences between unfractionated and low molecular weight heparin (LMWH).

	Heparin	LMWH
Bioavailablility	<30%	>90%
Protein binding	Yes	No
Half-life	Shorter	Longer
Drug interactions	Yes	No
Risk of HIT	Higher	Lower
IV cannula required*	Generally yes	No
Monitoring of blood levels	Daily	Often unnecessary
Risk of osteopaenia[†]	Higher	Lower
Reversibility with protamine	Better	Not as good

* The disadvantage of using an IV cannula is the risk of infection. Also, if a cannula tissues and needs replacement, the delay might reduce the efficacy of anticoagulation. On a busy overtime shift, such delays are not uncommon.

† Heparin-induced osteoporosis or osteopaenia tends to occur in the setting of long-term anticoagulation with heparin at high doses. A typical scenario would be a pregnant woman requiring anticoagulation. Because warfarin is teratogenic, the alternative is many months of high-dose heparin therapy.

Source: Adapted from Ageno and Turpie (2002).

Q: From where is protamine sulfate derived?

A: Would you believe from fish sperm? In fact, in people with a history of fish allergy, prior use of protamine-containing insulin or vasectomy are at higher risk of suffering a severe allergic reaction to protamine and can be pretreated with antihistamines and corticosteroids (Hirsh *et al.*, 2008).

Achievements

You now:
- know the mechanism of the action of heparin
- can initiate heparin therapy

- know how to monitor heparin therapy
- can make appropriate adjustments for subtherapeutic or overtherapeutic APTTs
- know to check the full blood count regularly to monitor for HIT
- can diagnose and treat HIT
- know how to commence warfarin therapy
- can make appropriate adjustments for subtherapeutic or overtherapeutic INRs
- can educate the patient about being on warfarin for a long period
- can manage a patient with a high INR
- are confident using LMWH
- know some differences between unfractionated heparin and LMWH
- are familiar with the NOACs (new oral anticoagulants).

References

Ageno, W. and Turpie, A.G. (2002), 'New advances in the management of acute coronary syndromes: 4. Low-molecular-weight heparins', *Canadian Medical Association Journal*, vol. 166, no. 7, pp. 919–924.

Ansell, J. *et al.* (2001), 'Managing oral anticoagulant therapy', *Chest*, vol. 119, 1 (suppl.), pp. 22S–38S.

Ansell, J., Hirsh, J., Hylek, E., Jacobson, A., Crowther, M. and Palareti, G. (2008), 'Pharmacology and management of vitamin K antagonists', *Chest*, vol. 133, no. 6 (suppl.), pp. 160S–198S.

Baker, R.I., Coughlin, P.B., Gallus, A.S. *et al.* (2004), 'Warfarin reversal: Consensus guidelines, on behalf of the Australasian Society of Thrombosis and Haemostasis', *Medical Journal of Australia*, vol. 181, no. 9, pp. 492–497.

Brieger, D. and Curnow, J. (2014), 'Anticoagulation: A GP primer on the new oral anticoagulants', *Australian Family Physician*, vol. 43, no. 5, pp. 254–259.

Chapman, N.H., Brighton, T., Harris, M.F., Caplan, G.A., Braithwaite, J. and Chong, B.H. (2009), 'Venous thromboembolism—management in general practice', *Australian Family Physician*, vol. 38, no. 1–2, pp. 38–40.

Gallus, A. *et al.* (2000), 'Consensus guidelines for warfarin therapy', *Medical Journal of Australia*, vol. 172, no. 12, pp. 600–605.

Haematology and Pharmacy Departments (2005), 'TCH intravenous heparin prescribing guidelines', The Canberra Hospital, at <http://acthealth/c/healthi ntranet?a=glob&object=902608962&did=5000441&sid=>

Hirsh, J., Bauer, K.A., Donati, M.B., Gould, M., Samama, M.M. and Weitz, J.I. (2008), 'Parenteral anticoagulants: American College of Chest Physicians Evidence-Based Clinical Practice Guidelines (8th edition)', *Chest*, vol. 133, no. 6 (suppl.), pp. 141S–159S.

Hirsh, J. *et al.* (2001), 'Guide to anticoagulant therapy. Heparin: A statement for healthcare professionals from the American Heart Association', *Circulation*, vol. 103, no. 24, pp. 2994–3018.

National Prescribing Service Limited (2009), 'Rivaroxaban (Xarelto) for preventing venous thromboembolism after hip or knee replacement surgery', at <www.nps.org.au/health_professionals/publications/nps_radar/issues/current/august_2009/rivaroxaban>

Nazario, R., Delorenzo, L.J. and Maguire, A.G. (2002), 'Treatment of venous thromboembolism', Cardiology in Review, vol. 10, no. 4, pp. 249–259.

Salem, D.N., O'Gara, P.T., Madias, C. and Pauker, S.G. (2008), 'Valvular and structural heart disease', Chest, vol. 133, no. 6 (suppl.), pp. 593S–629S.

Sivakumaran, M. et al. (1996), 'Osteoporosis and vertebral collapse following low-dose, low molecular weight heparin therapy in a young patient', Clinical & Laboratory Haematology, vol. 18, no. 1, pp. 55–57.

Tran, H.A., Chunilal, S.D. and Harper, P.L. et al. (2013), 'An update of consensus guidelines for warfarin reversal', Medical Journal of Australia, vol. 198, no. 4, pp. 1–7.

Tran, H., Young, J.L. and McRae, S. et al. (2014), 'New oral anticoagulants: a practical guide on prescription, laboratory testing and peri-procedural/bleeding management', Internal Medicine Journal, vol. 44, no. 6, pp. 525–536.

Warkentin, T.E. (2002), 'Current agents for the treatment of patients with heparin-induced thrombocytopenia', Current Opinion in Pulmonary Medicine, vol. 8, no. 5, pp. 405–412.

Warkentin, T.E., Greinacher, A., Koster, A. and Lincoff, A.M. (2008), 'Treatment and prevention of heparin-induced thrombocytopenia', Chest, vol. 133, no. 6 (suppl.), pp. 340S–380S.

Chapter 33
Intravenous fluids

Scenario

It is another overtime shift on the wards. You are accompanied by Maddy, one of the final year medical students, as you wander back down to ward 10 North towards midnight. On arrival there, one of the nurses asks you to chart IV fluids for Mr Tikolo, a 45-year-old man awaiting an elective right hemicolectomy. He has been added to tomorrow's theatre list, but could be the first or last case of the day. Therefore, the surgical registrar wants him to be made nil by mouth and charted for IV fluids to last until tomorrow evening.

Q: What is your approach?

A: One of the most common tasks junior doctors are asked to perform is charting IV fluids. It is important to realise that this is not an exact art; sometimes you will get it wrong. It is therefore always important to assess regularly a patient's fluid status and electrolytes.

You can make a reasonable estimate of a patient's daily fluid requirements using the following formula:

daily fluid requirements = maintenance fluids + excess losses

'Maintenance fluids' refer to a person's normal daily fluid requirements. 'Excess losses' occur in situations where patients require fluid beyond their normal daily requirements, including where there is:
- third-space loss of fluid into the peritoneal cavity (e.g. acute pancreatitis, bowel obstruction)
- nasogastric tube losses (again in bowel obstruction)
- dehydration (commonly seen in the elderly)
- loss of fluids through fistulae
- excess loss of fluid through the urine (e.g. the polyuric phase of acute tubular necrosis).

In Mr Tikolo's case, you only have to chart maintenance fluids, as he does not have excess losses to replace. (However, some people, especially the elderly, can get dehydrated from the preoperative bowel preparation.)

Q: What are an average adult's usual daily fluid requirements?

A: There are many ways to calculate the daily fluid requirements for an adult. One simple formula is 30–35 mL/kg/day. In other words, you need to know a patient's weight before calculating the fluid requirements. Although a lot of patients do get weighed in the Emergency Department or in a pre-admission clinic, often you will have to 'eyeball' a patient and estimate a weight or weigh the person on the ward.

Q: You go through Mr Tikolo's notes: he was not weighed during his admission. However, he tells you that he was 80 kg when he weighed himself at home last week. You also feel that he looks about 80 kg.

How much fluid does he need?

A: An 80 kg man would require 2400–2800 mL/day of fluid (30–35 × 80 kg). Let's pick 2800 mL as the daily requirement.

Because IV fluids are run through infusion machines at an hourly rate and because you will have to chart the fluids at an hourly rate on the IV fluid chart, you should divide the daily requirement by 24 hours: 2800/24 = approximately 115 mL/hour.

Q: But is this all you need to know before charting Mr Tikolo's fluids?

A: No. You now need to decide how much sodium and potassium Mr Tikolo requires in his IV fluids.

Q: What are the daily sodium and potassium requirements for an average adult?

A: Sodium: 1–2 mmol/kg/day; potassium: 0.7–1.0 mmol/kg/day. Therefore, our 80 kg man requires:
- 80–160 mmol/day of sodium (let's say 90 mmol/day)
- 56–80 mmol/day of potassium (let's say 60 mmol/day)
- 2800 mL/day of fluid (115 mL/hour).

Q: What are the common types of IV fluid formulations?

A: The most common types are:
- normal saline
- 4% dextrose and 1/5 normal saline ('4% and a 1/5' or '4% D and N/5')
- 5% dextrose (5% D)
- Hartmann's solution.

Q: What do these formulations contain?
A:

	Sodium (mmol/L)	Potassium (mmol/L)
Normal saline	150	0
4% D and N/5*	30	0[†]
5% D	0	0
Hartmann's	131	5

* Because normal saline contains 150 mmol/L of sodium, it makes sense that 1/5 normal saline (as in '4% D and N/5') contains 30 mmol/L of sodium.
[†] Some formulations of '4% D and N/5' come with 30 mmol/L of potassium.

Q: Should we give our 80 kg patient 2800 mL of normal saline over 24 hours to meet his daily requirement?
A: This would give him sufficient fluid to meet his daily requirement, which is 2800 mL. But he would receive far too much sodium (almost 450 mmol instead of 90 mmol) and no potassium. This is why it can be a problem to use normal saline as a maintenance fluid.

Therefore, you should use 2800 mL of '4% and a 1/5' over 24 hours. The first and third litres of fluid should be bags of fluid with premixed 30 mmol potassium. Now, using '4% and a 1/5' with potassium supplements over 24 hours, our 80 kg man will receive:

- 2800 mL of fluid
- 84 mmol of sodium (close to our estimated 90 mmol of sodium)
- 54 mmol of potassium (close to our estimated 60 mmol of potassium).

This formulation is close to ideal for Mr Tikolo.

Q: How would you write this on the IV fluid chart?
A:

Date	Fluid type	Volume	Additives	Rate	Signature
10 Oct	4% D + N/5	1 litre	30 mmol KCl	115 mL/hour	KLM
10 Oct	4% D + N/5	1 litre		115 mL/hour	KLM
10 Oct	4% D + N/5	1 litre	30 mmol KCl	115 mL/hour	KLM

It is worth familiarising yourself with the fluid chart used in your teaching hospital. It will have a similar format to the preceding example.

Q: How would you approach Mr Tikolo's fluid management if he had gastrointestinal losses (vomiting, fistulae losses, etc.)?

A: Again, you would apply the formula of:

maintenance fluids + excess losses

In the case of gastrointestinal losses, you must account for excess fluid losses as well as maintenance fluids.

In the hospitalised patient, nursing staff can measure the volume of vomiting and fistula losses, so you will know how much excess fluid loss there has been. But, as with maintenance fluids, you must remember to account for the electrolyte loss through vomiting, fistulae and other gastrointestinal losses. Worthley (1997) described this as follows:

- gastric losses (vomiting, nasogastric suction)
- pancreatic and biliary losses (fistulae)
- intestinal losses (diarrhoea, ileus, fistulae, ileostomy).

In all cases, the differing losses of potassium, chloride and sodium will need to be replaced. In the case of pancreatic and biliary losses, the loss of bicarbonate must be taken into account (serum bicarbonate is routinely measured as part of the 'EUC' electrolyte blood test and can be replaced either orally or intravenously).

Q: 'But what about patients with severe heart failure?' Maddy asks.

A: Maddy has highlighted one of the limitations of our calculations. Imagine trying to give 2800 mL of fluid over 24 hours to a patient with heart failure and severe systolic dysfunction—the unfortunate recipient would almost certainly go into acute pulmonary oedema! It is therefore crucial to check a patient's history for any underlying comorbidities—such as heart, liver or renal failure—that would affect the ability to tolerate large volumes of fluid. A specialist may have already restricted such a patient's daily fluid intake.

If our 80 kg man does have such a condition (e.g. heart failure with moderately severe left ventricular systolic dysfunction), you may have to compromise on the amount of fluid you give. For example, you may decide to give 2000 mL/day rather than 2800 mL/day. But this is just an estimate. The key to success lies in regularly assessing the patient through daily electrolytes (this should be routinely performed for any patient who is nil by mouth) and daily physical examination to look for dehydration or fluid overload. You can then adjust the fluid volumes accordingly.

Q: Would you give Mr Tikolo potassium supplementation in his IV fluids immediately after surgery?

A: Some surgeons advise against giving potassium supplementation in the first 24 hours after surgery. This is because surgical trauma releases potassium into the bloodstream and aldosterone activity is increased postoperatively.

Q: Once Mr Tikolo shows evidence that his gastrointestinal function may be returning after surgery (e.g. the passage of flatus), the surgeon will commence him on 'clear oral fluids'. This usually means water and juices. How does this affect the way you will chart Mr Tikolo's IV fluids?

A: This 80 kg patient will still need a total of 2800 mL of fluid a day, regardless of whether it is given intravenously, orally or by both means. Therefore, if he takes 500 mL orally, you will need to reduce his IV intake to about 2300 mL of fluid.

Although the whole process sounds complicated, you will soon be able rapidly to calculate a patient's fluid requirements using these basic calculations.

Q: Maddy then asks: 'I heard something about patients being fluid restricted 'perioperatively to promote better outcomes. Is that true?'

A: Maddy has raised an issue that eventually may change fluid management around abdominal surgery. Brandstrup *et al.* (2003) demonstrated that the current standard fluid administration after colorectal surgery results in weight gain, which can be associated with increased cardiorespiratory and surgical-site-healing complications. Furthermore, fluid restriction aimed at avoiding such weight gain was associated with a significant reduction in these complications. Lobo *et al.* (2002) showed that fluid-restricted patients experienced a quicker return of gastrointestinal function and had a shorter hospital stay. But it's not so clear cut. A recent systematic review and meta-analysis concluded that perioperative fluid restriction did not reduce postoperative complications or length of stay (Boland *et al.*, 2013). Practice may vary among surgeons.

Nevertheless, even if they don't believe in fluid restriction, your knowledge is likely thoroughly to impress the surgeon and terrify the surgical registrar!

Achievements

You now:
- can calculate the daily fluid and electrolyte requirements of a patient on the ward
- know how to write up IV fluids on a fluid chart
- realise that the calculation of fluid and electrolyte requirements is not an exact art and requires constant reassessment

- appreciate that fluid requirements may have to be reduced in certain cases (heart failure)
- are aware that fluid restriction after colorectal surgery may be of benefit to the patient.

References

Boland, M.R., Noorani, A., Varty, K., Calvin Coffey, J., Agha, R. and Walsh, S.R. (2013), 'Perioperative fluid restriction in major abdominal surgery: Systematic review and meta-analysis of randomized clinical trials', *World Journal of Surgery*, vol. 37, no. 6, pp 1193-1202.

Brandstrup, B., Tonnesen, H., Beier-Holgersen, R. *et al.* (2003), 'Effects restriction on postoperative complications. Comparison of two perioperative fluid regimens: A randomised assessor-blinded multicenter trial', *Annals of Surgery*, vol. 238, no. 5, pp. 641–648.

Lobo, D.N., Bostock, K.A., Neal, K.R. *et al.* (2002), 'Effect of salt and water balance on recovery of gastrointestinal function after elective colonic resection: A randomised controlled trial', *Lancet*, vol. 359, no. 9320, pp. 1812–1818.

Worthley, L.I.G. (1997), 'Fluid and electrolyte therapy', in T.E. Oh (ed.), *Intensive Care Manual*, Butterworth–Heinemann, Oxford, pp. 700–710.

Chapter 34
Mrs Van Dyke takes an overdose

Scenario

It has been a busy day in the Emergency Department. Just as you finish a break, the department's specialist comes up to you and says, 'A woman has been brought in with a possible overdose. Could you please sort her out?'

Q: What is the first thing you must do?

A: You will almost certainly see at least one overdose patient as a junior doctor working in the Emergency Department. In all cases, the first thing you must do is assess the ABCs (airway, breathing, circulation), as some poisons can result in a compromised airway or circulatory collapse.

Q: The patient's name is Mrs Van Dyke. She is lying in bed, and is teary but clearly awake and breathing comfortably. The preliminary observations reveal normal oxygen saturation, pulse and blood pressure. You are satisfied that her ABCs are fine for now. You introduce yourself and proceed to take a history.

What are the important points to remember when taking a history from an overdose patient?

A: Find out what poison was used, the quantity, the route and the time it was taken. Keep in mind that you may not be able to trust the patient's response. If the patient is unconscious, you should ask any witnesses about medications found at the premises and Mrs Van Dyke's physician about any medications she takes, as well as other relevant information.

Try to determine the reason for the overdose: did Mrs Van Dyke say that she intended to kill herself? Is there evidence of an underlying mental illness (e.g. depression, a cry for help, attention-seeking behaviour)? You might need to gather this information from a number of sources, including the patient, any family or friends present, old hospital notes documenting a psychiatric history or previous suicide attempts.

Scenario

Mrs Van Dyke tells you that she is a 76-year-old woman who lives alone in a unit. She is a widow and has no family or friends nearby. Today is the first anniversary of her husband's death. She has been so lonely that she decided to end it all. She took around 20 × 500 mg paracetamol tablets 6 hours ago and went to bed to die, but then became afraid and called an ambulance. Mrs Van Dyke has had pulmonary emboli, for which she takes warfarin. She denies overdosing on warfarin today. She also denies previous suicide attempts or having been treated for depression. You speak to the ambulance officers who brought her to the hospital. They support Mrs Van Dyke's assertion that warfarin and paracetamol were the only medications they saw in her home.

Q: How does paracetamol cause toxicity?

A: Paracetamol normally produces a small amount of toxic metabolite (N-acetyl-p-benzoquinone imine [NAPQI]) in the liver, and glutathione usually neutralises this. However, during an overdose, glutathione stores cannot deal with the large amount of toxic metabolite produced. This leaves enough of the substance to cause hepatotoxicity.

Q: A final year medical student, Elijah, asks you if 10g paracetamol could cause hepatotoxicity. What do you tell him?

A: In adults and children older than 6 years, paracetamol toxicity can occur when (Daly *et al.*, 2008):

- >200 mg/kg or 10 g (whichever is less) is taken in a single dose over a period of less than 8 hours or over a single 24-hour period
- >150 mg/kg or 6 g (whichever is less) is ingested per 24-hour period for the preceding 48 hours
- >100 mg/kg or 4 g/day (whichever is less) in those with risk factors.

Mrs Van Dyke has ingested 10 g of paracetamol within the past 8 hours and is at risk of toxicity. Paracetamol overdose is fairly common, so you should be familiar with how to treat these patients.

Q: Elijah diligently listens to the criteria you previously outlined before saying, 'Wait a minute. Didn't you say that 4g/day of paracetamol can be hepatotoxic in certain risk groups? But isn't 4 g/day the normal dose we prescribe on the ward for people who need paracetamol for pain?'

A: He's right. On the wards, paracetamol is usually charted as '1 g qid'. In other words, 4 g/day shouldn't be a problem for the vast majority of people taking paracetamol. There are certain risk groups, in whom even this 'safe' dose could lead to hepatotoxicity. These groups are people with dehydration, chronic alcohol misuse, starvation or who are using enzyme-inducing drugs. It is thought that these risk factors predispose to increased production of NAPQI, reduced glutathione production or both. The clinical relevance of these risk factors to paracetamol toxicity remains controversial (Daly *et al.*, 2008) although such cases have been described (Lubel *et al.*, 2007).

Q: Returning to Mrs Van Dyke's case, Elijah asks, 'But shouldn't she have symptoms of paracetamol toxicity by now?'

A: Hung and Nelson (2000) divide paracetamol toxicity into 4 stages:
1. **Stage I** (first 24 hours): asymptomatic or minimal signs and symptoms.
2. **Stage II** (days 2–3): non-specific gastrointestinal clinical features and abnormal liver function tests.
3. **Stage III** (days 3–4): most recover, but some develop fulminant hepatic failure.
4. **Stage IV** (the following week): survivors tend to recover completely.

Although you do not need to learn these 4 stages, it is important to realise that overdose patients who eventually develop fatal hepatic failure were probably asymptomatic on presenting to the Emergency Department soon after their overdose. In other words, Mrs Van Dyke may be at risk of dying from hepatic failure and should be treated accordingly, even though she is asymptomatic now.

Q: You proceed to examine Mrs Van Dyke. Elijah is puzzled: 'You have just told me that Mrs Van Dyke is unlikely to have clinical features of paracetamol toxicity within 24 hours of her overdose. So what are you looking for on physical examination?'

A: In the setting of an overdose, the physical examination may reveal signs of an overdose of another medication that the patient has not told you about, either deliberately or unintentionally.

The following list (adapted from Hack and Hoffman, 2000) may be useful, but you do not need to memorise it! Just be aware that any physical sign in an overdose patient may point you towards the toxin that was taken. Once you have identified the sign (e.g. tachycardia), you can consult someone or refer to a text to determine the possible causes. With experience, you will come to recognise automatically the signs associated with overdose of different toxins.

- **Diaphoresis:**
  - sympathomimetics (cocaine, amphetamine)
  - hypoglycaemia (insulin, sulfonylurea)
  - cholinergics (organophosphate insecticides).

- **Dry skin or mucous membranes:**
  - anticholinergics.
- **Central nervous system depression:**
  - opioids (morphine, heroin)
  - benzodiazepines
  - tricyclics.
- **Altered mental status:**
  - nearly any medication overdose can alter mental status.
- **Tachycardia:**
  - sympathomimetics
  - anticholinergics
  - hypoglycaemia
  - salicylates
  - serotonin syndrome
  - tricyclic antidepressants.
- **Bradycardia:**
  - cholinergics
  - opioids
  - barbiturates
  - beta-blockers/calcium antagonists.
- **Hypertension:**
  - sympathomimetics
  - hypoglycaemia
  - anticholinergic
  - tricyclic antidepressants (see below)
  - serotonin syndrome.
- **Hypotension:**
  - opioids
  - oral antihypertensives
  - salicylates
  - tricyclics (more likely to cause hypotension than hypertension through alpha-effects and negative inotropy).
- **Hyperthermia:**
  - sympathomimetics
  - anticholinergics
  - salicylates.
- **Hypothermia:**
  - opioids.
- **Mydriasis:**
  - sympathomimetics
  - anticholinergics.

- **Miosis:**
  - opioids
  - cholinergics
  - serotonin syndrome.
- **Salivation/lacrimation/bronchorrhoea:**
  - cholinergic
  - respiratory depression
  - opioids
  - benzodiazepines.
- **Increased muscle tone/hyperreflexia:**
  - serotonin syndrome.
- **Urinary retention:**
  - anticholinergics.
- **Urination/defaecation:**
  - cholinergics.

Q: The physical examination is unremarkable, apart from Mrs Van Dyke being visibly upset. What investigations should you order at this stage?

A: If you were confident that Mrs Van Dyke had only taken paracetamol 6 hours ago and nothing else, you could justify only ordering a single blood test, namely a paracetamol level (Daly *et al.*, 2008)—even if she had taken a toxic dose, you wouldn't expect her liver function tests to be abnormal yet. However, she takes warfarin, is elderly and you are unsure if she really does have other underlying serious comorbidities. So it's not unreasonable to order a few more tests.

  1. **Full blood count, electrolytes, urea, creatinine, blood sugar, coagulation studies**. These are useful as baseline tests and may identify a metabolic derangement due to an overdose that must be corrected (e.g. metabolic acidosis, electrolyte abnormalities).
  2. **Paracetamol level**. This is the only way of determining whether Mrs Van Dyke is likely to suffer from paracetamol toxicity. But you will get a reliable indicator of toxicity only if the level is taken ≥ 4 hours after ingestion with a further level 4 hours later (Daly *et al.*, 2008).

     Every Emergency Department will have a nomogram for paracetamol toxicity. The y- and x-axes of the nomogram are the 'paracetamol level' and 'time after ingestion', respectively. Simply look at where the points intersect; this will tell you if your patient is likely to develop toxicity.
  3. **Liver function tests**. The main toxicity of paracetamol overdoses is in the liver. However, as noted earlier, patients who present

early are unlikely to have abnormal liver function tests at presentation. Nevertheless, the tests will provide a useful baseline if a patient goes on to develop hepatotoxicity.

4. **INR.** Given that Mrs Van Dyke takes warfarin, this is an easy way to exclude a warfarin overdose. Given that paracetamol toxicity itself can lead to a coagulopathy, Mrs Van Dyke's coagulation studies will have to be monitored regularly regardless of the initial result.

5. **12-lead electrocardiogram.** Overdose with a number of medications can cause cardiac toxicity (e.g. beta-blockers, digoxin, tricyclic antidepressants). In patients who are unhelpful or not capable of giving a history, an abnormal ECG might be the only indication of an overdose with a cardiotoxic substance.

6. **Chest X-ray.** This may be useful, especially in a drowsy patient, to exclude aspiration pneumonia.

It will take a little while for the test results to return.

Q: Elijah wonders if you should initiate gastrointestinal decontamination. But, first of all, what is gastrointestinal decontamination?

A: Gastrointestinal decontamination involves preventing a toxin that is already present in the gut from entering the bloodstream.

Hack and Hoffman (2000) identify 3 methods of gastrointestinal decontamination:

- gastric emptying (orogastric lavage)
- adsorption in the gut lumen (activated charcoal)
- elimination (whole bowel irrigation).

In the case of paracetamol overdose, the most commonly used method would be adsorption in the gut lumen using activated charcoal. In fact, activated charcoal will probably be the most common form of decontamination you will see as a junior doctor in the Emergency Department.

Q: So, returning to Elijah's question, would you give Mrs Van Dyke activated charcoal?

A: No. Mrs Van Dyke ingested the paracetamol more than 6 hours ago. To have been effective, the activated charcoal should have been given within 1–2 hours of ingestion of the paracetamol (Daly *et al.*, 2008). By now, it would already have been absorbed from the gut.

As a rule, there is little benefit in giving activated charcoal beyond 4 hours of ingestion of any toxin. However, if there is any uncertainty about the time of ingestion, you should give the charcoal, provided that the patient is alert and not at risk of vomiting and aspiration.

Q: Mrs Van Dyke's INR is therapeutic at 2.3. Her ECG and basic blood tests are unremarkable. The 6-hour paracetamol level, however, is 1000 μmol/L and is predictive of toxicity according to the nomogram. Apart from supportive therapy, how will you treat her?

A: N-acetylcysteine is the antidote for paracetamol toxicity. In Australia it is given intravenously as 3 separate infusions over 20–21 hours, but in other countries an oral formulation may also be available. N-acetylcysteine is a very effective agent that guarantees survival and prevents all serious hepatic damage if given within 8 hours of paracetamol ingestion. N-acetylcysteine is reasonably expensive and can have some serious side effects. In other words, it should only be given if necessary. Side effects include anaphylactoid reactions in 10–50% of cases which can manifest with wheezing, rash or mild hypotension. The treatment for such reactions is to cease or slow down the infusion and administer antihistamines (Daly et al., 2008).

Q: Elijah shakes his head in frustration. 'We knew that she took a toxic dose of paracetamol. Shouldn't we have just started N-acetylcysteine immediately instead of waiting for the paracetamol level from the lab? That wasted another 45 minutes. Surely starting the N-acetylcysteine earlier will lead to a better outcome?'

A: Interestingly, as long as the N-acetylcysteine is started within 8 hours of ingestion, then the outcome is the same regardless of when within that 8-hour period the antidote was commenced (Daly et al., 2008). Therefore, starting Mrs Van Dyke on N-acetylcysteine at 6 hours and 45 minutes post-ingestion instead of 6 hours post-ingestion (when she presented to the Emergency Department) has not affected her outcome, which should be excellent. However, Elijah's concerns are justified if the N-acetylcysteine is given >8–10 hours post-ingestion—the efficacy of the antidote starts to drop. But even if used late in established fulminant hepatic failure from paracetamol, N-acetylcysteine can have a beneficial effect in reducing inotrope requirements and the degree of cerebral oedema and improving survival by 30% (Daly et al., 2008).

Q: The Emergency registrar agrees with your assessment and commences Mrs Van Dyke on an N-acetylcysteine infusion. Is there anyone else who needs to know about this overdose?

A: In most hospitals, the psychiatry team is always informed about every overdose. You should therefore contact the psychiatry registrar about Mrs Van Dyke's case.

You return after 4 days off, and are pleased to hear that Mrs Van Dyke did not develop hepatotoxicity. After an interview, the psychiatry registrar diagnosed her with depression and felt that she was at high risk of suicide. He has therefore admitted her to the acute psychiatric ward to be treated for depression.

Achievements

You now:
- know the important points in taking a history from an overdose patient
- know how much paracetamol is required to cause toxicity
- know how paracetamol causes toxicity
- can correlate abnormalities on physical examination with different drug overdoses
- know which investigations to order in overdose patients
- know how to use paracetamol levels and the nomogram to predict hepatotoxicity
- understand the role of gastrointestinal decontamination in overdose
- know that N-acetylcysteine is the antidote for paracetamol toxicity
- realise the importance of consulting the psychiatry team for any overdose.

References

Daly, F.F., Fountain, J.S., Murray, L., Graudins, A. and Buckley, N.A. (Panel of Australian and New Zealand clinical toxicologists) (2008), 'Guidelines for the management of paracetamol poisoning in Australia and New Zealand—explanation and elaboration. A consensus statement from clinical toxicologists consulting to the Australasian poisons information centres', *Medical Journal of Australia*, vol. 188, no. 5, pp. 296–301.

Hack, J.B. and Hoffman, R.S. (2000), 'General management of poisoned patients', in J.E. Tintinalli, G.D. Kelen and J.S. Stapczynski (eds), *Emergency Medicine*, McGraw-Hill, New York, pp. 1057–1063.

Hung, O. and Nelson, L.S. (2000), 'Acetaminophen', in J.E. Tintinalli, G.D. Kelen and J.S. Stapczynski (eds), *Emergency Medicine*, McGraw-Hill, New York, pp. 1125–1132.

Lubel, J.S., Angus, P.W. and Gow, P.J. (2007), 'Accidental paracetamol poisoning', *Medical Journal of Australia*, vol. 186, no. 7, pp. 371–372.

Chapter 35
Mr Wilson presents with an acutely painful leg

Scenario

You have had a busy day in the Emergency Department. Just as you discharge a patient and are about to have a late lunch, the triage nurse approaches you: 'I have just seen a 60-year-old man with a very painful leg. Could you please see him now?'

You agree and are led to Mr Wilson, who is grimacing in pain. He tells you that he woke up about an hour ago with severe pain in his right leg. He has never experienced anything like this before.

Q: Does he really need to be seen right now? Surely you can give him some analgesia to settle the pain, have some lunch and see him later?

A: Wrong! Go to the back of the class and call your medical defence lawyer. An acutely painful limb is the classical presentation for acute limb ischaemia. Therefore, the first thing you must do is exclude this diagnosis. And if Mr Wilson is suffering from acute limb ischaemia, it may be only hours before the damage becomes irreversible. An early diagnosis will save the limb, while a late diagnosis will result in amputation.

Q: By the end of your history and examination of Mr Wilson, what should you have worked out?

A: You should know:
- whether he does have an acutely ischaemic limb
- if so, the likely cause of this.

Q: What features on history and examination will support the diagnosis of an acutely ischaemic limb?

A: Easy! All you have to do is remember the '6 Ps':
- pain
- pallor
- pulselessness
- perishing cold (also known as poikilothermia)

- paraesthesias (ischaemia to nerves)
- paralysis[1] (ischaemia to nerves).

Pain is the most common symptom but this can become less severe as paraesthesia sets in; however, this is a bad sign as the onset of paraesthesia means that the ischaemia has progressed, damaging nerves. Pallor occurs early on and represents emptying of the arteries and vasospasm. Then mottling of the skin appears due to stagnant blood in the capillaries. This is initially blanching which represents reversible ischaemia; however, when the ischaemia becomes irreversible, the mottling becomes non-blanching (O'Connell and Quinones-Baldrich, 2009).

Q: What are the most common causes of acute limb ischaemia?

A: Although there are a number of causes, the ones you are most likely to encounter as a junior doctor are:

- embolus—cardiogenic in 80–90% of cases (O'Connell and Quinones-Baldrich, 2009)
- thrombosis of a native vessel or a graft
- trauma.

Q: Can you differentiate between an embolic or thrombotic cause of acute limb ischaemia on the basis of history and examination? Does it matter?

A: The answer to the second question is that it does matter because different management strategies can be used for the 2 causes.

There will be clues on the history or examination that will point to either an embolus or thrombosis. These are set out in the following table.

Clue	Embolus	Thrombosis
Onset of limb pain	Sudden	More gradual
History of ischaemic heart disease (mural thrombus)	More likely	
Clue	Embolus	Thrombosis
History of AF	More likely	
History of PVD (intermittent claudication, bypass surgery)		More likely
Examination reveals AF	More likely	
Examination reveals normal pulses on opposite limb	More likely	
Examination reveals arterial bruits		More likely

---

[1] Once an acutely ischaemic limb becomes paralysed, it is likely that the damage will be irreversible.

In an ideal situation, you may find a patient with an acutely ischaemic limb who fits neatly into one of these categories (e.g. in a 35-year-old woman with untreated atrial fibrillation [AF] and no other medical problems it will almost certainly be an embolic cause). Unfortunately, however, in real life the distinction is often not that clear because a single patient may have all these conditions at once.

Q: Mr Wilson has a 4-month history consistent with intermittent claudication of both legs. Furthermore, he has been developing palpitations intermittently for the past 3 months, but has not been concerned enough to seek medical advice. He has smoked a packet of cigarettes a day for 30 years.

This morning he woke up with severe pain in his leg. It appeared suddenly. His only concern was getting to a hospital as soon as possible.

On examination, you find that Mr Wilson has the following characteristics:

- irregularly irregular pulse
- pale and cool right lower limb below the knee
- sluggish capillary return
- femoral artery is palpable but you cannot detect any other pulses
- sensation is still normal and he has a full range of movement in the limb on the left lower limb.

Does Mr Wilson have an acutely ischaemic limb?

A: Yes. The pain, pallor, pulselessness and coolness (perishing cold) all support acute ischaemia of his right leg.

Q: Is Mr Wilson's ischaemia due to an embolus or thrombosis?

A: He clinically has AF, which is a risk factor for embolism according to the above table. But Mr Wilson also has clinical evidence of peripheral vascular disease (i.e. intermittent claudication, reduced pulses in the 'normal' limb), which is a risk factor for thrombosis. This highlights the fact that patients will often have risk factors for both embolism and thrombosis, making the underlying reason for the acute ischaemia uncertain.

Q: What is the most important thing to do now?

A: You have efficiently assessed that Mr Wilson has an acutely ischaemic limb. The most important thing to do now is inform the vascular surgery registrar immediately. Remember that your prompt referral may be the only difference between Mr Wilson's leg being saved or amputated.

Q: Brenda, the vascular surgery registrar, rushes down to the Emergency Department to see Mr Wilson. She agrees with your assessment and thanks you for your prompt referral. In addition, she also performs arterial and venous Dopplers during which she hears blood flow. Then she says, 'I'm going to call my consultant. While I'm doing that, please order the appropriate investigations'. What should you order?

A: Mr Wilson's management may well involve urgent surgery. You should therefore order a standard preoperative work-up as follows:
- full blood count
- electrolytes, urea, creatinine
- coagulation studies
- group and hold
- 12-lead ECG
- chest X-ray.

Mr Wilson also has newly diagnosed AF. It would therefore be worth initiating some basic investigations for this condition (see Chapter 4).

Q: Brenda returns and agrees with the investigations that you have ordered. 'You're doing a pretty good job at the moment. Before we definitively deal with the ischaemic limb, is there anything else we can do for Mr Wilson?'

What do you tell her?

A: Two simple measures that you can initiate at this stage are:
1. **Analgesia**. An acutely ischaemic limb is extremely painful. It is essential to make the patient comfortable.
2. **Commence IV heparin**. Talk to the vascular registrar before administering heparin. If the patient is about to have an angiogram, the heparin might be delayed until after the procedure. However, heparin is reversible with protamine and has a short half-life, so it is not usually a problem if it is administered beforehand. Then again, you will never get into trouble for checking. (Refer back to Chapter 32 for how to initiate heparin.)

Q: Brenda agrees with your plan. 'Now how do we treat the ischaemic leg itself?'

A: This practice may vary from hospital to hospital but one approach is to manage the ischaemic limb according to its clinical stage.

Stage	Sensation	Motor function	Arterial Doppler	Venous Doppler	Management
I: Viable	Intact	Intact	Audible	Audible	Usually arteriography and invasive therapy

Stage	Sensation	Motor function	Arterial Doppler	Venous Doppler	Management
II: Marginally threatened	Minimal loss (toes) or none	Intact	Inaudible	Audible	Arteriography* and invasive therapy
III: Immediately threatened	More loss than toes, rest pain	Mild/ moderate loss	Inaudible	Audible	Invasive therapy
IV: Irreversible (a bit of a misnomer as early-onset cases due to a large embolus can be cured)	Profound loss, anaesthetic	Profound, paralysis	Inaudible	Inaudible	1. If early onset (<1–2 hours), consider invasive therapy 2. If >1–2 hours, then delayed amputation

*Arteriography can help differentiate between an embolus and thrombosis. Some centres perform arteriograms on all acutely ischaemic limbs; others perform them only if the origin of the ischaemia is uncertain. If the limb is still viable, an arteriogram can be performed in the radiology department. If there is very little time to save the limb, it can be performed on the operating table.
Source: Adapted from Rutherford (2009).

Q: In general, what sort of invasive therapy can be used to revascularise the ischaemic limb?

A:

1. **Thrombotic cause:**
   a. **Catheter-directed thrombolysis.** A catheter is inserted directly into a thrombus before a thrombolytic agent is infused. Urokinase and rt-PA may be preferable to streptokinase (Alonso-Coello *et al.*, 2012). As with thrombolysis for acute MI, contraindications must be excluded before commencing therapy.
   b. **Bypass surgery.** Surgery will be undertaken if thrombolysis is not appropriate.
2. **Embolic cause:**
   a. **Embolectomy** (using a balloon, or Fogarty, catheter).
   b. **Balloon catheter embolectomy** (sometimes followed by thrombolysis to clear distal thrombus).
   c. **Bypass surgery** (used where other measures are not possible).
   The American College of Chest Physicians also agrees that reperfusion therapy (intra-arterial thrombolysis or surgery) should

be undertaken in acute limb ischaemia; however, they quote a meta-analysis which suggests that surgery is superior to intra-arterial thrombolysis. But the quality of the data was only moderate (Alonso-Coello *et al.*, 2012).

Q: Brenda is impressed with your knowledge. Mr Wilson is given a bolus of IV heparin. An arteriogram is performed in the radiology department because the cause of the ischaemia is unclear. It reveals that the ischaemia is due to acute thrombosis of the popliteal artery. Mr Wilson receives catheter-directed urokinase and a heparin infusion. By 6 hours, he has clinically reperfused.

A few more hours pass and the end of your shift is approaching. The nurse looking after Mr Wilson looks concerned. He has now developed severe calf pain in the reperfused limb after being pain-free since reperfusion. You quickly assess him: all the limb pulses are present, but his leg is quite swollen and the calf muscles are tense and tender.

What might be happening?

A: Mr Wilson could have 'reperfusion injury', which occurs when perfusion is restored to an acutely ischaemic limb. Ischaemia-reperfusion injury is multifactorial in origin. Causes include cytokine release (e.g. TNF-alpha and IL-1 beta), complement cascade and the formation of toxic oxygen metabolites. Furthermore, the consequences of injury to muscle from the initial ischaemic insult (e.g. release of potassium, myoglobin, creatine kinase, etc.) are exacerbated by reperfusion (Eliason and Wakefield, 2009). Ischaemia reperfusion can also be associated with lactic acidosis.

Anyway, the implications of ischaemia reperfusion in the previously ischaemic muscle is that interstitial and muscle oedema occur potentially leading to compartment syndrome.

As mentioned above, the return of blood flow to a limb can result in a 'washout' of inflammatory mediators, myoglobin, hydrogen and potassium ions and oxygen free radicals. This can lead to:

- life-threatening hyperkalaemia (see Chapter 16)
- metabolic acidosis
- acute kidney injury (myoglobinuria)
- non-cardiogenic pulmonary oedema
- depressed myocardial function.

To avoid these effects, you need to:

- observe the limb closely for compartment syndrome
- monitor pH, serum creatinine and potassium levels
- regularly measure oxygen saturation.

Brenda rushes down from the operating theatre. She agrees that Mr Wilson is suffering from compartment syndrome. Your blood tests and oxygen saturations reveal no systemic effects of reperfusion injury. Mr Wilson is rushed to the operating theatre, where a fasciotomy is urgently performed to decompress the muscle compartments.

After a 4-day break, you return to work and find Brenda. She tells you that Mr Wilson is doing well and that his compartment syndrome is under control.

Achievements

You now:

- can recognise an acutely ischaemic limb
- recognise the urgency of treating an acutely ischaemic limb
- know some of the differences between an embolic and thrombotic cause of an acutely ischaemic limb
- know how important it is to inform the vascular surgery team as soon as you recognise an acutely ischaemic limb
- can investigate an acutely ischaemic limb
- know the principles of treating an acutely ischaemic limb
- are aware of the dangers and manifestations of reperfusion injury.

References

Alonso-Coello, P., Bellmunt, S., Gorrian, C., *et al.* (2012), 'Antithrombotic therapy in peripheral artery disease: antithrombotic therapy and prevention of thrombosis, 9th edition: American College of Chest Physicians evidence-based clinical practice guidelines', *Chest*, vol. 141, no. 2_suppl, e669S–e690S. doi:10.1378/chest.11-2307.

Eliason, J.L. and Wakefield, T.W. (2009), 'Metabolic consequences of acute limb ischemia and their clinical implications', *Seminars in Vascular Surgery*, vol. 22, no. 1, pp. 29–33.

Engledow, A.H. and Crinnion, J.N. (2002), 'Acute lower limb ischaemia', *Hospital Medicine*, vol. 63, no. 7, pp. 412–415.

O'Connell, J.B. and Quinones-Baldrich, W.J. (2009), 'Proper evaluation and management of acute embolic versus thrombotic limb ischemia', *Seminars in Vascular Surgery*, vol. 22, no. 1, pp. 10–16.

Rutherford, R.B. (2009), 'Clinical staging of acute limb ischemia as the basis for choice of revascularization method: When and how to intervene', *Seminars in Vascular Surgery*, vol. 22, no. 1, pp. 5–9.

The Royal Free Hospital Vascular Unit (2003), 'Arterial disease: Acute limb ischaemia/ALI (= acute arterial occlusion)', at <www.freevas.demon.co.uk/ Freevas_frameset.html>

Chapter 36
Bruno presents with acute flank pain

Scenario

You are currently enjoying your term as the urology intern. As you finish assisting with another transurethral resection of the prostate, your registrar's pager goes off. It turns out to be a consult from the Emergency Department—a possible case of renal colic. Your registrar has to scrub up for another case, so he asks you to assess this patient.

You are directed to the clinics section of the Emergency Department, where you meet Bruno, a 45-year-old man in obvious distress. You ask him what is wrong.

You learn that Bruno has been experiencing terrible pain for the past 3 hours. It starts in the left flank and radiates down to the groin. It is coming in waves and is the worst pain he has ever known. It is so bad that he has vomited 3 times. He denies fevers, rigors or pain on passing urine. He has never had this pain before.

Apart from high cholesterol that is well controlled with statins, Bruno is in excellent health. He denies gout (around 20% of patients with uric acid stones have gout). The only abnormality on examination is left flank tenderness.

Q: What is the most likely diagnosis?
A: The history and examination support a diagnosis of renal or ureteric colic. The pain Bruno reports is the classical 'loin to groin' pain.

Q: Antoine is the medical student in the Emergency Department. 'Acute flank pain from the loin to groin—it has to be renal colic', he asserts. Do you agree with him?
A: No. It is very important to remember that there are other causes of acute flank pain radiating down to the groin. In particular, a ruptured abdominal aortic aneurysm can mimic the pain of renal colic and must not be missed. Other possibilities include acute appendicitis, acute diverticulitis and, in women, pelvic inflammatory disease.

Q: In what other 'non-organic' situation will people present with this type of pain?

A: Unfortunately, during your career, you will encounter individuals pretending to have renal colic in order to receive opiate analgesia. There is no easy way to manage this problem. Even if a person is known to Emergency Department staff as a seeker of narcotic analgesia, no one can be sure that their next presentation will not be a genuine episode of renal colic or even a ruptured aortic aneurysm. In that case, dismissing such an episode as fraud and sending the person home may be a fatal mistake. Consequently, you should carefully assess each episode objectively on its merits.

Q: What simple and cheap bedside test will provide further support for a diagnosis of renal colic?

A: A dipstick analysis of a midstream urine specimen usually reveals microscopic haematuria.

Q: Bruno provides you with a midstream urine specimen. It does indeed demonstrate microscopic haematuria. Can you say that he definitely has renal colic?

A: Although you cannot be absolutely certain at this stage, the diagnosis is very likely. In fact, Sandhu *et al.* (2003) cited a study by Eskelinen *et al.* (1998) that showed that a diagnosis of renal colic can be made with a sensitivity of 84% and a specificity of 99% through the combination of:
- classical history
- flank tenderness
- microscopic haematuria.

It is worth noting, however, that 10% of patients with renal colic don't have microscopic haematuria; therefore, don't dismiss the diagnosis if microscopic haematuria isn't present (Masarani and Dinneen, 2007).

Q: Antoine asks: 'Given that renal colic is the likely diagnosis in this patient, do we need to order imaging to make a definitive diagnosis? Can't we just treat him?'

A: Although Antoine has asked a good question, it is still worth pursuing a definitive diagnosis of renal colic because:
- investigations may reveal another cause of acute flank pain (e.g. aortic aneurysm, acute diverticulitis, appendicitis or, in a woman, pelvic inflammatory disease)
- investigations may reveal an indication for urgent intervention (e.g. obstruction proximal to the stone)
- diagnosis of renal colic will often necessitate lifestyle changes for the individual to prevent further episodes

- diagnosis of renal colic may preclude the individual from certain occupations (e.g. airline pilots) and therefore have an enormous impact on lifestyle.

Q: You convince Antoine that you should investigate further to try and make a definitive diagnosis. What imaging investigations should you order?

A: You should order:

1. **a plain 'kidney–ureter–bladder' radiograph** (more commonly known as a 'KUB') AND
2. **a non-contrast helical CT of the abdomen and pelvis** (also known as a 'CT urogram').

Although it is not a very good test for identifying stones (sensitivity 45–58%), a KUB can be performed in minutes in the Emergency Department and is non-invasive. Furthermore, a KUB plays a role in identifying uric acid stones. Radiolucent uric acid stones are not normally visible on a KUB, but they will be visible on a CT. Stones that are visible on both a KUB and a CT are likely to be calcium stones. The importance of seeing a calcium stone on both CT and KUB is that only KUB X-rays can be used to follow up passage of the stone, thereby reducing the amount of radiation to which the patient is exposed (Masarani and Dinneen, 2007).

An unenhanced (non-contrast) helical CT of the abdomen and pelvis is probably the best radiological investigation to identify renal or ureteric calculi. It has sensitivities of 96% and specificities of 100% and will identify all types of calculi. A CT will identify an extra-urinary cause of acute flank pain in 6–12% of cases, for example appendicitis. And the fact that there is no need for contrast is an added bonus. Although it can't demonstrate the excretory function of the kidney as well as an intravenous pyelogram, a CT can demonstrate other features of obstruction such as hydronephrosis and hydroureter that indicate dysfunction (Masarani and Dinneen, 2007). You should be able to order this investigation in nearly all metropolitan hospitals in Australia. Even if you see a calculus on the KUB, you should still order the unenhanced helical CT because of all the information it provides.

If required, other investigations for identifying renal calculi include ultrasound and intravenous pyelogram (IVP). An ultrasound can identify calculi in the renal pelvis, calyces, pelviureteric junction (PUJ) and vesicoureteric junction (VUJ) but is poor at picking up calculi between the PUJ and the VUJ (Masarani and Dinneen, 2007).

Q: You order a KUB and a CT. The former is performed within minutes. There appears to be a tiny radio-opaque opacity where the distal ureter should be, but you cannot be certain. Radiology can only do the unenhanced helical CT in 2 hours. What should you do in the meantime?

A:
1. Provide analgesia.
2. Take some appropriate blood tests.
3. Commence IV fluids.

Q: Renal colic is an extremely painful condition. You must provide Bruno with adequate analgesia. Antoine says, 'Let's give him morphine!' What do you think about that?

A: Both opiates and non-steroidal anti-inflammatory drugs (NSAIDs) are commonly used to treat renal colic; however, NSAIDs are probably the favourite with opiates used if NSAIDs fail to provide adequate relief. Renal colic stimulates local prostaglandin production with resultant increased renal-pelvic pressures and ureteral smooth muscle spasm (Micali *et al.*, 2006). NSAIDs counter this prostaglandin effect and reduce local oedema and inflammation (Masarani and Dinneen, 2007).

Routes of administration are:
- parenteral (ketorolac, the only NSAID given parenterally, at a loading dose 30–60 mg IV/IM, then 15 mg IV/IM q6h up to 90 mg/day in an adult with normal renal function)
- suppository (indomethacin)
- oral (e.g. diclofenac, indomethacin).

The first 2 means of delivery are useful in nauseated patients who cannot tolerate oral medication.

If NSAIDs are insufficient, morphine can be used. Administer metoclopramide 10 mg IV/IM with morphine to prevent nausea.

Q: Antoine asks, 'Is there anything else we can give?'

A: Both calcium channel blockers (e.g. nifedipine) or alpha-receptor blockers (e.g. tamsulosin) may reduce ureteral muscle spasm to facilitate passage of ureteric calculi. Patients on either of these drugs have a 65% higher chance of passing a stone than those not taking them. There may also be a benefit if oral corticosteroids are added (Masarani and Dinneen, 2007). Most of the studies with nifedipine or tamsulosin were performed on distal ureteric calculi (Micali *et al.*, 2006).

Q: Since he appears to have a distal ureteric calculus, Bruno is given tamsulosin 400 mg/day in addition to IV ketorolac and metoclopramide. Fortunately, his pain largely settles soon after giving this combination of medications. What laboratory tests are you going to order and why?

A:

1. **Dipstick urinalysis plus or minus a midstream urine specimen.** It is important to exclude a UTI in the setting of renal colic because a UTI will require antibiotic treatment and it can be another indication for urgent intervention.

   Perform a dipstick urinalysis first (as you have already done for Bruno). If the results suggest infection (i.e. positive for white cells or nitrites), send a midstream urine specimen to the laboratory for microscopy, culture and sensitivities.

2. **Electrolytes, urea and creatinine.** These will identify any renal impairment caused by an obstructing calculus. Renal impairment due to a calculus is another indication for urgent intervention.

3. **Calcium and serum urate.** If Bruno does have renal colic, he will have to be investigated at a later stage for an underlying metabolic cause. However, even at this acute stage, you can order these simple tests to identify hypercalcaemia or hyperuricaemia, which could lead to the formation of calcium oxalate and urate stones, respectively.

4. **Lipase, amylase and liver function tests.** Although renal colic is the most likely cause, you still don't know for sure. Therefore, order these tests as you would for anyone with acute abdominal pain.

5. **Full blood count and coagulation studies.** These provide a baseline and may identify any abnormalities that might affect the outcome of invasive therapy.

6. **Neutrophilic leukocytosis.** This may support the presence of urinary sepsis.

7. **Blood cultures.** These should be ordered if the patient has a picture suggestive of a UTI.

Q: The non-contrast helical CT abdomen is performed and demonstrates a 4 mm stone in the distal left ureter. This matches up with the radio-opaque abnormality you saw on the plain KUB. No obstruction is seen. Bruno's pain is controlled after the medication. His IV fluids continue.

   Antoine wants to know if Bruno needs urgent invasive intervention to remove the stone. What do you tell him?

A: The indications for urgent intervention in renal colic, as discussed earlier, include:
- an obstructed upper urinary tract
- an infected upper urinary tract
- acute renal failure
- intractable pain and vomiting
- anuria.

We know that Bruno's case does not meet any of these criteria, so urgent intervention is not required. Where it is required, the 2 most common methods are extracorporeal shock wave lithotripsy (ESWL) and ureteroscopy. A Cochrane review comparing these 2 modalities concluded that ureteroscopy achieves a higher stone-free state than ESWL but at the expense of a longer hospital stay and higher complication rates (Nabi *et al.*, 2007).

Q: 'So will Bruno just pass the stone spontaneously?' asks Antoine. What do you tell him?

A: Ninety-five per cent of stones less than 5 mm in diameter are likely to pass spontaneously but may take up to 40 days to do so. Fifty per cent of stones greater than 5 mm will require intervention to remove them (Miller and Kane, 1999).

Q: 'Should we alkalinise his urine?' asks Antoine.

A: Alkalinisation of the urine with potassium citrate (or potassium magnesium citrate) is a useful therapy to dissolve uric acid, calcium and cystine stones. It is reportedly successful in 80% of uric acid stones. Interestingly, hypocitraturia is found in up to 20% of people with stones. In those patients who can't tolerate the citrate supplement, increased consumption of citrus fruits or juices can also have a beneficial effect. Oral sodium bicarbonate is another supplement for alkalinising the urine for treating uric acid stones; however, the high sodium content can lead to fluid overload in people with predisposing conditions (e.g. cardiac and renal failure) and can even lead to increased formation of calcium oxalate stones (Micali *et al.*, 2006).

In summary, Bruno's calcium stone (radio-opaque on KUB) may benefit from alkalinisation of the urine with citrate but not sodium bicarbonate. Bruno is admitted under the care of your team for 24 hours. He is completely asymptomatic and all his blood tests are unremarkable. Your registrar discharges him home with instructions to:
- drink plenty of fluids to keep well hydrated
- strain his urine to try and catch the stone so it can be analysed

- repeat the CT and KUB in 4 weeks to see if the stone has been passed, then see the urologist in his rooms.

Achievements

You now:
- know the importance of trying to make a definitive diagnosis of renal colic
- know that combined KUB and helical CT are the best imaging tests for renal colic
- know what analgesia to give a patient with renal colic
- appreciate the role of calcium antagonists and alpha-receptor antagonists in stone expulsion
- know what pathology tests to order for a patient with renal colic
- are aware of the indications for urgent intervention and the common methods used
- know that alkalinisation of urine is a useful way to dissolve ureteric stones
- know that nearly all stones less than 5 mm in diameter are likely to pass spontaneously.

References

Masarani, M. and Dinneen, M. (2007), 'Ureteric colic: New trends in diagnosis and treatment', *Postgraduate Medical Journal*, vol. 83, no. 981, pp. 469–472.

Micali, S., Grande, M., Sighinolfi, M.C., De Carne, C., De Stefani, S. and Bianchi, G. (2006), 'Medical therapy of urolithiasis', *Journal of Endourology*, vol. 20, no. 11, pp. 841–847.

Miller, O.F. and Kane, C.J. (1999), 'Time to stone passage for observed ureteral calculi: A guide for patient education', *Journal of Urology*, vol. 162, no. 3 pt 1, pp. 688–690.

Nabi, G., Downey, P., Keeley, F., Watson, G. and McClinton, S. (2007), 'Extracorporeal shock wave lithotripsy (ESWL) versus ureteroscopic management for ureteric calculi', *Cochrane Database of Systematic Reviews*, 1, CD006029.

Sandhu, C., Anson, K.M. and Patel, U. (2003), 'Urinary tract stones—Part I: Role of radiological imaging in diagnosis and treatment planning', *Clinical Radiology*, vol. 58, no. 6, pp. 415–421.

Teichman, J.M.H. (2004), 'Acute renal colic from ureteral calculus', *New England Journal of Medicine*, vol. 350, no. 7, pp. 684–693.

Chapter 37
Indiana returns from overseas with fever

Scenario

You are one of the Emergency Department interns. Your first patient of the shift is a 44-year-old man, Indiana, who returned from a 3-week trip to Thailand 5 days ago. He became unwell 3 days ago with high fevers and presented to the Emergency Department for the second day in a row because he isn't getting any better. His only concurrent medical problem is hypertension for which he takes perindopril. A medical student, Byron, is keen to see this patient with you.

Q: How should you approach history taking in a febrile traveller?

A: While a thorough history should be performed on every patient that you see, this is especially so for the returned traveller with fever. Important areas to cover include:

1. **A detailed travel itinerary**—certain diseases may be prevalent in some countries and not in others. Even within the same country, disease prevalence may vary; for example, malaria is less commonly found in major cities or high-altitude regions.

2. **Onset of the illness after returning to Australia**—some infections such as dengue have a short incubation period (usually less than 7 days); therefore if the patient became ill more than 14 days after returning, dengue would be most unlikely. Conversely, malaria can first manifest months after returning from an endemic area.

3. **Prophylaxis**—this includes malaria prophylaxis, travel vaccines and a general immunisation history.

4. **Sexual activity**—5–50% of short-term travellers engage in casual sexual activity and sexually transmitted infections are well described in travellers (Matteelli and Carosi, 2001).

5. **Recreational activities**—these could lead to being exposed to a number of infections, for example swimming in fresh water

could lead to leptospirosis or tick bites while bushwalking could lead to a rickettsial infection.

6. **Dietary history**—consumption of unusual items might point to a particular disease; for example, a patient with neurological signs who had recently eaten frog may have gnathostomiasis or a patient with fever who ate unpasteurised dairy products may have brucellosis.

7. **Animal exposures**—visiting farms, hunting, animal bites.

8. **Previous travel history**—some infections can have a long latent period, for example malaria and tuberculosis; therefore, although his recent time overseas may not be responsible for his presentation, a previous trip might be.

Q: Indiana tells you that he went to Thailand on business and spent most of the time in Bangkok itself; however, after the business negotiations had been completed, he spent about 2 weeks travelling to various rural areas. Indiana concedes that he did have 2 unprotected sexual encounters during his trip. One was with a local woman that he met at a bar but he denies that she was a sex worker. The other was an American businesswoman with whom he was negotiating. He denied any extensive outdoor activities and can't recall any animal encounters although he was bitten by mosquitoes in the rural areas. He ate hotel and restaurant food in Bangkok. Even in the rural areas, he tried to ensure that everything was freshly cooked. Certainly, he didn't eat any 'unusual' foods. He has only travelled to the USA and France previously. Prior to this trip, he was vaccinated against hepatitis A and B infection and typhoid. He has also been on malaria prophylaxis (atovaquone-proguanil) which he has been taking correctly and still continues with. What have you learnt from the history so far?

A: The history so far has been useful. Indiana has had unprotected sexual encounters and suffered mosquito bites in malarious areas. The history of hepatitis A and B vaccination makes those infections highly unlikely.

Q: With regard to his illness, he first felt hot with slight chills and his temperature was around 37.7–37.8 °C. Over the next few days, he developed a frontal headache with generalised myalgias and dry cough. The shivers and fevers seem to have worsened in the past couple of days and he now is measuring temperatures between 38.7 °C and 39 °C. He presented yesterday to the Emergency Department when his wife noticed a fine rash over his chest and abdomen. His blood tests that day demonstrated a mild leukopenia and mildly elevated liver function tests. He was reviewed by an intern who assessed him as having 'a viral illness' and suggested resting at home. The intern thought that the rash was a viral exanthem; however, it had disappeared by the time that Indiana returned home from the Emergency Department.

He specifically denies shortness of breath, urinary symptoms and diarrhoea; in fact, he has been constipated for the last few days.

On examination, Indiana looks tired. He has a fever of 39 °C and a regular pulse rate of 85/minute. Despite the headache, he has no neck stiffness. The only other positive findings are a white coated tongue and mild splenomegaly.

His blood tests today, like yesterday, again show a mild leukopenia and mildly elevated liver function tests (mixed picture).

What are the possible diagnoses?

A: There is a broad differential diagnosis although one diagnosis seems more likely than others, as we shall discuss below. Generally with fevers in the returned traveller, infectious diseases physicians immediately consider 3 diagnoses (also known as the 'Big Three', 'Terrible Threesome' or 'Unholy Trinity'), namely:

- malaria
- enteric fever (of which typhoid fever is a subgroup)
- dengue.

On the basis of further information, for example areas visited, incubation period, clinical and lab features, some or all of these 3 may be dismissed as diagnoses—but they are always considered. Certainly, in Indiana, the 'Unholy Trinity' is possible in that they all occur in Thailand, fit into the incubation period and can all cause a non-specific febrile presentation.

There is a broad list of possible causes of fever in Indiana including:

- malaria—caused by *Plasmodium* species transmitted by the *Anopheles* mosquito
- dengue—caused by a flavivirus transmitted mainly by the *Aedes aegypti* mosquito
- enteric fever (typhoid fever or paratyphoid fever)—a purely human infection transmitted faeco-orally
- influenza
- meningococcal disease
- HIV seroconversion[1]
- syphilis[1]
- disseminated gonococcal infection[1]

---

[1]Indiana's sexual encounters make these sexually transmitted infections more likely than other travellers without a history of casual travel sex.

- amoebic liver abscess
- melioidosis
- locally acquired illness.[2]

Q: Byron listens to your list of differential diagnoses. He looks puzzled. 'But Indiana has been compliant with appropriate malaria prophylaxis. He's also been vaccinated against typhoid fever. So surely malaria and typhoid fever can be ruled out?' Is he right?

A: No. With regard to typhoid fever (due to *Salmonella enterica* serotype Typhi), the vaccines are only 50–80% effective. Furthermore, their benefit is only short lived (Basnyat *et al.*, 2005) and they don't provide immunity against *Salmonella enterica* serotype Paratyphi A (a cause of paratyphoid fever [there are also paratyphi B and C], which is the other subgroup of enteric fever); therefore, Indiana could still have enteric fever despite being vaccinated.

Similarly, taking malaria prophylaxis is no guarantee of preventing infection with malaria, especially if occasional doses have been missed; however, it clearly reduces the risk.

Q: Byron persists with his scepticism though. 'But enteric fever is due to *Salmonella* and I thought that *Salmonella* causes diarrhoea. If anything, this man has been constipated. Explain that please.'

What is your response?

A: There are many *Salmonella* species other than those that cause enteric fever. Many of them cause diarrhoeal illnesses but enteric fever is largely an exception to this rule. This will be discussed overleaf.

Q: You tell Byron that enteric fever (either due to typhoid fever or paratyphoid fever) is the most likely diagnosis here although you can't be sure. What features of the illness have swayed you towards enteric fever?

A: There are a few features suggestive of enteric fever (Senanayake, 2007):

1. **The 'stepladder' fever pattern**—in classical enteric fever, the fever increases in a stepwise fashion during the first week, before plateauing in the second week and decreasing in the third and fourth weeks (Bal and Czarnowski, 2004).

2. **Coated tongue**—this is another feature of enteric fever; although, by itself, it is not a particularly sensitive or specific sign. In combination with bradycardia, loose bowel motions and

---

[2]Just because Indiana has travelled overseas doesn't have to mean that he has an overseas-acquired or exotic illness. This might still end up being community-acquired pneumonia, infectious mononucleosis (although the absence of lymphadenopathy is surprising), *Staphylococcus aureus* sepsis, bacterial endocarditis, etc.

a stepladder rise in fever, one study found that a coated tongue had a specificity of 94% for enteric fever (Haq *et al.*, 1997).

3. **Transient truncal rash**—these sound like 'rose spots'. These are red-pink spots, 2–4 mm in diameter, which are usually found on the chest and abdomen in enteric fever. Its usefulness as a diagnostic sign is limited by its transient appearance and the difficulty of finding them on people with darker skin. For these reasons, it is only recognised in less than 30% of cases of enteric fever (Parry *et al.*, 2002; Thisyakorn *et al.*, 1987; Klotz *et al.*, 1984).

4. **Constipation**—due to the association of various *Salmonella* species with acute diarrhoeal illnesses, many health care workers assume that patients with enteric fever will also have loose bowel motions. This is a common misconception, since many patients with enteric fever become constipated (30% in one study [Tran *et al.*, 1995]); however, diarrhoea can occur and is more common in young children and in HIV-positive individuals with typhoid fever (Parry *et al.*, 2002).

5. **Myalgias, dry cough and headache**—these are non-specific but common symptoms in enteric fever (Basnyat *et al.*, 2005). One study found that they occurred around 20%, 33% and 70% respectively in patients with enteric fever (Tran *et al.*, 1995).

6. **Relative bradycardia**—normally, people mount an increasing heart rate in response to a fever. This association may be confounded by other factors, for example medications to slow the heart rate. But certain infections are associated with an inappropriately low heart rate in the presence of a fever. Both enteric fever and dengue are causes of relative bradycardia (Senanayake, 2006; Basnyat *et al.*, 2005).

7. **Splenomegaly**—this is common in enteric fever but alone is a non-specific sign as it is found in many of the differential diagnoses, including dengue and malaria.

8. **Leukopenia and abnormal liver function tests**—these are common laboratory features of typhoid fever. The full blood count tends to be normal or reduced (anaemia, leukopenia, thrombocytopenia) and hepatic enzymes are elevated usually no more than 2–3 times above baseline levels (Parry *et al.*, 2002). In children, though, leukocytosis is not uncommon (Bhutta, 2006).

Q: Apart from the basic blood tests (FBC, EUC LFT) that have been ordered so far, what specific tests will you order to determine the cause of the fevers?

A: A reasonable approach would be to order the following:
1. **Thick and thin blood films for malaria.** To feel fairly confident of excluding malaria, you should have 3 negative films, each about 8–12 hours apart. The first film is positive in the vast majority of cases of malaria.
2. **Rapid dipstick tests for malaria.** Most labs will do this test automatically if malaria films have been ordered; however, just in case, you should specifically ask for it. Similar to testing urine with a urinalysis strip, blood can be tested with these dipsticks. There are 2 kinds (Fairhurst and Wellems, 2005):
   a. Histidine-rich protein-2 (HRP-2)—very sensitive for *Plasmodium falciparum* but can't identify the other species of malaria, such as *P. vivax, P. ovale, P. malariae* and *P. knowlesi*.
   b. Plasmodium lactate dehydrogenase (pLDH)—this has the advantage over the HRP-2 dipstick in that it can detect other plasmodial species in addition to *P. falciparum*.
3. Glucose-6-phosphate dehydrogenase (G6PDH) level on blood (for malaria but this is discussed later).
4. **Dengue viral antigen (e.g. NS1) of blood.** Antigen tests such as NS1 are often more accessible than polymerase chain reaction (PCR) testing of blood. NS1 assays are over 90% sensitive in primary dengue illnesses during the febrile phase (Heilman *et al.*, 2014).
5. **Dengue polymerase chain reaction (PCR) of blood.** In the early part of dengue, patients are viraemic and the PCR will identify the viraemia. The difficulties here are that the viraemia wouldn't be as pronounced now (Indiana is in day 3 of his illness) as in the first 2 days of the illness, leading to a negative result. Also, this isn't a readily available test; therefore, it may have to be sent interstate for testing, meaning that it may be days before you get a result (Senanayake, 2006).
6. **Dengue IgM.** Dengue serology can be quite confusing, especially if this is not the patient's first dengue illness (there are 4 dengue serotypes and illness with one doesn't protect from the others. In fact, repeat dengue infections are often worse than the preceding infection and are a risk factor for developing dengue haemorrhagic fever). But assuming that this is Indiana's first dengue infection, a dengue IgM is a very sensitive test; however, it is reliably positive at day 5 of illness and Indiana is in day 3 of his illness so he may still not have developed detectable IgM to dengue (Senanayake, 2006).

7. **Two sets of blood cultures from different sites** (ideally before antibiotics are given). Blood cultures have a 60–80% sensitivity of identifying the *Salmonella* species responsible for causing enteric fever (Basnyat *et al.*, 2005; Parry *et al.*, 2002). Furthermore, they will identify other bacterial causes of infection.

8. **Influenza tests.** Ideally this would involve a nasal flocked swab (swab with lots of little knobs on top to pick up more viral particles) which then undergoes a rapid immunochromatographic test +/− influenza PCR. It will often detect a number of different respiratory viruses.

9. **Tests to identify sexually transmitted infections.** You wouldn't always ask for these tests unless the clinical picture was suspicious for a sexually transmitted infection or you identified risk factors in the history. Certainly, Indiana warrants these tests due to his unprotected sexual encounters.

   - HIV antigen-antibody test
   - syphilis serology
   - early morning urine PCR for gonococcus and *Chlamydia trachomatis*
   - hepatitis B and C serology (hepatitis B infection is unlikely if he was vaccinated properly. Also, these tests will have to be repeated for some months as it may be too early for them to become positive).

10. **Amoebic serology.**

11. **Plain chest X-ray (for community-acquired pneumonia).**

12. **Midstream urine.**

13. **ESR and C-reactive protein.**

14. **Consider an abdominal ultrasound to exclude an amoebic liver abscess.**

Q: Byron helps you organise these tests. He also asks you about stool cultures to help diagnose enteric fever. What do you think?

A: Byron is certainly correct in that stool cultures can be used to diagnose enteric fever; however, the sensitivity is low (25%) and the organism usually isn't found in the stool till after the first week of illness and Indiana is only in day 3 of his infection (Basnyat *et al.*, 2005; Parry *et al.*, 2002). If you are ordering stool cultures, you should order 1 stool specimen/day for 3 days to optimise the sensitivity of the test. On the request form, write 'stool M/C/S O/C/P'. The O/C/P is to look for ova, cysts and parasites which the lab won't look for unless you specifically request it.

Just out of interest, the most sensitive test for diagnosing enteric fever is a bone marrow biopsy (80–95% even with prior antibiotic use) (Basnyat *et al.*, 2005; Parry *et al.*, 2002); however, this invasive investigation is not commonly used in the initial work-up for a returned traveller with fever.

Q: The first malaria results return a couple of hours later. Both the HRP-2 dipstick test and examination of the blood films were negative. Malaria is still a possibility and you will need to order a second blood film in about 8 hours; however, you are more confident of your diagnosis of enteric fever. You decide to commence empirical antibiotic therapy for enteric fever.

What should you begin?

A: A reasonable choice for empirical treatment of enteric fever in an adult would be oral azithromycin 1 g daily for 5 days or IV ceftriaxone 2 g daily. Due to high rates of fluoroquinolone resistance in many parts of the world, ciprofloxacin shouldn't be used empirically (Antibiotic Expert Group, 2014; Senanayake, 2007). The infectious diseases registrar reviews the patient and commences oral azithromycin.

And note ...

If you were uncertain about your diagnosis at this stage and the patient was very unwell, then it may not be unreasonable to add broader antibiotic cover to the azithromycin to cover more common causes of sepsis such as *Staphylococcus aureus* or other Gram-negative bacteria. But this should first be discussed with a more senior colleague.

Q: 'What about antibiotics for dengue?' asks Byron.

What do you think?

A: There is no specific antiviral therapy for dengue. The management is supportive.

Q: If the malaria tests had confirmed a diagnosis of malaria, in broad terms how would you have treated the patient?

A: The intricacies of antimalarial therapy are beyond the scope of this section; however, in broad terms, all malaria patients will need medications to clear the parasitaemia. But *P. vivax* and *P. ovale* have a latent phase in the liver (hypnozoites). Thus, patients infected by *P. vivax* and *P. ovale* need to have a medication to specifically clear the parasites from the liver, in addition to the agent to clear the parasitaemia, otherwise the organism will lie latent in the liver and lead to a relapse at a later date. The medication used to treat the liver forms is primaquine.

It can cause haemolytic anaemia in people with G6PDH deficiency; therefore, G6PDH activity should be assessed on blood tests prior to using primaquine.

Q: After 12 hours, Indiana's blood cultures flag positive. A Gram stain shows Gram-negative bacilli which are subsequently identified as *S. enterica* serotype Typhi. Your diagnosis of enteric fever was correct. Indiana is still having fevers (which isn't surprising this early into treatment) but overall he is feeling better. Does anyone else need to be informed of your diagnosis of enteric fever?

A: Yes. Enteric fever is a notifiable infection, therefore the Public Health Unit needs to be informed. This will have particular implications for Indiana if he is a food handler, for example waiter, cook, food factory worker or Masterchef contestant because of the faeco-oral transmission. Incidentally, malaria and dengue are notifiable infections too in Australia.

Scenario

Over the next few days, Indiana dramatically improves and is ready for discharge. His urinary PCR for chlamydia infection is positive but the azithromycin for his enteric fever will also treat the chlamydia. The remainder of his sexually transmitted infection screen is thankfully negative. He will continue to have hepatitis B and C and HIV serology for some time to come which his GP will arrange.

Achievements

You now:
- know the importance of taking a detailed history in a febrile traveller
- know always to consider the triad of malaria, dengue and enteric fever in a traveller with fevers
- know some of the key clinical features of enteric fever
- can order appropriate investigations for the febrile traveller
- know that typhoid vaccination and malaria prophylaxis aren't a guarantee of immunity from these infections
- broadly understand the treatment for malaria, dengue and enteric fever.

References

Antibiotic Expert Group (2014), *Therapeutic Guidelines: Antibiotic*, Version 15, Therapeutic Guidelines Ltd, Melbourne.

Bal, S.K. and Czarnowski, C. (2004), 'A man with fever, cough, diarrhea and a coated tongue', *Canadian Medical Association Journal*, vol. 170, no. 7, p. 1095.

Basnyat, B., Maskey, A.P., Zimmerman, M.D. and Murdoch, D.R. (2005), 'Enteric (typhoid) fever in travelers', *Clinical Infectious Diseases*, vol. 41, no. 10, pp. 1467–1472.

Bhutta, Z.A. (2006), 'Current concepts in the diagnosis and treatment of typhoid fever', *British Medical Journal*, vol. 333, no. 7558, pp. 78–82.

Fairhurst, R.M. and Wellems, T.E. (2005), 'Plasmodium species (malaria)', in G. L. Mandell, J.E. Bennett and R. Dolin (eds), *Principles and Practice of Infectious Diseases*, Philadelphia, Churchill Livingstone, pp. 3121–3144.

Haq, S.A., Alam, M.N., Hossain, S.M., Ahmed, T. and Tahir, M. (1997), 'Value of clinical features in the diagnosis of enteric fever', *Bangladesh Medical Research Council Bulletin*, vol. 23, no. 2, pp. 42–46.

Heilman, J.M., Wolff, J.D., Beards, G.M. and Basden, B.J. (2014), 'Dengue fever: A Wikipedia clinical review', *Open Medicine*, vol. 8, no. 4, e105–e115.

Klotz, S.A., Jorgensen, J.H., Buckwold, F.J. and Craven, P.C. (1984), 'Typhoid fever: An epidemic with remarkably few clinical signs and symptoms', *Archives of Internal Medicine*, vol. 144, no. 3, pp. 533–537.

Matteelli, A. and Carosi, G. (2001), 'Sexually transmitted diseases in travelers', *Clinical Infectious Diseases*, vol. 32, no. 7, pp. 1063–1067.

Parry, C.M., Hien, T.T., Dougan, G., White, N.J. and Farrar, J.J. (2002), 'Typhoid fever', *New England Journal of Medicine*, vol. 347, no. 22, pp. 1770–1782.

Senanayake, S.N. (2006), 'Dengue fever and dengue haemorrhagic fever—a diagnostic challenge', *Australian Family Physician*, vol. 35, no. 8, pp. 609–612.

Senanayake, S.N. (2007). 'Case 7: Enteric fever', in *Clinical Cases in Infectious Diseases: A Public Health Approach*, McGraw-Hill, Sydney, pp. 105–129.

Thisyakorn, U., Mansuwan, P. and Taylor, D.N. (1987), 'Typhoid and paratyphoid fever in 192 hospitalized children in Thailand', *American Journal of Diseases of Children*, vol. 141, no. 8, pp. 862–865.

Tran, T.H., Bethell, D.B., Nguyen, T.T. *et al.* (1995), 'Short course of ofloxacin for treatment of multidrug-resistant typhoid', *Clinical Infectious Diseases*, vol. 20, no. 4, pp. 917–923.

Chapter 38
A red leg in a very sick person

Scenario

You are one of the interns experiencing a busy winter evening in the Emergency Department. Luckily, there are some eager medical students around willing to 'scout ahead' and see some patients. Ellie is one of the students who has just seen someone for you. Though very proactive, you have noticed that she can be a touch overconfident. She comes back with her report.

'I've just seen a 58-year-old woman with cellulitis of the leg. I just wanted to check that the usual causes are group A strep and *Staph aureus*.'

Q: Is Ellie correct?

A: Yes. In the vast majority of cases of cellulitis of the leg, group A streptococcus (*Streptococcus pyogenes*) and *Staphylococcus aureus* are the commonest causes. 'Oh good,' she says. 'And isn't the usual antibiotic IV flucloxacillin?'

Q: Is that true?

A: Yes, for cellulitis requiring IV therapy where group A streptococcus or *S. aureus* (non-MRSA) are the likely pathogens, the following would be reasonable (eTG, 2013):

1. IV flucloxacillin 2 g q6h OR
2. IV cephazolin 2 g q8h (if hypersensitive to penicillin, excluding immediate hypersensitivity) OR
3. PO clindamycin 450 mg tds (if immediate hypersensitivity to penicillin) (due to its excellent oral bioavailability, clindamycin can be given orally).

'Great!' says Ellie. 'I'll go and get that organised. By the way, what's the dose for noradrenaline?'

Your ears prick up at that last remark as you ask Ellie to describe the case in more detail. Your suspicions that she had failed to mention 1 or 2 relevant details turn out to be true.

Scenario

The patient is a 58-year-old diabetic woman named Maria. She cut herself against a table 5 days earlier, causing a small laceration on her lower left leg. She thought nothing of it and went for a dip in the lake on the following day (despite the winter, she is an ardent swimmer). Everything was fine until yesterday when the leg became red and painful. She describes overnight sweats and rigors. Today, her husband found her to be lethargic and very unwell so he called an ambulance to bring her to hospital.

On examination, Maria is sick. She is awake and oriented but is very restless and clearly in a lot of pain. She has a high fever, is tachypnoeic, tachycardic and her BP is 85/60. Her whole body looks flushed. The lower half of her left leg is erythematous, hot, swollen and tender with indistinct margins. The area proximal to the cellulitis is also tender. A small superficial dry laceration is visible just above the lateral malleolus. Above the laceration are 2 large, tense bullae. She has no lymphangitis and no inguinal lymphadenitis. The remainder of the examination is normal.

Her blood test show a neutrophilia, an elevated CRP, deranged liver functions tests, acute kidney injury and thrombocytopenia.

Q: You tell Ellie that she should have mentioned how sick the patient was. She apologises but still says that a group A streptococcal or staphylococcal infection is most likely even though Maria is so sick. Is she right?

A: While it is certainly possible for a group A streptococcal or *S. aureus* infection to cause severe cellulitis, it is important to look at the history. Maria stated that 1 day after suffering the laceration, she went swimming in the lake. This raises the possibility of other organisms found in the water. Such organisms will often need different antibiotics to the standard flucloxacillin.

Q: 'What bacteria from water can cause cellulitis?'
A: There is a variety (Diaz, 2014):
   1. Gram-negative rods (*Aeromonas hydrophila, Chromobacterium violaceum, Edwardsiella tarda, Shewanella, Vibrio vulnificus*)
   2. Gram-positive cocci (*Streptococcus iniae*)
   3. Gram-positive bacilli (*Erysipelothrix rhusiopathiae*)
   4. *Mycobacterium marinum.*

Q: Ellie says, 'I've seen quite a few cases of leg cellulitis, especially in my general practice rotation. But they've never been this sick. What's going on?'

A: You tell Ellie that a *systemic* process and a *local* process may be the problem here. You are concerned that the local process may be necrotising fasciitis.

'No way! But what makes you think of necrotising fasciitis? Isn't that really rare?'

Necrotising fasciitis is uncommon. Only around 500 cases occur annually in the UK (Sultan *et al.*, 2012) and between 500 and 1000 in the USA. Ellie's question is valid as it is a difficult condition to diagnose (Lancerotto *et al.*, 2012).

The features of Maria's presentation that suggest necrotising fasciitis are (Wang *et al.*, 2007):

- pain out of proportion to the physical signs (this is because the fascial inflammation and necrosis is deep and not visible: only the cutaneous changes are apparent)
- the presence of bullae (about 40% present on day 0 and 77% by day 4)
- the indistinct cutaneous margins of inflammation
- the presence of tenderness beyond the margins of the cellulitis in the more proximal leg
- the absence of lymphangitis (since the inflammatory process is in the deep fascia).

Q: 'But shouldn't she have crepitus and the skin be anaesthetic?'

A: While very helpful in diagnosing necrotising fasciitis, signs such as crepitus, necrosis and skin anaesthesia are late signs. If present, these signs suggest Stage 3 disease with a mortality of almost 50% (Wang *et al.*, 2007)

Q: Ellie looks stumped. 'But isn't there a test to confirm the diagnosis?'

A: There are unfortunately no easy roads to diagnosing necrotising fasciitis. With regard to blood tests, there may be a raised creatine kinase, leukocytosis, hypoalbuminaemia, hyponatraemia, all of which are fairly nonspecific (Lancerotto *et al.*, 2012).

Interestingly, a group devised a scoring system based on laboratory tests to try to identify necrotising fasciitis: CRP, white cell count, haemoglobin, sodium, creatinine and glucose. While it provided great sensitivity and specificity in a Singaporean population (93% and 92% respectively), it was less specific in other populations (74% and 81% respectively) (Sultan *et al.*, 2012). Also, the investigators did not regard an intermediate score (6–7) or even a high score (≥8) as sufficient to make a definitive diagnosis of necrotising fasciitis but rather an indication to perform further investigations to confirm the diagnosis.

Q: 'What about radiology?' asks Ellie. 'An X-ray with gas in the soft tissue will confirm it, surely?'

A: Once again, imaging is limited in its capacity to confirm a diagnosis of necrotising fasciitis. There are pros and cons to each modality (see table on the role of imaging in diagnosing necrotising fasciitis below):

	Features	Comment
X-ray	Soft tissue gas	Low sensitivity and specificity
CT	Soft tissue gas Fascial swelling, inflammation	Better than X-ray
Ultrasound	Superficial abscesses	Low sensitivity and specificity
MRI	High intensity signal on T2-weighted images at deep fascia and in muscles	Best investigation but not perfect and difficult to get at short notice

Source: Adapted from Lancerotto *et al.*, 2012; Sultan *et al.*, 2012

Q: A mobile X-ray is performed, which is unremarkable. Ellie asks, 'Is there anything else we can do?'

A: There are bedside tests but these aren't commonly done. They include the 'finger test', where a 2 cm incision is made down to deep fascia to look for a lack of bleeding, lack of resistance to blunt finger dissection and the presence of dishwater pus. While there, a frozen section, culture and Gram stain can be performed. A noninvasive test with a 100% sensitivity and 97% specificity is near-infrared spectroscopy to identify the presence of low tissue oxygen saturation (at a cut-off of <70%).

Q: Ellie asks, 'So then: what do we do?'

A: Given the seriousness of the condition, even suspected necrotising fasciitis should be referred urgently to the surgeons. Surgery is not only the mainstay of therapy but will also confirm the diagnosis.

Q: Ellie asks, 'It's an infection, so aren't antibiotics more important than surgery?'

A: In necrotising fasciitis, antibiotics do have a role, but surgery is the most important intervention. Delayed surgical debridement is associated with an increased mortality. The surgery involves extensive debridement of all infected tissues, with patients often needing multiple operations (Lancerotto *et al.*, 2012; Shimizu and Tokuda, 2010).

But antibiotics serve as an important adjunct to surgery. As the microbiological cause is uncertain, it is reasonable to commence meropenem IV 1 g q8h (adjust for abnormal renal function) and clindamycin IV 600 mg q8h and vancomycin IV (loading dose 25–30 mg/kg and then 15–20 mg/kg q12h) (Antibiotic Expert Group, 2014).

Q: You suspect that group A streptococcus is the causative agent, but you can't be 100% sure, especially given Maria's history of water exposure; therefore, you commence her on IV meropenem 1 g q12h (renally adjusted) and IV clindamycin 600 mg q8h. The surgical registrar, Earl, reviews the patient and agrees that necrotising fasciitis is very likely. But Earl is puzzled by one thing: 'Why is her whole body red?'

A: Early on, you told Ellie that Maria was suffering from two processes: a systemic one and a local one. The local one is necrotising fasciitis. You suspect that the systemic process is toxic shock syndrome (TSS) due to group A streptococcus (*Streptococcus pyogenes* or GAS). TSS occurs when bacterial proteins called superantigens generate a massive immune response that is deleterious to the host.

TSS is usually due to *S. aureus* or GAS. Staphylococcal TSS was first associated with tampon carriage in young women in the 1980s as *S. aureus* colonises the vagina in about 5% of women. But nonmenstrual cases due to *S. aureus* infections elsewhere can also lead to TSS (Lappin and Ferguson, 2009).

Streptococcal TSS was first reported in 1987. It is more common in people with chronic conditions, in people after varicella infections and with the use of non-steroidal anti-inflammatory drug. The risk of streptococcal TSS is 13% with any streptococcal infection; therefore, it is not surprising to see it in Maria with necrotising fasciitis. TSS is a dangerous condition with a 7-day mortality of 44% with TSS due to GAS having a higher mortality than TSS due to *S. aureus* (Lappin and Ferguson, 2009).

Q: 'So is the rash part of TSS?'

Both staphylococcal and streptococcal TSS are associated with a diffuse macular, erythematous rash that gives a flushed appearance and will often desquamate days later. They also cause hypotension and can lead to multi-organ impairment, as evidenced by abnormal blood tests or clinical features (Lappin and Ferguson, 2009).

A: Maria has probable necrotising fasciitis, is hypotensive with erythroderma, acute kidney injury and abnormal liver function; therefore, TSS from GAS is likely.

Q: Ellie wants to know if you should change the antibiotics.

A: No. The combination you have chosen for Maria (meropenem and clindamycin) is fine. But make sure that two sets of blood cultures have been taken from two different sites before starting antibiotics. This is because 60% of patients with GAS TSS will be bacteraemic, which will aid in narrowing down the microbiological diagnosis. In addition, in TSS, clindamycin is used due to its inhibitory effect on superantigens and its ability to deal with a large inoculum of bacteria in a stationary growth phase (Lappin and Ferguson, 2009).

Scenario

Q: Maria's family arrive just as she is about to be wheeled to the operating theatre for urgent surgery. They have heard about necrotising fasciitis in the media as the 'flesh-eating bacteria' and can't understand how she could have got it. What do you tell them?

A: Maria is diabetic, which is a risk factor for necrotising fasciitis. Other risk factors for necrotising fasciitis include (Lancerotto *et al.*, 2012; Sultan *et al.*, 2012):

- chronic hepatitis
- malignancy
- immunosuppression
- end-stage renal failure
- pulmonary disease
- blunt trauma
- injecting drug use
- sepsis
- varicella (in children, although necrotising fasciitis is rare in childhood)
- surgical procedure or puncture.

Even if Maria wasn't diabetic, about 25% of cases of necrotising fasciitis occur in people without any risk factors.

Q: Maria's family asks, 'But with antibiotics and the surgery, she'll definitely be fine, won't she?'

A: Unfortunately, that is an outcome you can't guarantee. Necrotising fasciitis alone has a mortality of 25%, but in patients with TSS as well as necrotising fasciitis, the mortality rate is closer to 70% (Shimizu and Tokuda, 2010).

Scenario

Maria undergoes surgery, which confirms a diagnosis of necrotising fasciitis. An extensive debridement is performed and intraoperative cultures are taken. Maria is brought to the intensitve care unit postoperatively. You go to ICU to follow up the case and listen to a discussion between the intensivist and the infectious diseases physician. The intensivist asks the infectious diseases physician about using intravenous immunoglobulin (IVIG) for Maria's TSS.

Q: Why would she ask this?

A: Although studies haven't definitively shown a benefit from IVIG in TSS, many have suggested it. It is reasonable to give IVIG very early in the course of managing TSS (Lappin and Ferguson, 2009).

Q: The infectious diseases physician advises giving 2 doses of IVIG. Then the issue of hyperbaric oxygen comes up for Maria's necrotising fasciitis. Is it useful?

A: While studies show that postsurgical hyperbaric oxygen therapy increases oxygen tension levels in subcutaneous tissue in necrotising fasciitis, there's no definitive clinical data confirming its role in necrotising fasciitis (Lancerotto *et al.*, 2012). The micro registrar, who is also present, provides everyone with the news that Maria's blood cultures have grown group A streptococcus. This confirms the diagnosis of GAS TSS and necrotising fasciitis. As you leave the intensive care unit, you see the surgeons returning to assess Maria for further surgery. Maria has a long, uncertain road ahead. You wish her well as you return to the Emergency Department.

Achievements

You now:
- know the organisms commonly associated with cellulitis
- can empirically treat cellulitis due to group A streptococcus and *Staphylococcus aureus* (non-MRSA)
- are aware that water exposure means that different pathogens may be responsible for cellulitis
- know the difficulties in diagnosing necrotising fasciitis
- know that surgery is the mainstay of treatment for necrotising fasciitis
- know how to diagnose and treat toxic shock syndrome.

References

Antibiotic Expert Group (2014), *Therapeutic Guidelines: Antibiotic*, Version 15, Therapeutic Guidelines Ltd, Melbourne.

Diaz, J.H. (2014), 'Skin and soft tissue infections following marine injuries and exposures in travelers', *Journal of Travel Medicine*, vol. 21, no 3, pp. 207–213.

Lancerotto, L., Tocco, I., Salmaso, R., Vindigni, V. and Bassetto, F. (2012), 'Necrotizing fasciitis: Classification, diagnosis, and management', *Journal of Trauma and Acute Care Surgery*, vol. 72, no. 3, pp. 560–566.

Lappin, E. and Ferguson, A.J. (2009), 'Gram-positive toxic shock syndrome', *Lancet Infectious Diseases*, vol. 9, no. 5, pp. 281–290.

Shmizu, T. and Tokuda, Y. (2010), 'Necrotizing fasciitis', *Internal Medicine*, vol. 49, no. 12, pp. 1051–1057.

Sultan, H.Y., Boyle, A.A. and Sheppard, N. (2012), 'Necrotising fasciitis', *British Medical Journal*, vol. 345, e4274.

Wang, Y.S., Wong, C.H. and Tay, Y.K. (2007), 'Staging of necrotizing fasciitis based on the evolving cutaneous features', *International Journal of Dermatology*, vol. 46, no. 10, pp. 1036–1041.

Wong, C.H., Khin, L.W., Heng, K.S., Tan, K.C. and Low, C.O. (2004), 'The LRINEC (Laboratory Risk Indicator for Necrotizing Fasciitis) score: A tool for distinguishing necrotizing fasciitis from other soft tissue infections', *Critical Care Medicine*, vol. 32, no. 7, pp. 1535–1541.

Chapter 39
Peter collapses at a wedding

Scenario

It is a sublime summery Saturday that provides the opportunity for a number of outdoor activities. Unfortunately, you are working in the Emergency Department today. With a wistful gaze out of the window, you click on the next patient to be seen. You are being shadowed by Reshmi, a final-year medical student.

You and Reshmi read the triage nurse's summary. Peter Walsh is a 49-year-old man who is normally healthy. His only medication is metoprolol for hypertension. Mr Walsh is here today because he collapsed. A blood sugar taken by the paramedics was 6.3 mmol/L.

'Collapse,' says Reshmi. 'Must be syncope.'

Is Reshmi right?

A: She could be. But syncope is only one possible cause of collapse. Syncope has a very specific definition (Jamalyan and Khachatryan, 2010): **a transient loss of consciousness with rapid onset, short duration and spontaneous full recovery that is due to transient global hypoperfusion.**

Therefore, if someone collapses without losing consciousness, it is not syncope.

Q: Reshmi absorbs the definition that you told her. 'Transient global hypoperfusion? How do you diagnose that at the bedside?'

A: It's a good point—you can't. You will have to rely on the clinical features within the definition to assist you (i.e. rapid onset, short duration and spontaneous, full recovery).

Q: You go to see Mr Walsh. He is awake, lying in bed and attached to a monitor. His concerned wife is with him. What are your objectives with the history and examination in a patient with a collapse?

A: You need to establish:

- Did he actually lose consciousness?
- If this is syncope, what is the cause?

Q: You ascertain from Mrs Walsh that there was a definite loss of consciousness for about 10 seconds before he awoke. He had a few twitches in his hands for a couple of seconds. After about 3–5 minutes, he seemed fine. Mr Walsh recalls feeling some nausea and being a bit sweaty just before he blacked out, but nothing else. The back of his head is sore from the fall. Reshmi picks up on one part of the history. 'Twitches? It sounds like syncope. And clearly, epilepsy is the cause of the syncopal episode.' Is Reshmi right about the syncope being due to epilepsy?

A: Partly. Let's dissect Reshmi's response. First of all, Mr Walsh definitely lost consciousness. Although this would support a diagnosis of syncope, it is important to realise that there are a few causes of a nontraumatic loss of consciousness, namely (Jamalyan and Khachatryan, 2010; Sutton *et al.*, 2010):

- syncope (transient global hypoperfusion)
- epilepsy
- factitious
- rare causes (complex migraine, subclavian steal syndrome, transient ischaemic attack).

So, the first thing to realise from this list is that epilepsy is *not* a form of syncope, even though it can lead to a transient loss of consciousness.

Does the history of Mr Walsh's loss of consciousness fit with syncope? Yes—it was rapid onset, of short duration and he had a spontaneous full recovery.

Q: But what about the twitches? Doesn't that imply epilepsy?

A: This can be difficult to distinguish. Around 5–15% of patients with supposed syncopal episodes end up being diagnosed with seizures (Jamalyan and Khachatryan, 2010). But the presence of twitches alone does not mean that Mr Walsh had a seizure.

Some features that distinguish seizures from syncope include (Hanna, 2014; TDMS *et al.*, 2009):

- an aura prior to the seizure (e.g. odd smells) (seizures)
- tongue-biting (seizures)
- lip-smacking and other automatisms (seizures)
- blue face (seizures)
- confusion for a prolonged period after waking up (seizures)
- tonic–clonic movements that are limited and last under 15 seconds (syncope)
- urinary incontinence (unhelpful as can occur with both syncope and seizures).

Q: Given all of the above information, you feel that it is more likely that Mr Walsh's transient loss of consciousness was due to syncope. It is now your task to try to determine the cause of the syncope. What are the common causes of syncope?

A: There are three broad groups of syncope (Hanna, 2014):
- neurally mediated 60–70% (vasovagal, situational, post-exertional, carotid sinus hypersensitivity)
- cardiac 10–20%
- orthostatic 10%.

Q: How will the history help you determine the cause of syncope?

A: There are certain aspects of the history that will be very useful (Jamalyan and Khachatryan, 2010):

1. **Posture**
   - Syncope with prolonged standing (reflex syncope [e.g. vasovagal] more likely)
   - Syncope while changing positions (e.g. sitting to standing) (orthostatic hypotension more likely)
   - Syncope while seated or lying down (cardiac arrhythmia more likely)

2. **Onset**
   - Syncope associated with exertion (cardiac arrhythmia, cardiac outflow obstruction or postexertional syncope*)
   - Syncope with preceding nausea, lightheadedness, visual changes, sweating, dizziness (reflex syncope more likely)
   - Syncope associated with chest pain, shortness of breath, palpitations (cardiac cause more likely)
   - Syncope with no warning or preceding symptoms (arrhythmia more likely)
   - Syncope associated with certain situations (e.g. cough, micturition) (neurally mediated situational syncope highly likely)
   - Syncope following stimulation of the carotid sinuses (e.g. shaving, wearing a tight collar, extending or rotating the head) (carotid sinus syncope)

---

*Postexertional syncope is a form of vasovagal syncope that occurs on cessation of exercise due to a combination of reduced venous return from peripheral muscle contraction and the relatively empty heart still hypercontracting due to the exercise-related release of catecholamines. This leads to a vagal reflex with vasodilatation and reflex bradycardia (Hanna, 2014).

3. Medications

Up to 15% of medications contribute to syncope, typically through orthostatic hypotension or arrhythmias. The usual suspects include the 'blockers' (calcium, alpha, beta), antiarrhythmics, tricyclic antidepressants and diuretics. Pay close attention to the recent introduction of a medication or a recent change in dose.

4. Comorbidities

The presence of cardiac disease, previous syncopal episodes, a heavy menstrual cycle (not in Mr Walsh) and diabetes (a cause of orthostatic hypotension through autonomic neuropathy) are some medical problems that need to be ascertained.

5. Family history

A history of family members who suffered from sudden deaths, early cardiac deaths, or had cardiomyopathies may be very important if the cause of the syncope is unclear or thought to be cardiac in origin. Interestingly, a large proportion of children with syncope secondary to orthostatic hypotension or reflex syncope have a strong family history of these conditions.

Q: Mr Walsh tells you that he arrived at the wedding feeling fine. Prior to fainting, he had been standing with the other wedding guests for at least 15 minutes. He recalls feeling a bit sweaty and nauseous just before he blacked out. There is no family history of note. He has been taking metoprolol for hypertension for 3 years and the dose hasn't been changed for at least 18 months. What is the most likely diagnosis at this time?

A: The syncopal episode occurred following prolonged standing and was preceded by nausea and sweating. A vasovagal episode seems most likely.

Q: You begin to examine Mr Walsh. What are the important parts of the examination?

A: Mr Walsh should undergo a standard physical examination, in particular looking for any evidence of heart disease (e.g. murmurs, extra heart sounds, peripheral signs of heart failure). In addition, his postural blood pressure should be checked.

Q: How do you test for orthostatic hypotension?

A: Normally, on standing, almost a third of the blood volume pools in the lower limbs and pelvis, leading to reduced venous return and stroke volume. The cardiovascular system eventually compensates in a number of ways, including an increase in vascular resistance and a 10–15 beat/minute increase in heart rate while still maintaining the blood pressure. When these mechanisms fail, orthostatic hypotension occurs.

Orthostatic hypotension is defined as having a drop in blood pressure (systolic $\geq$ 20 mm Hg or diastolic $\geq$ 10 mm Hg) between 30 seconds and 5 minutes of taking an upright posture. The blood pressure should be checked on standing at 0, 3 and 5 minutes (Hanna, 2014).

The presence of orthostatic hypotension in someone with a syncopal episode must be taken extremely seriously. One study found, however, that orthostatic hypotension in people aged $\geq$ 75 was quite common (55%) and only caused symptoms in 33% (Poon and Braun, 2005).

Q: Mr Walsh's blood pressure on lying down is 110/60 and on standing at 3 and 5 minutes is 115/65. His heart rate is regular at 65 beats/minute and there are no murmurs, extra heart sounds or signs of heart failure. He has a tender haematoma over his occiput where he fell.

Are there any other bedside tests that should be performed for syncope?

A: A simple but important investigation is a 12-lead ECG. This can identify a variety of abnormalities relevant to a syncopal episode (e.g. nonsinus rhythm, bradycardia < 50 beats/minute, signs of injured myocardium, prolonged QT intervals, signs of left ventricular hypertrophy and strain, T wave changes consistent with arrhythmogenic right ventricular cardiomyopathy (Jamalyan and Khachatryan, 2010).

Q: Would any further tests be of use?

A: A noncontrast brain CT may be reasonable, not so much for the cause of the syncope, but rather to ensure that the heavy knock to Mr Walsh's occiput didn't lead to any fractures or haemorrhage.

Basic blood tests (full blood count, electrolytes, pregnancy test in a woman of childbearing age, drug screen in certain patients) are easy to perform and may identify a precipitant for the syncope (e.g. electrolyte abnormality leading to an arrhythmia or anaemia), but they are often not helpful in the setting of syncope (Jamalyan and Khachatryan, 2010).

Q: The CT brain comes back as normal, as do the blood tests. You are confident on the basis of all the evidence that Mr Walsh suffered from a vasovagal episode due to prolonged standing on a hot day during the wedding ceremony.

What is vasovagal syncope?

A: Vasovagal syncope occurs when an aroused sympathetic nervous system leads to a hypercontractile heart with a reduced ventricular activity. This results in a vagal response with reflex bradycardia and vasodilatation. Triggers for this include emotional stress, prolonged standing, dehydration and heat (Hanna, 2014).

Q: Reshmi asks, 'Shouldn't he undergo tilt-table testing and carotid sinus massage before we clear him?' Are these tests necessary?

A: **Tilt-table testing** was first used to determine the cause of unexplained syncope. It can simulate the conditions that result in reflex syncope (e.g. vasovagal syncope). The typical indication for tilt testing is to confirm reflex syncope when the initial evaluation leaves the diagnosis unclear (TDMS *et al.*, 2009). In Mr Walsh's case, this is only his first episode of syncope. Also, the history, examination and the normal 12-lead ECG are consistent with vasovagal syncope; therefore, he does not need further evaluation. A tilt-table test involves strapping a patient to a table that is moved into the vertical position for up to 45 minutes. In order to accentuate the conditions, IV isoproterenol or sublingual nitroglycerin can be given. The blood pressure is usually continuously monitored. Contraindications to the test include severe carotid and coronary artery disease as well as recent strokes or myocardial infarctions (Hanna, 2014).

    Carotid sinus massage is usually performed in people > 40 years with syncope of unknown origin despite an initial evaluation. Therefore, Mr Walsh does not need it. It is contraindicated in those with a history of transient ischaemic attacks or stroke or myocardial infarction within the last 3 months or in those with carotid bruits (unless dopplers exclude significant stenoses). Each carotid sinus (found just below the angle of the mandible) is consecutively massaged for 10 seconds in supine and erect positions, with the latter position being the most sensitive. A positive response occurs when CSM leads to syncope in the presence of a fall in the systolic blood pressure >50 mm Hg and/or asystole >3 seconds. A positive test may be indicative of sinoatrial or atrioventricular nodal disease (Hanna, 2014; TDMS *et al.*, 2009).

Q: If you had been concerned about an arrhythmia in someone with unexplained syncope after initial evaluation, what are some common types of monitoring that can be used?

A: They include (TDMS *et al.*, 2009):
- Holter monitoring (often for 24–48 hours): only 1–2% yield but may be useful if an arrhythmia is not documented during a symptomatic episode
- external loop recorders: these can be worn for some weeks
- implantable loop recorders: these are implanted subcutaneously for almost 2 years.

Q: You reassure Mr Walsh that his syncope was due to a vasovagal with clear triggers. He is happy about this. 'My friend had one of these drop attacks recently when he stood up. They tested him like you tested me and found that his blood pressure dropped a lot on standing. Is there much you can do about that?'

A: It sounds like Mr Walsh's friend had syncope secondary to orthostatic hypotension. If so, the general approach to managing orthostatic hypotension is (Arnold and Shibao, 2013):

- Cease the culprit medications.
- Reduce venous pooling (e.g. avoiding getting up too quickly or standing still, using waist-high compression stockings) (30–40 mm Hg).
- Increase central volume (e.g. by increasing salt and fluid intake).
- Use medications that promote sodium and fluid retention (e.g. fludrocortisone 0.1–0.3 mg/day orally).
- Use vasoconstrictor medications (e.g. midodrine 2.5–10 mg orally).

Achievements

You now:
- know the definition of syncope
- recognise that syncope isn't the only cause of a loss of consciousness
- can distinguish between syncope and loss of consciousness due to epilepsy
- know the different causes of syncope
- can target particular areas of the history and examination to determine the cause of syncope
- know the utility of certain investigations in identifying the cause of syncope
- know the management of orthostatic hypotension.

References

Arnold, A.C. and Shibao, C. (2013), 'Current concepts in orthostatic hypotension management', *Current Hypertension Reports*, vol. 15, no. 4, pp. 304–312.

Hanna, E.B. (2014), 'Syncope: etiology and diagnostic approach', *Cleveland Clinic of Medicine*, vol. 81, no. 12, pp. 755–766.

Jamalyan, S.V. and Khachatryan, L.A. (2010), 'Emerging risk stratification in syncope', *European Journal of Cardiovascular Medicine*, vol. 1, no. 2, pp. 38–48.

Poon, I.O. and Braun, U. (2005), 'High prevalence of orthostatic hypotension and its correlation with potentially causative medications among elderly veterans', *Journal of Clinical Pharmacy and Therapeutics*, vol. 30, no. 2, pp. 173–178.

Sutton, R., Benditt, D., Brignole, M. and Moya, A. (2010), 'Syncope: Diagnosis and management according to the 2009 guidelines of the European Society of Cardiology', *Polskie Archiwum Medycyny Wewnetrznej*, vol. 120, no. 1–2, pp. 42–47.

Taskforce for the Diagnosis and Management of Syncope (TDMS), European Society of Cardiology, European Heart Rhythm Association, *et al.* (2009), 'Guidelines for the diagnosis and management of syncope', *European Heart Journal*, vol. 30, no. 21, pp. 2631–2671.

Chapter 40
Christine is feeling under the weather

Scenario

You are a GP registrar and your first patient is Christine, a 45-year-old woman who is here to get the results from a work-up from 3 weeks ago for fatigue. The fatigue had been present for some months. She is otherwise healthy and takes no regular medications. All the tests are normal except for:
- TSH – 50 mIU/L (range 0.4–4.0)
- fT4 – 5 pmol/L (range 9–20).

Q: What is the most likely diagnosis?

A: She has primary hypothyroidism, as evidenced by the high TSH and low fT4 (free thyroxine).

Q: She is surprised. 'My friend had an underactive thyroid and she was much sicker than me. Are you sure about the diagnosis?'

A: Primary hypothyroidism has a number of clinical manifestations; however, they will vary between patients. Even the degree of TSH elevation doesn't correlate with clinical features: some patients with a mildly elevated TSH may feel much sicker than someone with a much higher TSH. The clinical features of hypothyroidism are shown in the box below:

System	Clinical features
Nutrition and metabolism	Cold intolerance
	Reduced appetite
	Increase in body weight
Cardiovascular	Reduced heart rate
	Reduced exercise tolerance
	Increased diastolic blood pressure
	Pericardial (and pleural) effusions

System	Clinical features
Skin, hair, nails	Nonpitting oedema (accumulated glycosaminoglycans)
	Coarse and fragile hair
	Brittle nails
	Pretibial myxoedema
	Decreased sweating
Nervous system	Somnolence
	Slowing of thinking
	Delayed relaxation of deep tendon reflexes
	Carpal tunnel syndrome
Respiratory	Hypoventilation
	Hypercapnia
Gastrointestinal	Constipation
Reproductive	Oligo-amenorrhoea
	Hypermenorrhoea: menorrhagia
	Reduced fertility
	Increased risk of miscarriage
Pregnancy	Spontaneous abortion
	Pre-eclampsia
	Miscarriage
	Still birth
	Pre-term birth
	Postpartum haemorrhage

Source: Adapted from Devdhar *et al.* (2007).

Q: Despite the fatigue being Christine's main complaint, you take a focused history and examination. You discover that she is also constipated and more cold intolerant than usual and has a slower heart rate than on her previous check-ups. There is no thyroid mass. You explain these findings to her. She is worried. 'But I thought that you had to be iodine deficient. I have a healthy diet. Why should I have an underactive thyroid?'

A: While the commonest cause of hypothyroidism worldwide is iodine deficiency, in developed countries like Australia, the commonest cause of hypothyroidism is autoimmune chronic lymphocytic thyroiditis, also known as Hashimoto's disease. This is usually associated with positive antithyroid antibodies, with the antithyroid peroxidase (anti-TPO) antibody being the most sensitive and specific (Garber *et al.*, 2012).

Q: 'Do I need an X-ray or scan of my thyroid?'

A: No. Imaging of the thyroid is not required for primary hypothyroidism in the absence of thyroid nodules or a mass (So *et al.*, 2012).

Q: How will you treat Christine's hypothyroidism?

A: Christine requires replacement with synthetic thyroxine at a starting dose of 1.0–1.6 ug/kg/day. But in the elderly or those with significant coronary artery disease, start at a lower dose of 25–50 ug/day (Devdhar *et al.*, 2007). Thyroxine should be taken on an empty stomach to maximise absorption (Liwanpo and Hershman, 2009).

Q: You prescribe 125 ug/day of thyroxine for Christine. When should you check her TSH?

A: The half-life of thyroxine is 7 days; therefore, check the serum TSH when a steady state is reached at about the 4–6 week mark. Then check the TSH every 4–6 weeks until a normal serum level is reached. After this, check the serum TSH and fT4 once a year (Devdhar *et al.*, 2007).

Q: You go on some well-deserved leave for 3 months. When you return, Christine is your first patient of the day. She arrives with a recent blood test showing a rise in her TSH level. The blood test was prompted by reduced energy levels. She is very disappointed because she started on iron supplements a few weeks ago to deal with heavy periods and was hoping for her energy levels to improve rather than decrease. The haemoglobin and iron studies are normal. Christine has been compliant with her thyroxine. What could be happening?

A: It appears that despite being compliant with her thyroxine dose, Christine has become hypothyroid, hence her reduced energy levels. This may be due to a drug interaction. A number of medications can affect thyroxine absorption. It is therefore important to counsel patients before starting thyroxine that any new supplement or medication could interfere with the absorption of thyroxine; therefore, closer monitoring of the TSH level may be required for a time.

In this case, ferrous sulfate is known to interfere with thyroxine's absorption, which may account for Christine's rise in TSH and clinical deterioration.

Other medications implicated in interfering with thyroxine absorption include calcium carbonate, raloxifene, phosphate binders, aluminium-containing antacids and proton pump inhibitors (Liwanpo and Hershman, 2009).

Scenario

Q: The following week you meet Ben, a 52-year-old public servant. He is well and takes no regular medications. Last month, he underwent a series of blood tests before applying for income protection insurance. The only abnormality was his thyroid results: TSH 7 mIU/L (range 0.4–4.0) and fT4 11 pmol/L (range 9–20).
You take a history and find that he is asymptomatic. In fact, he has never felt fitter. What does Ben have?

A: The presence of a mildly elevated TSH (between 5 and 10) and normal fT4 are consistent with a condition known as 'subclinical hypothyroidism'. It is a controversial area although it appears people with this are more likely to progress to frank hypothyroidism, especially if they have anti-TPO antibodies. One approach in managing this condition would be to repeat the test within 3 months and then do the following:

TSH (mIU/L)	fT4 (pmol/L)	Plan
>10	Low or normal	Thyroxine
5–10	Low	Thyroxine
5–10	Normal	If hypothyroid symptoms, give 3–6 month trial of thyroxine
5–10	Normal	If no hypothyroid symptoms, repeat TSH every year (if anti-TPO+) or every 3 years (if anti-TPO−)

Source: Adapted from Vaidya and Pearce (2008).

Scenario

Q: A couple of weeks later, you are in a private hospital doing an overtime shift. You are asked to review results for a patient, Mrs Flower, with *E. coli* bacteraemia following pyelonephritis. She is much better than on admission 3 days earlier. Today, following a low-grade fever, blood tests were performed. The results overall are pleasing with improvements in her white cell count and CRP; however, her thyroid function tests are abnormal:
- TSH 0.3 mIU/L (range 0.4–4.0)
- fT4 10 pmol/L (range 9–20)
- fT3 2.4 pmol/L (range 2.6–5.7).

You are able to access Mrs Flower's thyroid function tests from 6 months earlier when she had blood taken as part of a routine checkup. At that time, they were all within normal limits. What could be causing her abnormal thyroid function tests now?

A: Although there are a few possibilities, it is most likely that Mrs Flower has 'nonthyroidal illness syndrome' (also known as 'euthyroid sick syndrome') arising from sepsis (Adler and Wartofsky, 2007).

Nonthyroidal illness syndrome is a change in thyroid function tests due to various clinical situations such as starvation, sepsis, renal, hepatic or cardiac disease. It can be seen in up to three-quarters of patients in hospital. The most common changes include (Adler and Wartofsky, 2007):

- low serum T3
- normal fT4, but it may be low or increased
- elevated serum reverse T3
- normal TSH, but it may be slightly low, especially in sepsis, where there is reduced TSH production from the pituitary.

There is debate as to whether or not nonthyroidal illness syndrome is a euthyroid state and whether it should be treated with thyroid hormone replacement. As discussed above, thyroid hormone administration can lead to serious side effects (Adler and Wartofsky, 2007).

You speak to Mrs Flower's physician, who agrees that the thyroid function tests probably represent nonthyroidal illness syndrome. Since Mrs Flower is doing so well, the physician suggests repeating the thyroid function tests in a month.

Q: She also says, 'And of course, she may have received IV glucocorticoids in ICU when she was first admitted'. What is the basis of this cryptic comment?

A: She is probably referring to the fact that a number of medications can lead to abnormal thyroid function tests. These include medications given in critical illness such as glucocorticoids and dopamine. In addition, drugs such as frusemide, salicylates, amiodarone, iodine, beta-blockers and phenytoin can affect thyroid function tests (Adler and Wartofsky, 2007).

Achievements

You now know:
- the clinical and laboratory parameters for diagnosing hypothyroidism

- how to prescribe thyroxine and monitor thyroid function tests
- how other medications can affect absorption of thyroxine
- how to diagnose subclinical hypothyroidism
- that nonthyroidal illness syndrome is a common cause of abnormal thyroid function tests in hospitalised patients
- that a number of medications can affect thyroid function tests.

References

Adler, S.M. and Wartofsky, L. (2007), 'The nonthyroidal illness syndrome', *Endocrinology and Metabolism Clinics of North America*, vol. 36, no. 3, pp. 657–672.

Devdhar, M., Ousman, Y.H. and Burman, K.D. (2007), 'Hypothyroidism', *Endocrinology and Metabolism Clinics of North America*, vol. 36, no. 3, pp. 595–615.

Garber, J.R., Cobin, R.H., Gharib, H., Hennessey, J.V., Klein, I., Mechanick, J.I., *et al.* (2012), 'Clinical practice guidelines for hypothyroidism in adults: Cosponsored by the American Association of Clinical Endocrinologists and the American Thyroid Association', *Endocrine Practice*, vol. 18, no. 6, pp. 988–1028.

Liwanpo L. and Hershman J.M. (2009), 'Conditions and drugs interfering with thyroxine absorption', *Best Practice & Research Clinical Endocrinology & Metabolism*, vol. 23, no. 6, pp. 781–792.

So, M., MacIsaac, R.J. and Grossman, M. (2012), 'Hypothyroidism', *Australian Family Physician*, vol. 41, no. 8, pp. 556–562.

Vaidya, B. and Pearce, S.H.S. (2008), 'Management of hypothyroidism in adults', *British Medical Journal*, vol. 337, no. a801.

Chapter 41
Saesha calls in sick

Scenario

It is a chilly June Sunday. You were meant to be having a day off after a week of evenings in the Emergency Department but got called in because one of your colleagues is 'sick'. 'Probably hung over from Friday night partying,' you keep muttering to yourself. Somewhat disgruntled at having to return to the Emergency Department but pacified at the thought of the double-time pay, you pick up the first patient for this shift. You are shocked to find that it is Saesha, your intern colleague, who called in sick in the first place! The triage nurse sees you with Saesha's file and says, 'Poor thing's probably got flu: after all, it's flu season. Anyway, I've put her in precautions'.

Q: When is 'flu season'?

A: In temperate climates, influenza season peaks during winter when it is cold. In tropical climates, however, there is background influenza all year round with epidemics occurring in intermediate periods between the influenza season of temperate nations of both the northern and southern hemispheres (Viboud *et al.*, 2006).

Q: What 'precautions' should be used if Saesha has influenza?

A: People with suspected or proven influenza should be placed in *droplet precautions*. Infections that spread via droplets cannot travel more than 1–2 metres; therefore, Saesha does not need to be in a negative pressure room. But she should be isolated in a single room. People entering the room should wear gloves, gowns and facemasks. If Saesha leaves the room for a test or another reason, she should also wear a facemask (Centers for Disease Control and Prevention, 2013).

Q: Saesha looks awful. She is 24 years old and is otherwise healthy. Yesterday, she suddenly developed chills, fevers, generalised myalgias and a sore throat. By this morning, she also had a runny nose and dry cough on top of the other symptoms. The fevers have persisted despite regular paracetamol. Her oral intake is poor and she is too sick to get out of bed. She lives alone and felt that she needed to be in hospital. Looking at her woeful state, you agree. 'At least you know I wasn't faking when I called in sick,' she says, managing a tired smile. 'The thought never crossed my mind,' you lie shamelessly.

The physical examination is only remarkable for a red, congested nose, fever and tachycardia. The lungs, in particular, are clear.

Q: The triage nurse comes up to you. 'She's got an ILI during flu season. It's got to be influenza, don't you think?'

Is the triage nurse right? And what does she mean by an 'ILI'?

A: An 'ILI' stands for 'influenza-like illness'. It is a syndrome consisting of various symptoms that could be due to influenza. The definition for an ILI varies but typically will require 4–6 of 9 criteria (Michiels *et al.*, 2011):

- cough
- fever
- rigors/chills
- headache
- weakness and prostration
- myalgias
- widespread aches and pains
- abrupt onset
- influenza in a close contact.

Saesha has 5 of these (abrupt onset, cough, fevers, chills, myalgias, cough) and would therefore meet the definition for an ILI.

The limitation of the definition for an ILI is that it is nonspecific and can apply to so many other infections. For example, a study of Polish armed forces with ILIs during an influenza season found that only 40% of specimens were positive for viruses. Of those positive for viruses, influenza only accounted for 6% of them, with coronaviruses, rhinoviruses/enteroviruses and parainfluenza viruses making up the vast majority (Kocik *et al.*, 2014).

This distribution will vary according to population, location and season, but it demonstrates that influenza isn't the only cause of an ILI. With regard to Saesha, she has an ILI during influenza season; therefore, influenza must be high on your list of differential diagnoses.

Q: How can you confirm a diagnosis of influenza in Saesha?

A: It would be reasonable to perform basic blood tests and a chest X-ray, but results commonly seen in influenza, such as lymphopaenia, are nonspecific.

The 'money' is in viral testing. The 2 most commonly used tests that you are likely to see in hospital are (Centers for Disease Control and Prevention, 2014a; Centers for Disease Control and Prevention, 2014b):

1. **Rapid influenza diagnostic tests (RIDT)**
   - Can use a nasal swab, throat swab, nasopharyngeal swab, nasal aspirate.
   - Is best performed within 5 days of symptom onset in adults (longer in children).
   - Has low sensitivity (50–70%), so it's not great at ruling out influenza.
   - Has high specificity (90–95%) so a positive result is reliable for influenza.
   - As the name implies, it gives a rapid result (within 15 minutes).

2. **Reverse transcriptase polymerase chain reaction (RT-PCR assay)**
   - Can use similar specimens as with RIDT (see above) as well as bronchial and endotracheal washings.
   - Is best performed within 2–3 days of testing.
   - Is extremely sensitive and specific.
   - Can get a same-day result, depending on lab testing schedules.
   - Will often be part of a multiplex assay which tests for other viruses and therefore might provide an alternative diagnosis (e.g. enterovirus, parainfluenza virus, respiratory syncytial virus, human metapneumovirus, *Bordetella pertussis*, coronavirus).

Q: Saesha has a normal chest X-ray and her blood tests are unremarkable apart from a CRP of 40 mg/L (normal < 5 mg/L) and a lymphopaenia. The RIDT comes back negative. The RT-PCR from a nasal swab will be available in a few hours so you still can't rule out influenza. Should Saesha be treated?

A: All patients in hospital with suspected or confirmed influenza should be given antiviral agents (Centers for Disease Control and Prevention, 2015).

Q: What antiviral agents are available against influenza?

A: There are two main groups of antiviral drugs for influenza (Krol *et al.*, 2014):

1. **Neuraminidase inhibitors**
   - These are the most widely used in Australia.
   - They prevent the release of virus from infected cells.

- They include oseltamivir (oral), zanamivir (inhaled) and peramivir (intravenous).
2. **M2 ion channel inhibitors**
   - These include amantidine and rimantidine.
   - They only work against influenza A (not B) but now, there are high circulating levels of resistance.
   A number of novel agents are also being developed (e.g. hemagglutinin inhibitors, endocytosis inhibitors).

Q: You speak to the ED Registrar who agrees that Saesha should be admitted. If the tests confirm influenza, how long should she remain in droplet precautions for?

A: The idea of droplet precautions is to minimise transmission of influenza from the patient to others. Swine flu (influenza A, H1N1), for example, is typically shed for 4–8.5 days after the onset of illness (Punpanich and Chotpitayasunondh, 2012). The Centers for Disease Control and Prevention (2013) recommend that influenza patients be kept in droplet precautions until 1 week after symptom onset or 1 day after fever and respiratory symptoms have gone, whichever is longer.

Q: You tell Saesha that it is best for her to be admitted; however, Saesha politely refuses. 'I feel much better after the IV fluids. I'd rather recover at my sister's place. And please don't give me the antiviral: I've seen it cause nausea.'

Despite your pleas, Saesha discharges herself, promising to return if she gets worse. At the end of your shift, you check with the lab and find that Saesha is positive for influenza A, subtype H1N1 (swine). What does this mean?

A: Influenza is an RNA virus from the family orthomyxoviridae. There are three types of influenza virus: A, B and C. Of these, A and B are responsible for flu; therefore, we only test for influenza A and B in patients with suspected influenza (Chen and Deng, 2009).

Saesha has an infection due to influenza A. This can be further classified according to 2 glycoproteins of the influenza A virus: hemagglutinin (H) and neuraminidase (N). There are various combinations of hemagglutinins and neuraminidases (e.g. H1N1, H5N1, H7N7), many of which do not cause disease in humans. In Saesha's case, her influenza A strain is H1N1, which caused the 2009 swine flu pandemic, and continues to circulate.

Q: You call Saesha, both to update her and check on how she is. Saesha is able to answer the phone and sounds okay; however, she is annoyed with the diagnosis. 'But that's not fair! I got my flu shot, just like I was meant to. How did I get flu?' What do you tell her?

A: There are three broad groups of influenza vaccines: inactivated intramuscular vaccines (used in Australia), inactivated intradermal vaccines (used in Australia) and live intranasal vaccines (not used in Australia). The inactivated vaccine that Saesha would have received isn't perfect: its efficacy in preventing lab-confirmed influenza in healthy adults under 65 years of age is about 60%. Therefore, cases of influenza can occur despite immunisation. But the vaccine does have an impact on hospitalisations due to pneumonia and influenza and on all-cause mortality in people over 65 years in nursing homes (Department of Health, 2013).

Q: Saesha is still miffed. 'But I haven't treated anyone with a flu-like illness recently or had any sick family or friends. How could I have been infected?'

A: As a doctor, Saesha may have been infected either in the community or in a healthcare setting. Influenza has an incubation period of around 1–4 days but people begin to shed the virus about 1 day before they develop symptoms; furthermore, about 1/3 of influenza infections are asymptomatic (Punpanich and Chotpitayasunondh, 2012). Therefore, Saesha's infectious contact may have been asymptomatic. Also, inanimate objects or surfaces contaminated with virus can be a source of infection (Centers for Disease Control and Prevention, 2013). In other words, Saesha may not have needed direct contact with an influenza victim to have become infected.

Q: Three days pass and you are in the Emergency Department again. You look on the computer list and are shocked to see that Saesha is back. This time, she looks even more unwell. She tells you that she had slowly improved and felt quite good yesterday: the fevers had resolved and the myalgias were settling. But today, she developed right-sided pleuritic chest pain, a worsening cough and shortness of breath. Her physical examination and chest X-ray is consistent with right lower lobe consolidation. What could have happened?

A: Saesha almost certainly has a bacterial co-infection with her influenza. This is a well-recognised phenomenon strongly associated with influenza A. It is thought that the preceding viral infection creates an environment conducive to a bacterial infection. The bacterial infection can be concurrent or secondary, occurring 7–21 days following influenza. The commonest causes of bacterial community-acquired pneumonia associated with influenza are *Streptococcus pneumoniae*, *Staphylococcus aureus* and *Haemophilus influenzae*. Even *Legionella pneumophila* infection has been associated with influenza (Joseph *et al.*, 2013).

Q: Saesha is admitted to hospital for both oseltamivir 75 mg bd po, azithromycin 500 mg daily po and piperacillin-tazobactam 4.5 g q8h IV. You are confident that this time she will be fine.

Scenario

Your next patient is a 75-year-old man with community-acquired left lower lobe pneumonia. Apart from hypertension and hypercholesterolaemia, he is otherwise well. His history is consistent with an ILI preceding the pneumonia by a few days.

Q: He hasn't been immunised against influenza. Should he have been?
A: Yes. The influenza vaccine contains 3 influenza viruses: 2 types of influenza A and 1 type of influenza B. Immunisation is recommended for a number of groups, some of which are (Department of Health, 2013):
- people ≥ 65 years (immunisation reduces hospitalisations for pneumonia and all-cause mortality)
- people at risk of complicated or severe influenza (pregnancy, immunocompromised, chronic lung or heart or renal or neurological disease, Down syndrome, obesity)
- Aboriginal or Torres Strait Islander people ≥15 years
- residents of long-term residential or aged care facilities
- people who can transmit influenza to those at increased risk of severe/complicated infection (e.g. healthcare workers).

Due to regular changes in influenza surface antigens, the influenza vaccine is usually changed annually. These changes are typically minor and are known as 'antigenic drift'. Major changes known as 'antigenic shift' can lead to a new virus subtype forming, potentially leading to a pandemic (Chen and Deng, 2009).

Achievements

You now know:
- the subtypes of influenza
- the definition and broad differential diagnosis of an influenza-like illness
- how influenza is transmitted, including asymptomatically
- what droplet precautions are
- how to diagnose influenza

- how to treat influenza
- that bacterial co-infection or secondary infections are serious complications of influenza
- the indications, types and efficacy of influenza vaccines.

References

Centers for Disease Control and Prevention (2015), 'Use of antivirals', at <www.cdc.gov/flu/professionals/antivirals/antiviral-use-influenza.htm>, accessed 14 January 2015.

Centers for Disease Control and Prevention (2014a), 'Guidance for clinicians on the use of RT-PCR and other molecular assays for diagnosis of influenza virus infection', at <www.cdc.gov/flu/professionals/diagnosis/molecular-assays.htm>, accessed 13 January 2015.

Centers for Disease Control and Prevention (2014b), 'Rapid diagnostic testing for influenza: Information for clinical laboratory directors', at <www.cdc.gov/flu/professionals/diagnosis/rapidlab.htm>, accessed 13 January 2015.

Centers for Disease Control and Prevention (2013), 'Prevention strategies for seasonal influenza in healthcare settings', at <www.cdc.gov/flu/professionals/infectioncontrol/healthcaresettings.htm>, accessed 12 January 2015.

Chen, J. and Deng, Y.M. (2009), 'Influenza virus antigenic variation, host antibody production and new approach to control epidemics', *Virology Journal*, vol. 6, no. 30, doi:10.1186/1743-422X-6-30.

Department of Health (2013), *The Australian Immunisation Handbook*, 10th edition, Canberra: Department of Health, at <www.immunise.health.gov.au/internet/immunise/publishing.nsf/Content/handbook10-4-7>, accessed 14 January 2015.

Joseph, C., Togawa, Y. and Shindo, N. (2013), 'Bacterial and viral infections associated with influenza', *Influenza and Other Respiratory Viruses*, vol. 7, suppl. 2, pp. 105–113.

Kocik, J., Niemcewicz, M., Winnicka, I., *et al.* (2014), 'Diversity of influenza-like illness etiology in Polish Armed Forces in influenza epidemic season', *Acta Biochimica Polonica*, vol. 61, no. 3, pp. 489–494.

Krol, E., Rychlowska, M. and Szewczyk, B. (2014), 'Antivirals – current trends in fighting influenza', *Acta Biochimica Polonica*, vol. 61, no. 3, pp. 495–504.

Michiels, B., Thomas, I., Van Royen, P., Coenen, S. (2011), 'Clinical prediction rules combining signs, symptoms and epidemiological context to distinguish influenza from influenza-like illnesses', *BMC Family Practice*, vol. 12, no. 4, doi: 10.1186/1471-2296-12-4.

Punpanich, W. and Chotpitayasunondh, T. (2012), 'A review on the clinical spectrum and natural history of human influenza', *International Journal of Infectious Diseases*', e714–723.

Viboud, C., Alonso, W.J. and Simonsen, L. (2006), 'Influenza in tropical regions', *PLoS Medicine*, vol. 3, no. 4, e89.

Chapter 42
Grace presents with urinary tract symptoms

Scenario

It is Thursday evening in the Emergency Department. You, the intern, have been allocated to the clinics section. One of your patients is a 25-year-old woman named Grace. She apologises for coming to the Emergency Department but says that her GP is booked out till the end of the week. Her concern is that she might have a urinary tract infection. You ask her about her symptoms. She describes 3 days of burning on passing urine and urinary frequency. Today, she developed some pain on the left flank. She has been systemically well. Her examination reveals a well-looking afebrile woman with mild left costovertebral tenderness.

Q: What is the likely clinical diagnosis?

A: Grace appears to have acute pyelonephritis.

Q: 'Pyelonephritis? What's that?' she asks with concern.

A: Acute pyelonephritis is an infection of the renal pelvis and kidney that typically is a result of infection ascending to the kidney from the bladder via the ureter (Colgan *et al.*, 2011).

Q: 'Is it common? I've never heard of it before.'

A: It is very common. In the USA, there are around 250 000 cases per year with 100 000 hospitalisations (Rollino *et al.* 2012).

Q: You explain to Grace that she most likely developed a bladder infection that has ascended to the kidneys. 'But why me? I'm normally so healthy.'

A: Women aged 15–29 have the highest incidence of the disease, which puts Grace in the target age group. There are other risk factors worth asking about, which includes (Colgan *et al.*, 2011):
- urinary tract infection (UTI) within the past 12 months
- maternal history of UTI
- new sexual partner within the last year
- sexual intercourse ≥3 times/week in the last 30 days

- use of spermicide
- diabetes mellitus.

Q: Grace tells you that she does have a new sexual partner and they've been together quite frequently in the last few weeks. Now that you've established a clinical diagnosis of pyelonephritis and potential risk factors, what else should you establish from the history?

A: You need to know if this is 'uncomplicated' or 'complicated' pyelonephritis. Regard pyelonephritis as complicated if the following criteria are met (Mandelll *et al.* 2010):

- structurally or functionally abnormal urinary tracts (including catheters and calculi)
- diabetes mellitus
- infection in pregnancy
- infection in children or men
- infection in hospital or the healthcare-associated setting.

Q: Is it just being pedantic to know whether this is complicated or uncomplicated pyelonephritis? Or does it have serve some practical purpose?

A: Patients with complicated pyelonephritis are more likely to have resistant bacteria causing their infection (Sobel and Kaye, 2010). In addition, they are more likely to progress to a severe complication such as an intrarenal abscess.

Q: You establish that Grace is otherwise healthy and unlikely to be pregnant. Your clinical assessment is that she has uncomplicated pyelonephritis. What tests should be performed?

A:

1. **Midstream urine (MSU).** The MSU should undergo dipstick analysis, which will usually be positive for leukocytes, nitrites (resulting from chemical reactions due to bacteria) and sometimes microscopic haematuria. It should then be sent for microscopy, culture and sensitivity.
2. **Blood cultures**.
3. **Full blood count.** Elevated leukocytes may be present.
4. **EUCs.** Acute kidney injury may be present.
5. **CRP.**
6. **Pregnancy test** (serum beta-HCG).

   It is both courteous and a good idea to copy Grace's GP into the blood and urine results (there is usually an area of the form that says 'Copy to:') as her GP will need to follow her up and check her urine results.

Q: Grace asks, 'What are the bugs that cause this?'

A: In 95% of cases, a single organism is responsible (Mandell *et al.*, 2010). In around 80% of cases, *E. coli* is the causative organism. *Klebsiella, Enterococcus, Proteus, Enterobacter, Pseudomonas, Staphylococcus saprophyticus* and *Candida* are less common organisms (Colgan *et al.*, 2011).

Q: 'And the urine should tell us what the bug is?'

A: In an ideal setting, yes. Since the urethra and periurethral areas can get contaminated, it is not uncommon for bacteria to be found in MSU samples, which can make interpretation difficult. To overcome this problem, guidelines have been established on the basis that the higher the bacterial count in the urine, the more likely true infection is. For example, in premenopausal, nonpregnant women, guidelines for diagnosis are (Grabe *et al.*, 2009):

- $\geq 10^4$ colony-forming units/mL for acute pyelonephritis
- $\geq 10^3$ colony-forming units/mL for acute cystitis.

Having said that, a recent series of hospitalised patients with pyelonephritis found a low rate of urine positivity of less than 25%. The reasons were unclear. In some cases, blood cultures were positive where urine cultures were not and there was not always concordance between positive urine and blood culture results (Rollino *et al.*, 2012). In other words, it is a good idea and a simple measure to take BOTH blood and urine cultures in patients with pyelonephritis.

Q: The urinalysis demonstrates leucocytes and nitrites, making you more confident of a diagnosis of acute pyelonephritis. Grace asks, 'Could it be anything else?'

A: In patients with acute flank pain, especially without urinary symptoms, there is a broad differential diagnosis. Some of the diseases include (Colgan *et al.*, 2011):

- intra-abdominal abscess
- acute appendicitis
- acute diverticulitis
- acute pancreatitis
- splenic abscess or infarct
- pelvic inflammatory disease
- endometriosis
- noninfectious renal disorders
- retroperitoneal haemorrhage
- zoster (shingles)

- lower rib fractures
- pulmonary lung pathology.

But Grace's clinical picture, especially with the dysuria and urinary frequency, make acute pyelonephritis the most likely diagnosis.

Scenario

You ask Grace to sit in the waiting room until her pregnancy test and basic bloods return. When they become available, apart from a mildly elevated CRP and white cell count, the blood tests are unremarkable. She is not pregnant. The cultures won't be back for 1–2 days but you wish to commence treatment now.

Q: What should you start?

A: For empiric treatment of patients with acute pyelonephritis not requiring hospitalisation, treatment with oral ciprofloxacin 500 mg bd for 7 days is reasonable (Gupta *et al.*, 2011).

This is on the assumption that local fluoroquinolone resistance is not over 10%. While this is not an issue for Australia, it is a problem in other parts of the world, especially in Asia and Southern Europe. Therefore, you should ask Grace if she has travelled in the last 6 months or so. If so, you should seek advice from a more senior colleague or an infectious diseases physician.

If the organism is known to be sensitive to cotrimoxazole (trimethoprim-sulfamethoxazole), then a 14-day course of cotrimoxazole DS (160/800) T bd can be used (Gupta *et al.*, 2011).

The Therapeutic Guidelines : Antibiotic also recommend trimethoprim 300 mg daily or cephalexin 500 mg q6h or amoxycillin-clavulanate 875/125 mg q12h (Antibiotic Expert Group, 2014); however, Gupta *et al.* (2011) note that oral beta-lactam agents are less effective for treating pyelonephritis than other agents.

Grace has not been overseas for years so you are happy to prescribe ciprofloxacin for her. You discuss the side effects of ciprofloxacin with her, including Achilles tendinitis and peripheral neuropathy, and write a letter for her GP, who she will see in 2 days. You tell her to return to hospital if she doesn't improve on the antibiotics.

Q: Before she leaves, she asks whether you need to do an X-ray of her kidneys. What do you tell her?

A: In uncomplicated infections, it is unnecessary to image the kidneys (Colgan *et al.*, 2011; Sobel and Kaye, 2010).

Scenario

Two days later, you are working again in the Emergency Department. Grace has returned. Although she is feeling a lot better, her GP was sick today so she couldn't see him. She is therefore following up on the culture results. You check for her and discover that the blood cultures were negative but the MSU isolated an *E. coli* sensitive to ciprofloxacin, resistant to amoxycillin-clavulanate, cephalexin and amoxicillin, intermediate resistance to cotrimoxazole. You tell her to continue the ciprofloxacin.

Q: Grace wants to know if it is necessary to repeat the urine test after she has finished treatment. What do you tell her?

A: No. If she is clinically cured, she doesn't need a repeat urine culture (Sobel and Kaye, 2010).

Scenario

A few days later, you see a 45-year-old woman named Linda who has no co-morbidities and no allergies. She was admitted with pyelonephritis that hasn't responded to 3 days of cotrimoxazole started by her GP. She recalls her GP doing a dipstick analysis of an MSU but not sending it for culture. She comes to hospital today with the onset of fevers, rigors, vomiting and worsening right flank pain. On examination, she is febrile, tachycardic and hypotensive, although alert. Her inflammatory markers are high but her creatinine is normal.

Q: What antibiotics should you give her, empirically?

A: This patient has urinary sepsis. According to the Therapeutic Guidelines: Antibiotic (2014), you can give her IV gentamicin 4–6 mg/kg for 1 dose (basing subsequent doses on levels and renal function) AND IV ampicillin 2 g q6h.

Q: Does Linda require imaging?

A: In someone with sepsis or a severe infection from the urinary tract, it is reasonable to image the urinary tract to look for underlying abnormalities and complications (e.g. obstruction or abscesses).

A sensitive combination of tests, which is rapid and involves little radiation, is a kidney/ureter/bladder (KUB) X-ray with a renal ultrasound. If the patient fails to improve despite normal imaging, the next step would be a contrast-enhanced CT (Sobel and Kaye, 2010).

Scenario

Linda improves rapidly with a combination of IV fluid resuscitation and antibiotics. The KUB X-ray is normal but the renal ultrasound shows an abnormality on the right kidney consistent with focal pyelonephritis. Her blood and urine cultures identify a fully sensitive *E. coli* so you continue IV ampicillin alone.

Q: At this time, one of your intern colleagues, Jeff, rushes to you carrying an X-ray. 'You've got to see this!' he exclaims. 'This is a 43-year-old woman with sepsis and acute flank pain. She is really unwell. This is her CT scan.' What does it show (Figure 42.1)?

A: The CT scan shows gas in the renal parenchyma. This patient almost certainly has an uncommon condition called 'emphysematous pyelo-nephritis'. It has a high mortality rate of 20% but in the past, it used to be much higher (around 80%) (Ubee *et al.*, 2011).

Q: What underlying condition is this patient most likely to have?

A: Around 95% of patients with emphysematous pyelonephritis will have diabetes mellitus, which is the major risk factor. Other associations include neurogenic bladder, alcoholism, drug abuse and renal tract anatomic abnormalities (Ubee *et al.*, 2011).

Q: Jeff says, 'I guess the gas means some anaerobe like *Clostridium* must be the cause'. Is he right?

A: Although different organisms have been implicated, *E. coli* is the main culprit, having been cultured in 70% of cases. In fact, anaerobes like

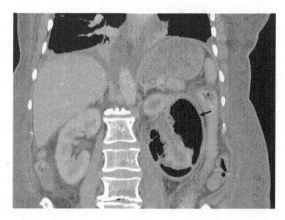

Figure 42.1 This coronal image shows abnormal gas in a swollen left kidney (black arrow).

Clostridium have only rarely been associated with this infection (Ubee *et al.*, 2011).

Q: Will a nephrectomy have to be performed?

A: Previously, emergency nephrectomy was often the accepted treatment for this condition. Now, better outcomes can be achieved with a combination of IV antibiotics and percutaneous drainage (Ubee *et al.*, 2011).

Achievements

You now:
- know the definition of acute pyelonephritis
- know the risk factors for acute pyelonephritis
- can differentiate between complicated and uncomplicated pyelonephritis
- know how to investigate and treat both uncomplicated and complicated cases
- have a differential diagnosis for acute flank pain
- have an overview of emphysematous pyelonephritis.

References

Antibiotic Expert Group (2014), *Therapeutic Guidelines: Antibiotic*, Version 15, Therapeutic Guidelines Ltd, Melbourne.

Colgan, R., Williams, M. and Johnson, J.R. (2011), 'Diagnosis and treatment of acute pyelonephritis in women', *American Family Physician*, vol. 84, no. 5, pp. 519–526.

Grabe, M., Bishop, M.C., Bjerklund-Johansen, T.E., *et al.* (2009), 'Guidelines on urological infections', at <www.uroweb.org/fileadmin/tx_eauguidelines/2009/Full/Urological_Infections.pdf>, accessed 19 September 2014.

Gupta, K., Hooton, T.M., Naber, K.G., *et al.* (2011), 'International clinical practice guidelines for the treatment of acute uncomplicated cystitis and pyelonephritis in women: A 2010 update by the Infectious Diseases Society of America and the European Society for Microbiology and Infectious Diseases', *Clinical Infectious Diseases*, vol. 52, no. 5, e103–120.

Rollino, C., Beltrame, G., Ferro, M., *et al.* (2012), 'Acute pyelonephritis in adults: A case series of 223 patients', *Nephrology, Dialysis, Transplantation*, vol. 27, no. 9, pp. 3488–3493.

Ubee, S.S., McGlynn, L. and Fordham, M. (2011), 'Emphysematous pyelonephritis', *BJU International*, vol. 107, no. 9, pp. 1474–1478.

Sobel J. and Kaye, D. (2010), 'Urinary tract infections', in G.L. Mandell, J.E. Bennett and R. Dolin (eds), *Principles and Practice of Infectious Diseases*, 7th edition, Churchill Livingstone, pp. 957–985.

Chapter 43
Mr Ecks presents with fever and generalised muscle aches

Scenario

You are working in clinics in the Emergency Department with a third-year medical student, Monica. She has just come to tell you about a patient she has seen. It is a 55-year-old man who has been unwell for 24 hours with fevers, shivers, generalised muscle aches and a sore throat. His background history includes abdominal surgery 2 months ago following a motor vehicle accident. He drinks 60 g alcohol per day. Monica says, 'I've examined him and there's nothing to find, not even pharyngitis, only his abdominal surgery scar. He came here because he doesn't have a regular GP. We've sent off some basic bloods and blood cultures, and I've asked my friend in haematology to call me as soon as his blood tests are back. If they are okay, shall I just send him home?'

Monica's assessment seems reasonable but she is still only a medical student so you need to see the patient before you clear him. When you meet Mr Ecks, you find a tall, overweight, unkempt man who looks fairly well. He confirms the history that Monica conveyed. You ask Mr Ecks about his abdominal surgery 2 months ago. He tells you that he got hit by a car as he was leaving a pub. He needed surgery to fix 'a bleeding liver and other stuff'. When you press him for more information, he shrugs his shoulders. 'I wasn't interested in finding out. I just wanted to leave hospital, go home to my dog and have a drink.'

Q: You are about to clear him and send him home when Monica gets a text. She reads it and says, 'Debbie has just examined his blood results and wants me to have a look at something. Do you want to come?'

With your curiosity piqued, you walk to the laboratory next door where Debbie, one of the scientists, shows you Mr Eck's blood film. 'He's got a slightly elevated neutrophil and platelet count. But I wanted to show you this. Go on, have a look.'

A: When you look down the microscope, there are red cells containing nuclear remnants, which are called Howell Jolly bodies.

Q: Armed with this information, what question should you ask Mr Ecks about his abdominal surgery?

A: Howell Jolly bodies are specific for hyposplenism; therefore, you want to know if he had a splenectomy.

Scenario

Again Mr Ecks brushes off your inquiries about his surgery. 'I really don't know what they did. I wasn't interested. I just wanted to go home. In fact, I left on my own terms because I got fed up with all the waiting.'

You quickly find and read his old notes. They confirm that his recent surgery included a splenectomy.

Around this time, Mr Ecks suddenly gets worse. He becomes restless and less responsive. He is febrile and has become tachycardic at 120/minute, hypotensive 80/40 and tachypnoeic at 28 breaths/minute. His oxygen saturations remain stable. The JVP is not elevated. His heart sounds are clear and dual. The trachea is midline. His breath sounds are vesicular, of normal intensity with no added sounds. The lung fields are resonant. There is no neck stiffness. You call a Code Blue.

Q: What are the potential causes of his hypotension?

A: Think of the mnemonic 'AM CASH' for causes of hypotension:

A: Anaphylaxis

M: Medications

C: Cardiopulmonary (pulmonary embolism, cardiogenic, tension pneumothorax)

A: Addisonian crisis (in people on corticosteroids or in sepsis complicated by adrenal haemorrhage e.g. Waterhouse–Friderichsen syndrome)

S: Sepsis

H: Hypovolaemia (bleeding or dehydration)

Scenario

The resuscitation team gets IV access with 2 large-bore cannulae before taking blood tests, including further blood cultures, and then commencing IV fluids. A 12-lead ECG and mobile CXR are performed: both are normal apart from showing a sinus tachycardia. His FBC and EUCs are repeated: both are unremarkable apart from a worsening of the neutrophilia and a drop in the platelet count. Coagulation studies are pending.

The team leader goes through the differential diagnoses with you: 'Anaphylaxis: unlikely as there doesn't seem to be a trigger and he has no other features. Medication-induced hypotension: unlikely because he doesn't take regular meds. Cardiopulmonary: unlikely with that ECG and CXR. Hypovolaemia: unlikely with that normal haemoglobin. No history of corticosteroid use to suggest an Addisonian crisis. That leaves sepsis. This man has fevers and hypotension, which would fit perfectly with septic shock. But he's crashed so quickly.'

Q: Is there anything else in the history to explain what's going on?

A: Absolutely. Mr Ecks has developed septic shock in the presence of a recent splenectomy. He may well have overwhelming post-splenectomy infection (OPSI).

Q: Monica hears this and is surprised. 'Why would the absence of a spleen predispose someone to overwhelming sepsis? I thought it just cleared old red blood cells from the circulatory system.'

A: The spleen contributes to the immune response in the following ways (Rodeghiero and Ruggeri, 2012):

1. having the red pulp remove bloodborne pathogens from the bloodstream
2. phagocytosis of antibody-coated cells or organisms
3. getting memory B cells to produce IgM
4. producing opsonins such as properdin and tuftsin.

Q: Monica writes down your words of wisdom. 'So what's this "OPSI" thing you talked about?'

A: It was in 1952 that the presence of OPSI was first documented after observing episodes of sepsis in splenectomised children (King and Shumacker, 1952). But OPSI is not just restricted to those who have had their spleens removed. It can also occur in people with 'functional asplenia'(people who have a spleen that doesn't work well). An example of functional asplenia is in sickle cell anaemia, where autoinfarction of the spleen occurs as red blood cells are sequestered there (Rodeghiero and Ruggeri, 2012). Also, patients with functional asplenia may not be aware that their spleen isn't working; therefore, have a high index of suspicion for OPSI and functional asplenia in septic patients with haemoglobinopathies and bone marrow transplants (Morgan and Tomich, 2012).

Patients often present with a nonspecific flu-like illness with fevers and appear well. This mild illness, however, can rapidly deteriorate into septic shock, just as has happened with Mr Ecks. A rash may appear, which may be nonspecific or typical of the purpura seen in meningococcal disease (Morgan and Tomich, 2012).

The mortality rate can be as high as 50% (Rubin and Schaffner, 2014); therefore, this is a serious infection.

Scenario

The team leader speaks to the on-call infectious diseases physician and orders empiric IV antibiotic therapy. At this point, one of the nurses reports that Mr Ecks is haemodynamically more unstable and that he has developed a rash. You rush to look at the rash as the team leader begins inotrope therapy to address his hypotension. It is widespread, non-blanching and purpuric.

Q: Monica exclaims, 'Meningococcal disease! It's got to be!' Is she right?

A: She could be. Certainly, it is a rash typical of meningococcal disease and it is important that medical students think of meningococcal disease as soon as they see that rash.

But a number of organisms can cause OPSI, of which *Neisseria meningitidis* (meningococcus) is only one, and which are more strongly linked to OPSI than meningococcus (see table below: organisms associated with OPSI).

Strong association with OPSI	Weak association with OPSI
Streptococcus pneumoniae (pneumococcus)*†	*Neisseria meningitidis* (meningococcus)*
Haemophilus influenzae b*	*Staphylococcus aureus*
Capnocytophaga canimorsus and *C. cynodegmi* (animal bites)	*Escherichia coli*
Bordetella holmesii	
Babesia	

*Organisms you must learn
†Pneumococcus is the leading cause of OPSI

OPSI can be so severe as to cause disseminated intravascular coagulation (DIC) and the purpuric rash usually attributed to meningococcal disease (Rubin and Schaffner, 2014). So while Monica's assumption about meningococcus might be correct, the other pathogens could also cause a similar picture.

Q: Monica then asks, 'If the spectrum of organisms is so broad, what antibiotics did we just give him?'

A: A reasonable empiric combination would be IV meropenem 1 g q8h and IV vancomycin (in case of a resistant strain of pneumococcus). Meropenem (rather than ceftriaxone) can be used as bacteria like *B. holmesii* can be quite resistant (Pittet *et al.*, 2014).

Scenario

Mr Ecks is now in the resuscitation bay. Debbie from the haematology lab calls to confirm that Mr Ecks's coagulation studies are consistent with DIC. More worryingly, examination of the blood film reveals diplococci.

Q: Could she be right?
A: It is possible but it is a very bad sign. It indicates a massive burden of organisms in the bloodstream.

  Within minutes of the call, Mr Ecks suffers a cardiac arrest. Despite everyone's best attempts, he cannot be revived. You end your shift, shocked by his death and the rapidity of his demise.

Scenario

The following week, you are working in the surgical pre-admissions clinic. Mrs Bruni is a 60-year-old woman about to undergo a splenectomy for idiopathic thrombocytopaenic purpura. She has read on the internet that removing the spleen increases the risk of infection.

Q: 'So doctor, what can I do to prevent it?'
A: As an intern, you probably aren't in the best position to discuss this off the top of your head. You should ask the surgical registrar to come in and speak to Mrs Bruni; however, it is likely that your hospital will have a guideline for dealing with elective post-splenectomy patients. Such a document will be based on recommendations by national or international resources such as the *Australian Immunisation Handbook* (a very useful online resource for all issues related to immunisation). It is a good idea to give the patient and their GP a copy of this guideline.

Such a guideline is likely to do the following (Antibiotic Expert Group, 2014; Department of Health, 2010):

1. explain that there is an increased risk of infection following splenectomy
2. recommend the use of prophylactic antibiotics (usually phenoxymethylpenicillin 250 mg bd or amoxycillin 250 mg

daily; but, if allergic to penicillin, roxithromycin 150 mg daily or erythromycin 250 mg daily can be used) (eTG, 2013)
3. recommend vaccinations 2 weeks before the elective splenectomy or 1 week after an unanticipated splenectomy. The vaccines would be against pneumococcus, meningococcus, *H. influenzae* b as well as an annual influenza vaccine
4. discuss the importance of being vigilant for fevers and seeking medical attention if it occurs
5. discuss what to do in the event of an animal bite.

The surgical registrar goes through the guidelines with Mrs Bruni and gives her a copy. She is a little overwhelmed by all the information and wants to know if all people having a splenectomy will have the same risk of OPSI as her. What do you tell her?

The risk of OPSI will vary according to the following factors (Rubin and Schaffner, 2014):

- indication for splenectomy (lowest risk for healthy patients whose splenectomy is for trauma)
- age at the time of splenectomy (highest risk if age is < 5 years old)
- time since splenectomy (highest risk in the first 1–2 years postoperatively).

After the clinic, you go to the Emergency Department and speak to the physician who looked after Mr Ecks with you. He updates you that his blood cultures had grown pneumococcus and that Mr Ecks had never been vaccinated post-splenectomy or taken prophylactic antibiotics. Apparently, the surgical team had tried their best but he wasn't interested and had discharged himself against medical advice soon after surgery. You thank your colleague for the update and head home, hoping for a better outcome with Mrs Bruni and her splenectomy.

Achievements

You now:
- recognise the significance of Howell Jolly bodies on a blood film
- know the main causes of hypotension
- understand the spleen's role in fighting infection
- know what OPSI is and what the main pathogens are
- understand how immunisation and post-surgical prophylaxis can reduce the risk of OPSI after a splenectomy.

References

Antibiotic Expert Group (2014), *Therapeutic Guidelines: Antibiotic*, Version 15, Therapeutic Guidelines Ltd, Melbourne.

Department of Health (2013), 'Groups with special vaccination requirements', *The Australian Immunisation Handbook*, tenth edition, Canberra: Department of Health, at <www.immunise.health.gov.au/internet/immunise/publishing.nsf/Content/handbook10-3-3>, accessed 9 September 2014.

King, H. and Shumacker, H.B. Jr (1952), 'Splenic studies. I. Susceptibility to infection after splenectomy performed in infancy', *Annals of Surgery*, vol. 136, no. 2, pp. 239–242.

Morgan, T.L. and Tomich, E.B. (2012), 'Overwhelming post-splenectomy infection (OPSI): A case report and review of the literature', *Journal of Emergency Medicine*, vol. 43, no. 4, pp. 758–763.

Pittet, L.F., Emonet, S., Schrenzel, J., Siegrist, C.A. and Posfay-Barbe, K.M. (2014), 'Bordetella holmesii: An under-recognized Bordetella species', *Lancet Infectious Diseases*, vol. 14, no. 6, pp. 510–519.

Rodeghiero, F. and Ruggeri, M. (2012), 'Short- and long-term risks of splenectomy for benign haematological disorders: Should we revisit the indications?', *British Journal of Haematology*, vol. 158, no. 1, pp. 16–29.

Rubin, L.G. and Schaffner, W. (2014), 'Care of the asplenic patient', *New England Journal of Medicine*, vol. 371, no. 4, pp. 349–356.

Chapter 44
Mrs Daniels presents with tremor and a tachycardia

Scenario

You are a GP registrar in a bustling suburban practice working with Les, your GP intern. Mrs Daniels, a 42-year-old woman, is your next patient. She is an office worker with well-controlled type I diabetes and a 10-pack year history of smoking. She hasn't been herself for a couple of months. In particular, she has been more uptight than usual for no obvious reason and has found the mild spring weather to be uncomfortably hot. At night, she wakes up with transient palpitations. She has lost 5 kg in weight despite no change in her diet or exercise routine. She is opening her bowels more frequently.

You examine her. She has a fine tremor and a tachycardia. A nontender diffuse swelling in the midline of the neck is present. You aren't sure but you think that there might be lid lag; you're not very confident. A 12-lead ECG confirms sinus tachycardia.

Q: You tell her that you are concerned about thyrotoxicosis as the symptoms are typical. Mrs Daniels is worried. 'Has this got something to do with my diabetes?'

A: Her type I diabetes mellitus is a risk factor for Graves disease, which is an autoimmune endocrine disorder. Other risk factors for thyrotoxicosis include autoimmune disease, a family history of thyroid disease and use of medications such as amiodarone and lithium (McDermott, 2012).

Q: 'What's making my thyroid overactive?'

A: The commonest cause of thyrotoxicosis is Graves disease, especially in young women, accounting for 50–80% of cases with the prevalence varying according to regional iodine uptake. The next commonest causes are solitary toxic adenomas and toxic multinodular goitres with thyroiditis accounting for around 10% of cases. Uncommon causes include drug-induced hyperthyroidism, TSH-producing pituitary adenoma and human chorionic gonadotrophin secretion (Franklyn and Boelaert , 2012).

Q: What tests can you order?

A: The best screening test is a serum thyroid stimulating hormone (TSH). If low, then proceed to check the free T4 (FT4) and free T3 (FT3) (Campbell and Doogue, 2012).

Q: The serum TSH comes back as undetectable (< 0.01 mIU/L) with subsequent FT4 and FT3 levels being elevated. Mrs Daniels definitely has thyrotoxicosis. Les, your GP intern, is puzzled. 'Why bother checking the FT3? Surely the FT4 is enough?'

A: Although the FT4 can be elevated in thyrotoxicosis due to most causes, there are times when only the FT3 is elevated (Brent, 2008). Isolated T3 toxicosis may be seen in toxic nodular goitre, but may aslo be seen with mild Graves disease.

Scenario

Q: Les now says, 'We need to test for TSH-receptor antibodies to confirm a diagnosis of Graves disease'. Is he right?

A: The presence of TSH-receptor antibodies is a very sensitive test that is characteristic of Graves disease; however, they don't need to be tested to clinch the diagnosis as Graves disease can even be diagnosed on purely clinical grounds, for example, if Mrs Daniels had definite features of Graves ophthalmopathy along with the thyrotoxicosis, it would be reasonable make the diagnosis without further testing (Campbell and Doogue, 2012). However, as mentioned above, you aren't sure about the lid lag and periorbital oedema.

Q: You explain to Les and Mrs Daniels that she most likely has Graves disease but that the absence of definite eye problems means you need to do a test. What test should you do?

A: A radionuclide thyroid scan. There are 3 patterns that often appear (Campbell and Doogue, 2012):

1. raised homogeneous uptake – Graves disease
2. raised heterogeneous uptake – multinodular goitre or toxic adenoma
3. reduced uptake – thyroiditis.

Q: The radionuclide thyroid scan has the raised homogeneous uptake characteristic of Graves disease. You inform Mrs Daniels of the diagnosis.

'Does that mean the problem you thought I had with my eyes is likely to be there?'

A: Yes. Periorbital oedema is one of the features of Graves ophthalmopathy, which is clinically apparent in 30–50% of those with Graves disease. Other features include proptosis, photophobia and exposure keratitis. Over 80% will have evidence of Graves ophthalmopathy on imaging (Brent, 2008). Lid lag is non-specific in that it can occur in other causes of hyperthyroidism.

Q: You refer her to an endocrinologist who can see her later this week. But Mrs Daniels is anxious to know how she will be treated. What do you tell her?

A: A broad approach to the management of thyrotoxicosis is as follows:
- pharmacologic treatment of symptoms (beta-blockers)
- pharmacologic treatment of the thyroid (the thyroid peroxidase inhibitors, carbimazole or propylthiouracil, that reduce thyroid hormone synthesis)
- annihilation of the thyroid via radioactive iodine or surgery.

Q: What other factors may contribute to Graves disease?

A: There are lifestyle changes that can be made (McDermott, 2012):
- stopping smoking as it worsens Graves ophthalmopathy
- avoiding excessive iodine e.g. kelp*
- reduction in caffeine intake*
- avoiding oral decongestants*
- avoiding heavy exertion.*

Scenario

After going through the lifestyle adjustments and starting her on metoprolol for symptom control, Mrs Daniels leaves your practice. Two weeks later, you receive a letter from the endocrinologist who agrees that she does have a mild Graves ophthalmopathy and has commenced her on a 12-month course of carbimazole.

Q: Les reads the letter and says, 'A whole year of carbimazole? Wow, that should be more than enough to get rid of the thyrotoxicosis for good'. Is he right?

A: Although antithyroid drugs are reasonable first-line therapy, they aren't that effective. In Australia, long-term remission is achieved in approximately 50% of cases (Campbell and Doogue, 2012).

---

*Until the thyrotoxicosis is controlled.

Scenario

In 2 months, Mrs Daniels' TSH is back to normal on carbimazole and she is off the beta-blocker. All seems to be going well until she turns up to your practice, looking sick. She has had fevers, a sore throat and mouth ulcers for 3 days.

Q: You initially wonder about an upper respiratory tract infection but realise what's going on when her full blood count reveals a marked neutropenia. What's the most likely diagnosis?

A: She has probably developed agranulocytosis, which occurs in 0.1–0.3% of patients on antithyroid drugs. This side effect, along with hepatocellullar damage, are 2 of the most serious adverse reactions to occur with carbimazole or propylthiouracil (Brent, 2008). You must discontinue the drug immediately and possibly send her to hospital.

Scenario

Given how unwell she looks, you call an ambulance. After a few days in hospital with no further carbimazole, she improves and is sent home.

Q: Les is pleased to hear this. 'But what now? She can't have antithyroid drugs. And her ophthalmopathy means that radioactive iodine isn't an option. I guess it has to be surgery.' Is he right?

A: Not necessarily. In Graves disease, radioactive iodine is an effective therapy that achieves about a 90% remission rate. In fact, nearly all patients will be hypothyroid within 6 months of therapy.

But, as Les mentioned, it can worsen Graves ophthalmopathy and shouldn't be used in people with moderate to severe disease. It can be used in those with mild disease (like Mrs Daniels), sometimes with a course of corticosteroids beforehand (McDermott, 2012).

Scenario

Mrs Daniels' endocrinologist arranges for radioactive iodine therapy after ensuring she isn't pregnant. She responds well and is cured of her thyrotoxicosis but has to take thyroxine for the subsequent hypothyroidism.

Seven months later, you are doing a CMO shift in the local Emergency Department. One of the interns asks you to help with a 75-year-old woman who is extremely unwell with 2 days of new onset atrial fibrillation (AF) with a rapid ventricular rate, high fevers and confusion. Her daughter tells you that her mother has been tired and somewhat depressed for the last few weeks. Then yesterday, she began to develop burning on passing urine, vomiting and left flank pain. She was due to see her doctor this afternoon but became so unwell with fevers and palpitations that her daughter brought her to hospital. On examination, she has tachycardia, fevers, hypotension and left flank tenderness. The urinalysis is consistent with urinary sepsis.

Q: The RMO asks if this is just a bad case of urinary sepsis. What do you say?

A: It may simply be acute pyelonephritis precipitating AF. But the AF and preceding depression and tiredness could also represent untreated thyrotoxicosis.

Q: How common is AF in hyperthyroidism?

A: Studies have found a 5–15% prevalence of AF in hyperthyroidism, so it not uncommon. The treatment of hyperthyroidism in some patients with AF will lead to reversion to sinus rhythm (Osman *et al.*, 2007).

Q: The intern is surprised. 'But the patient's been depressed and tired for the past few weeks. That's more in keeping with hypothyroidism, isn't it?'

A: 'Apathetic hyperthyroidism' describes how hyperthyroidism in the elderly can manifest more subtly with a combination of depression, fatigue and AF (McDermott, 2012). So it is possible that she has undiagnosed hyperthyroidism.

Q: If this is untreated hyperthyroidism in such a sick patient, what condition do you have to consider?

A: She may be having a 'thyroid storm' or 'thyroid crisis'. This is an exaggerated or severe form of hyperthyroidism with multiorgan involvement (central nervous system and gastrointestinal) and end-organ damage that can be precipitated by any number of acute events, including surgery (thyroidal or not), infection, trauma, pulmonary embolism, seizures, diabetic ketoacidosis and aspirin overdosage (Klubo-Gwiezdzinska and Wartofsky, 2012).

Q: Is it easy to diagnose thyroid storm?

A: No. It is quite a challenge. The problem is that many of the clinical manifestations of thyroid storm are nonspecific (e.g. vomiting, high fevers, tachycardia, tachypnoea, and dyspnoea). A thyroid storm alone can even generate a peripheral blood neutrophilia. As you can see, sepsis could generate the same clinical and laboratory findings. To add to the confusion, sepsis can precipitate a thyroid storm! Even thyroid function tests may not be helpful because serum FT3 can be normal due to reduced peripheral conversion from FT4. Also abnormal thyroid function tests do not distinguish uncomplicated hyperthyroidism from a thyroid storm (Klubo-Gwiezdzinska and Wartofsky, 2012). To aid in the diagnosis of thyroid storm, a scoring system has been developed involving the history and examination findings without any laboratory parameters (McDermott, 2012).

Q: You consult the on-call endocrinologist, who comes and reviews the patient. The FT4 and TSH are both consistent with hyperthyroidism. She shakes her head with uncertainty. 'She clearly has urinary sepsis. But her tests confirm hyperthyroidism and she meets the scoring criteria for a thyroid storm. So we better treat her as if she has a thyroid storm.

How will you treat her?

A: The principles for treating a thyroid storm are as follows (Klubo-Gwiezdzinska and Wartofsky, 2012; McDermott, 2012):

1. Admit to HDU for circulatory system support and monitoring.
2. Treat the underlying cause (in this case, urinary sepsis).
3. Reduce thyroid hormone synthesis (e.g. with carbimazole, propylthiouracil).
4. Inhibit thyroid hormone release with Lugol's iodine or potassium iodide (given after a few hours of antithyroid medications).
5. Administer glucocorticoids (to support the circulation and reduce peripheral conversion of T4 to T3).
6. Reduce the heart rate with beta (e.g. esmolol or metoprolol) or calcium blockers (e.g. diltiazem).

The patient improves with the combination of antibiotics and antithyroid therapy. Outpatient tests later confirm that she is indeed suffering from hyperthyroidism.

Achievements

You now are familiar with:

- the clinical features of thyrotoxicosis, including apathetic hyperthyroidism and Graves ophthalmopathy
- how to use thyroid function tests to diagnoses thyrotoxicosis
- the common causes of thyrotoxicosis
- the use of radionuclide scans to determine the cause of thyrotoxicosis
- the lifestyle, medication, surgical and radioactive treatment options for thyrotoxicosis
- the clinical presentation of antithyroid drug-induced neutropenia
- the difficulties of identifying a thyroid storm.

References

Brent, G.A. (2008), 'Clinical practice: Graves' disease', *New England Journal of Medicine*, vol. 358, no. 24, pp. 2594–2605.

Campbell, K. and Doogue, M. (2012), 'Evaluating and managing patients with thyrotoxicosis', *Australian Family Physician*, vol. 41, no. 8, pp. 564–572.

Franklyn, J.A., Boelaert, K. (2012), 'Thyrotoxicosis', *Lancet*, vol. 379, no. 9821, pp. 1155–1166.

Klubo-Gwiezdzinska, J. and Wartofsky, L. (2012), 'Thyroid emergencies', *Medical Clinics of North America*, vol. 96, no. 2, pp. 385–403.

McDermott, M.T. (2012), 'Hyperthyroidism', *Annals of Internal Medicine*, vol. 157, no. 1, pp. ITC 1–16.

Osman, F., Franklyn, J.A., Holder, R.L., Sheppard, M.C., Gammage, M.D. (2007), 'Cardiovascular manifestations of hyperthyroidism before and after antithyroid therapy: a matched case study', *Journal of the American College of Cardiology*, vol. 49, no. 1, pp. 71–81.

Index

A

ABCD² tool 142
ABCs (airway, breathing, circulation) 362
abdominal aortic aneurysm 73, 79–80
abdominal mass 180
abdominal paracentesis 128
Aboriginal Liaison Officer (ALO) 271–272
acidosis 146
Acinetobacter baumanii 266
activated charcoal 367
active antiretroviral therapy 242, 243
active bleeding
    control 89
    from dabigatran 351
    evidence 350
acute abdominal pain 94–96
acute arthritis and meningococcal
    infection 258–264
acute bowel obstruction 95
acute cholangitis 95, 100
acute colitis
    causes 103–104
    infective *see* inflammatory bowel disease
    investigations 104–106
    ulcerative *see* ulcerative colitis
acute coronary syndrome
    determining level of risk 5–6
    early invasive therapy 8
    electrocardiograph for 1–2
    gaining consent for coronary
        angiogram 9–10
    managing low-, intermediate- and
        high-risk NSTEACS 6
    serum cardiac markers 3–4
    subarachnoid haemorrhage and 164
    therapeutic agents for 6–9
acute flank pain
    acute pyelonephritis 423
    diseases associated with 425–426

'loin to groin' pain 377 *see also* renal
    colic
acute hepatitis 95
acute infections and delirium 314n1
acute inflammatory demyelinating
    polyneuropathy (AIDP) 158, 159
acute kidney injury (AKI) 174
    contrast-induced 180
    definition and staging 176
    medication-induced 176
    rhabdomyolysis and 178
    urine tests 178–179
acute limb ischaemia
    causes 371
    compartment syndrome 375–376
    features 370–371
    investigations 373
    reperfusion injury 375–376
    treatment according to clinical
        stage 373–375
    vascular surgery registrar 372–373
acute meningitis
    causes 252–253
    diagnosing 249–252
    fatality rates 256
    meningococcal disease *vs* 258–259
    sources 255
    viral *vs* bacterial 251–253
acute monoarthritis
    causes 192–194
    diagnosis by joint aspirate 195–196
    physical examination 194–195
acute myocardial infarction 1–2, 6
    abdominal pain and 95
    antihypertensive medications 338
    basic measures 11
    blood tests 11
    criteria for ECG 10–11, 19, 29
    elegibility for reperfusion therapy 11–12
    transthoracic echo 32

Q

R

S